ORTHOPEDIC CLINICS OF NORTH AMERICA

www.orthopedic.theclinics.com

Infections

April 2024 • Volume 55 • Number 2

Editor-in-Chief
FREDERICK M. AZAR

Editorial Board
MICHAEL J. BEEBE
CLAYTON C. BETTIN
TYLER J. BROLIN
JAMES H. CALANDRUCCIO
CHRISTOPHER T. COSGROVE
MARCUS C. FORD
BENJAMIN J. GREAR
BENJAMIN M. MAUCK†
WILLIAM M. MIHALKO
BENJAMIN SHEFFER
KIRK M. THOMPSON
WILLIAM J. WELLER

ELSEVIER

1600 John F. Kennedy Boulevard • Suite 1800 • Philadelphia, Pennsylvania, 19103-2899.

http://www.orthopedic.theclinics.com

ORTHOPEDIC CLINICS OF NORTH AMERICA Volume 55, Number 2
April 2024 ISSN 0030-5898, ISBN-13: 978-0-443-12973-5

Editor: Megan Ashdown
Developmental Editor: Shivank Joshi

Orthopedic Clinics of North America (ISSN 0030-5898) is published quarterly by Elsevier Inc., 360 Park Avenue South, New York, NY 10010-1710. Months of issue are January, April, July, and October. Business and Editorial Offices: 1600 John F. Kennedy Blvd., Suite 1800, Philadelphia, PA 19103-2899. Customer Service Office: 3251 Riverport Lane, Maryland Heights, MO 63043. Periodicals postage paid at New York, NY and additional mailing offices. Subscription prices are $368.00 per year for (US individuals), $433.00 per year (Canadian individuals), $511.00 per year (international individuals), $100.00 per year (US students), $100.00 per year for (Canadian students), $220.00 per year for (international students). For institutional access pricing please contact Customer Service via the contact information below. Foreign air speed delivery is included in all *Clinics* subscription prices. All prices are subject to change without notice. **POSTMASTER:** Send change of address to *Orthopedic Clinics of North America,* **Elsevier Health Sciences Division, Subscription Customer Service, 3251 Riverport Lane, Maryland Heights, MO 63043. Customer Service (orders, claims, online, change of address): Elsevier Health Sciences Division, Subscription Customer Service, 3251 Riverport Lane, Maryland Heights, MO 63043. Tel: 1-800-654-2452 (U.S. and Canada); 314-447-8871 (outside U.S. and Canada). Fax: 314-447-8029. E-mail:** journalscustomerservice-usa@elsevier.com **(for print support);** journalsonlinesupport-usa@elsevier.com **(for online support).**

Reprints. For copies of 100 or more, of articles in this publication, please contact the Commercial Reprints Department, Elsevier Inc., 360 Park Avenue South, New York, NY 10010-1710. Tel.: 212-633-3874; Fax: 212-633-3820; E-mail: reprints@elsevier.com.

Orthopedic Clinics of North America is covered in *MEDLINE/PubMed* (*Index Medicus*), *Cinahl, Excerpta Medica,* and *Cumulative Index to Nursing and Allied Health Literature.*

EDITORIAL BOARD

CONTRIBUTORS

EDITOR

FREDERICK M. AZAR, MD
Department of Orthopaedic Surgery and
Biomedical Engineering, Campbell Clinic, Inc,
University of Tennessee–Campbell Clinic,
Memphis, Tennessee

AUTHORS

SAMUEL B. ADAMS, MD, FAOA, FAAOS
Associate Residency Program Director,
Director of Foot and Ankle Research,
Associate Professor, Department of
Orthopedic Surgery, Duke University Medical
Center, Raleigh, North Carolina

MALINI ANAND, BS
School of Medicine, Vanderbilt
University Medical Center, Nashville,
Tennessee

ARMIN ARSHI, MD
NYU Langone Orthopedic Hospital,
NYU Langone Health, New York,
New York

ITAY ASHKENAZI, MD
NYU Langone Orthopedic Hospital, NYU
Langone Health, New York, New York

COURTNEY E. BAKER, MD
Department of Orthopedics, Vanderbilt
University Medical Center, Nashville,
Tennessee

JAMES BARGER, MD
Fellow, Indiana Hand to Shoulder Center,
Indianapolis, Indiana

FRANCISCO BENGOA, MD
Division of Lower Limb Reconstruction and
Oncology, Department of Orthopaedics,
Vancouver General Hospital, University of
British Columbia, Vancouver, British
Columbia, Canada

CLAYTON C. BETTIN, MD
Orthopaedic Surgeon, Department of
Orthopaedic Surgery and Biomedical
Engineering, University of Tennessee Health
Science Center–Campbell Clinic, Memphis,
Tennessee

TYLER J. BROLIN, MD
Assistant Professor, Associate Director,
Shoulder and Sports Medicine Fellowship,
Medical Director, Campbell Clinic ASCs,
Department of Orthopaedic Surgery and
Biomedical Engineering, University of
Tennessee Health Science Center–Campbell
Clinic, Memphis, Tennessee

NICHOLAS M. BROWN, MD
Department of Orthopaedic Surgery and
Rehabilitation, Loyola University Medical
Center, Maywood, Illinois

ELIZABETH CHO, MD
Department of Orthopaedic Surgery and
Rehabilitation, Resident Physician, Loyola
University Medical Center, Maywood, Illinois

CHRISTOPHER F. DEANS, MD
Assistant Professor, Department of
Orthopaedic Surgery and Rehabilitation,
University of Nebraska Medical Center,
Omaha, Nebraska

CARLO EIKANI, BS
Department of Orthopaedic Surgery and
Rehabilitation, Medical Student, Loyola
University Stritch School of Medicine,
Research Assistant, Loyola University Medical
Center, Maywood, Illinois

ANDREW J. FREAR, BS
Arthritis and Arthroplasty Design Group,
Department of Orthopaedic Surgery, School
of Medicine, University of Pittsburgh,
Pittsburgh, Pennsylvania

KEVIN L. GARVIN, MD
Professor and Chair, Department of
Orthopaedic Surgery and Rehabilitation,
University of Nebraska Medical Center,
Omaha, Nebraska

AKRAM A. HABIBI, MD
NYU Langone Orthopedic Hospital, NYU Langone Health, New York, New York

BRANDON A. HAGHVERDIAN, MD
Foot and Ankle Fellow, Department of Orthopedic Surgery, Duke University Medical Center, Durham, North Carolina

KATHERINE S. HAJDU, BS
School of Medicine, Vanderbilt University Medical Center, Nashville, Tennessee

WILLIAM HEFLEY, BS
School of Medicine, Vanderbilt University Medical Center, Nashville, Tennessee

BRIAN Q. HOU, BA
School of Medicine, Vanderbilt University Medical Center, Nashville, Tennessee

LISA C. HOWARD, MD, MHSc, FRCSC
Division of Lower Limb Reconstruction and Oncology, Department of Orthopaedics, Vancouver General Hospital, University of British Columbia, Vancouver, British Columbia, Canada

REED W. HOYER, MD
Partner, Indiana Hand to Shoulder Center, Indianapolis, Indiana

AARON HOYT, MD
Department of Orthopaedic Surgery and Rehabilitation, Resident Physician, Loyola University Medical Center, Maywood, Illinois

ANTHONY KAMSON, DO
Arthritis and Arthroplasty Design Group, Department of Orthopaedic Surgery, School of Medicine, University of Pittsburgh, Pittsburgh, Pennsylvania; Department of Orthopaedic Surgery, UPMC Central PA, Harrisburg, Pennsylvania

BABAR KAYANI, MBBS, BSc, FRCS (Tr & Orth), PhD
Adult Reconstruction Fellow, Division of Lower Limb Reconstruction and Oncology, Department of Orthopaedics, Vancouver General Hospital, University of British Columbia, Vancouver, British Columbia, Canada

BEAU J. KILDOW, MD
Assistant Professor, Department of Orthopaedic Surgery and Rehabilitation, University of Nebraska Medical Center, Omaha, Nebraska

JEFFREY KLOTT, MD
Shoulder and Sports Medicine Fellow, Department of Orthopaedic Surgery and Biomedical Engineering, University of Tennessee Health Science Center–Campbell Clinic, Memphis, Tennessee

ASHLEY E. LEVACK, MD, MAS
Department of Orthopaedic Surgery and Rehabilitation, Assistant Professor of Orthopaedic Surgery, Loyola University Stritch School of Medicine, Attending Orthopaedic Trauma Surgeon, Loyola University Medical Center, Maywood, Illinois

ASHLEY E. MacCONNELL, MD
Department of Orthopaedic Surgery and Rehabilitation, Loyola University Medical Center, Maywood, Illinois

BASSAM A. MASRI, MD, FRCSC
Division of Lower Limb Reconstruction and Oncology, Department of Orthopaedics, Vancouver General Hospital, University of British Columbia, Vancouver, Canada

MORTEZA MEFTAH, MD
NYU Langone Orthopedic Hospital, NYU Langone Health, New York, New York

DEANA MERCER, MD
Medical Doctor, UNMHSC Department of Orthopedics and Rehabilitation, University of New Mexico, Albuquerque, New Mexico

HEATHER L. MERCER, PhD
Doctor of Philosophy in Biology, Institute of Microbiology and Infection, School of Biosciences, University of Birmingham, Birmingham, England, United Kingdom

ELIZABETH MIKOLA, MD
Medical Doctor, UNMHSC Department of Orthopedics and Rehabilitation, University of New Mexico, Albuquerque, New Mexico

STEPHANIE N. MOORE-LOTRIDGE, PhD
Department of Orthopedics, Vanderbilt Center for Bone Biology, Vanderbilt University Medical Center, Nashville, Tennessee

MICHAEL E. NEUFELD, MD, MSc, FRCSC
Division of Lower Limb Reconstruction and Oncology, Department of Orthopaedics, Vancouver General Hospital, University of British Columbia, Vancouver, British Columbia, Canada

RHIANA RIVAS, BS
Bachelors of Science, UNMHSC Department
of Orthopedics and Rehabilitation, The
University of New Mexico, Albuquerque, New
Mexico

ELIZABETH RIVENBARK, BS
Bachelors of Science, UNMHSC Department
of Orthopedics and Rehabilitation, The
University of New Mexico, Albuquerque, New
Mexico

DIEGO RODRIGUEZ, BS
Bachelor of Science in Chemical Engineering,
UNMHSC Department of Orthopaedics
and Rehabilitation, University of New Mexico,
Albuquerque, New Mexico

RYAN G. ROGERO, MD
Orthopaedic Surgery Resident, Department of
Orthopaedic Surgery and Biomedical
Engineering, University of Tennessee Health
Science Center–Campbell Clinic, Memphis,
Tennessee

NADINE SADAKA, BS, NRP
Arthritis and Arthroplasty Design
Group, Department of Orthopaedic
Surgery, School of Medicine, University of
Pittsburgh, Pittsburgh, Pennsylvania

SHAAN SADHWANI, DO
Arthritis and Arthroplasty Design
Group, Department of Orthopaedic
Surgery, School of Medicine, University
of Pittsburgh, Pittsburgh, Pennsylvania;
Department of Orthopaedic Surgery,
UPMC Central PA, Harrisburg,
Pennsylvania

JONATHAN G. SCHOENECKER, MD, PhD
Department of Orthopedics, Vanderbilt
Center for Bone Biology, Vanderbilt University

Medical Center, Department of Pathology,
Microbiology and Immunology, Vanderbilt
University Medical Center, Department of
Pharmacology, Vanderbilt University Medical
Center, Vanderbilt University, Department of
Pediatrics, Monroe Carell Jr. Children's
Hospital at Vanderbilt, Nashville,
Tennessee

RAN SCHWARZKOPF, MD, MSc
Professor of Orthopedic Surgery, NYU
Langone Orthopedic Hospital, NYU Langone
Health, New York, New York

KARL M. SCHWEITZER, MD
Orthopaedic Foot and Ankle Surgery,
Assistant Professor of Orthopaedic Surgery,
Duke University, Durham, North Carolina

SAMHITA SWAMY, BS
Medical Student, University of Tennessee
Health Science Center College of Medicine,
Memphis, Tennessee

BENJAMIN D. UMBEL, DO
Foot and Ankle Fellow, Department of
Orthopedic Surgery, Duke University Medical
Center, Durham, North Carolina

KENNETH L. URISH, MD, PhD
Arthritis and Arthroplasty Design Group,
Department of Orthopaedic Surgery, School
of Medicine, University of Pittsburgh, The
Bone and Joint Center, Magee Womens
Hospital of the University of Pittsburgh
Medical Center, Departments of Orthopaedic
Surgery and Bioengineering, Clinical and
Translational Science Institute, University of
Pittsburgh, Pittsburgh, Pennsylvania

SPENCER A. WARD, BS
NYU Langone Orthopedic Hospital,
NYU Langone Health, New York,
New York

CONTENTS

Knee and Hip Reconstruction

Total joint arthroplasty (TJA) is a common procedure performed throughout
the entire world in hopes of alleviating debilitating hip or knee pain. The projected number of TJAs performed in the United States alone is projected to
exceed 1.9 million by 2030 and 5 million by 2040. With the significant increase
in TJA performed, more periprosthetic joint infections (PJIs) are likely to be
encountered. PJIs are a devastating complication of TJA. The economic and
clinical burden must be understood and respected to minimize occurrence
and allow optimal patient outcomes.

Prosthetic joint infection following total joint arthroplasty is a devastating complication, resulting in increased morbidity and mortality for the patient. The formation of a biofilm on implanted hardware contributes to the difficulty in
successful identification and eradication of the infection. Antibiotic therapy
and surgical intervention are necessary for addressing this condition; we
present a discussion on different treatment options, including those that are
not yet routinely utilized in the clinical setting or are under investigation, to
highlight the present and future of PJI management.

Periprosthetic joint infections (PJIs) are a devastating complication of joint
arthroplasty surgeries that are often complicated by biofilm formation. The
development of biofilms makes PJI treatment challenging as they create a
barrier against antibiotics and host immune responses. This review article
provides an overview of the current understanding of biofilm formation, factors that contribute to their production, and the most common organisms
involved in this process. This article focuses on the identification of biofilms,
as well as current methodologies and emerging therapies in the management
of biofilms in PJI.

Although one-stage exchange arthroplasty is gaining popularity, two-stage
exchange arthroplasty remains the gold standard for the treatment of periprosthetic
joint infections. Use of an articulating spacer for this procedure offers an avenue for
maintaining hip motion and controlled weight-bearing, allowing local antibiotic elution. However, there is no uniform consensus on the optimal surgical protocol for
using articulating spacers. This review describes the surgical technique for undertaking a first-stage exchange arthroplasty using an articulating spacer and discusses
the pertinent literature on key concepts relating to periprosthetic joint infections
in total hip arthroplasty to guide effective surgical decision making in these patients.

Periprosthetic joint infection (PJI) remains one of the most common complications after total joint arthroplasty. It is challenging to manage, associated with
significant morbidity and mortality, and is a financial burden on the health care
system. Failure of 2-stage management for chronic PJI is not uncommon.
Repeat infections are oftentimes polymicrobial, multiple drug-resistant microorganisms, or new organisms. Optimizing the success of index 2-stage revision
is the greatest prevention against failure of any subsequent management
options and requires a robust team-based approach.

Trauma

Fracture-related infections are a challenging complication in orthopedic
trauma that often necessitates multiple surgeries. Early administration of systemic antibiotics and surgical intervention remains the gold standard of care,
but despite these measures, treatment failures can be as high as 35%. For
these reasons, the introduction of local antibiotics at the site of at-risk fractures
has increased over the past decade. This review looks at the various measures
being used clinically including local antibiotic powder, polymethylmethacrylate, biodegradable substances, antibiotic-coated implants, and novel methods such as hydrogels and nanoparticles that have the potential for use in
the future.

Pediatrics

Musculoskeletal infection (MSKI) in children is a critical condition in pediatric
orthopedics due to the potential for serious adverse outcomes, including multiorgan dysfunction syndrome, which can lead to death. The diagnosis and treatment of MSKI continue to evolve with advancements in infectious organisms,
diagnostic technologies, and pharmacologic treatments. It is imperative for
pediatric orthopedic surgeons and medical teams to remain up to date with
the latest MSKI practices.

Sequestration, a condition where a section of bone becomes necrotic due to a loss of vascularity or thrombosis, can be a challenging complication of osteo-myelitis. This review explores the pathophysiology of sequestration, highlighting the role of the periosteum in forming involucrum and creeping substitution which facilitate revascularization and bone formation. The authors also discuss the induced membrane technique, a two-stage surgical procedure for cases of failed healing of sequestration. Future directions include the potential use of prophylactic anticoagulation and novel drugs targeting immunocoagulopathy, as well as the development of advanced imaging techniques and single-stage surgical procedures.

Shoulder and Elbow

Septic arthritis of the elbow is a serious problem requiring prompt, accurate diagnosis and urgent surgical intervention. Achieving successful patient outcomes depends heavily on early diagnosis and efficient streamlined surgical treatment. Essential tactics for treating the septic elbow joint include immediate joint irrigation and debridement in addition to administration of appropriate antibiotics. This comprehensive review delves into the cause of the septic elbow joint, identifies associated risk factors, and provides a comprehensive approach encompassing the diagnosis and treatment of the septic elbow. The aim of this review is to optimize patient care and outcomes.

The total number of patients with a total shoulder arthroplasty (TSA) is increasing, and the number of patients experiencing a (TSA) prosthetic joint infection (PJI) also will increase. It is important that physicians know how to identify signs of infection, know the common pathogens, and know how to work up a shoulder PJI. This publication reviewed the current literature about presenting signs and symptoms, common shoulder pathogens and how they differ from total knee and hip pathogens, and what images, tests, and procedures can aid in identification of infection.

Hand and Wrist

The fingertip is the interface between humans and the world, including the various thorns, dirty needles, and other hazards to be found there. It is unsurprising that this is the site where hand infections most frequently occur. Although commonly encountered by hand surgeons and other physicians, fingertip infections have several mimics, and diagnosis and management is not always straightforward. Early diagnosis and treatment are key to success. As with all infections, they are more common and are more aggressive in immunosuppressed patients. This article reviews fingertip anatomy, common and uncommon fingertip infections and their mimics, and recommendations for management

Septic arthritis of the wrist can have severe deleterious effects on cartilage and bone if not promptly addressed. Expedient diagnosis and early medical intervention are important. The most effective strategy involves immediate arthrocentesis of the infected joint, enabling precise antibiotic selection based on joint fluid analysis. Diagnostic imaging is important in excluding fractures and identifying abscesses. This review explores the etiologic factors underlying septic wrist joint, identifying risk factors, and delineating optimal diagnosis and treatment approaches. The overarching goal is to impart valuable insights and guidance in the management of septic wrist joint, ensuring the highest quality patient care and optimal clinical outcomes.

Foot and Ankle

As the number of primary total ankle replacements increases for treatment of end-stage ankle arthritis, failures are also expected to rise. Periprosthetic joint infection is among the causes of failures and has been reported to be as high as 5%. Diagnosis is usually made by a combination of clinical examination findings, imaging, laboratory, and microbiological workup. Management is generally separated into limb salvage or amputation. Limb salvage can be challenging and may involve a single versus staged approach. Options include revision arthroplasty or arthrodesis procedures (ankle versus tibiotalocalcaneal), and a multidisciplinary approach is sought to eradicate infection before definitive management.

The differentiation between acute Charcot neuroarthropathy and infection in the foot and ankle should be supported by multiple criteria. A detailed history and physical examination should always be completed. Plain radiographs should be performed, though advanced imaging, currently MRI, is more helpful in diagnosis. Scintigraphy and PET may become the standard imaging modalities once they are more clinically available due to their reported increased accuracy. Laboratory analysis can also act as a helpful diagnostic tool. Histopathology with culturing should be performed if osteomyelitis is suspected. The prompt diagnosis and initiation of treatment is vital to reducing patient morbidity and mortality.

INFECTIONS

PREFACE

Infections

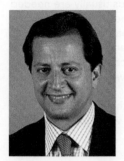

Frederick M. Azar, MD
Editor

Postoperative infections are becoming more prevalent, as the number of total joint arthroplasties (TJA) continues to rise worldwide, increasing readmissions and health care costs. This issue of *Orthopedic Clinics of North America* focuses on the challenges that such infections present and explores how to best deal with them to achieve optimal outcomes for patients.

By 2040, five million TJAs are expected to be performed in the United States each year, so more periprosthetic joint infections (PJIs) are expected to be encountered. Dr Shaan Sadhwani and team explain the current concepts about PJIs' clinical and economic impact. PJIs often are complicated by the formation of biofilm, which creates a barrier against antibiotics and host immune responses. Dr Spencer A. Ward and his colleagues focus on how the biofilms form, how to identify them, and current methodologies used in their treatment. Dr Ashley E. MacConnell and team, meanwhile, discuss the different treatment options for biofilm, including those not yet routinely used.

Two-stage exchange arthroscopy is considered the "gold standard" for treating PJIs, and using an articulated spacer for the procedure helps control weight-bearing and maintain hip motion. Dr Babar Kayani and team discuss the current literature regarding PJIs in total hip arthroplasty and describe the surgical technique for performing a first-stage exchange arthroscopy, which is gaining popularity.

Repeat PJIs are a scourge that often are drug-resistant, polymicrobial, or derived from new organisms. Dr Christopher F. Deans and colleagues write that a robust team approach is necessary to optimize index two-stage management for chronic PJI so that it succeeds; repeat two-stage is common with recurrent PJI, though success rates fall with each attempt. Other joint-salvage procedures may be considered depending on each individual's medical circumstances. Ultimately, novel therapeutic modalities and surgical protocols guided by high-quality research might be the key to successfully managing this problem, the Deans team writes.

Multiple surgeries often are needed to alleviate fracture-related infections, and treatment failures are common despite the often-early administration of systemic antibiotics. Consequently, local antibiotics are being used more often at the sites of at-risk fractures. Dr Carlo Eikani and colleagues review the delivery options as well as novel methods, such as hydrogels, that have potential for future use.

In pediatrics, the diagnosis and treatment of musculoskeletal infections (MSKI) continue to evolve. Dr Stephanie N. Moore-Lotridge and team explore current MSKI practices, the risk of deadly outcomes, and how to determine the appropriate treatment. Osteomyelitis, a bone inflammation that is more common in younger children, sometimes can trigger sequestration, where a piece of bone becomes necrotic because of thrombosis or a loss of

Orthop Clin N Am 55 (2024) xv–xvi
https://doi.org/10.1016/j.ocl.2023.12.001
0030-5898/24/© 2023 Published by Elsevier Inc.

vascularity. Dr Katherine S. Hajdu and colleagues delve into the pathophysiology of sequestration, the induced membrane technique, and potential treatments that are on the horizon, such as novel drugs that target immunocoagulopathy.

Septic arthritis of the elbow and wrist requires early diagnosis and efficient surgical treatment so that a successful patient outcome can be achieved. Immediate joint irrigation, debridement, and use of antibiotics are essential courses of action for the elbow, while joint aspiration and precise antibiotic selection are needed for the afflicted wrist. Dr Heather L. Mercer and her team discuss the cause of septic elbow and wrist joints, and what should be done to diagnose and treat them effectively.

Since the number of PJIs is increasing along with the number of total shoulder arthroplasties, physicians need to be able to recognize common shoulder pathogens and know the signs of infection. Drs Jeff Klott and Tyler J. Brolin review the current literature about presenting signs and discuss which tests can aid identification.

Diagnosis isn't always easy for infections of the fingertips, where most hand contamination occurs. Several maladies can be mistaken for them; Drs James Barger and Reed W. Hoyer explain how to diagnose and manage treatment of both common and rare fingertip infections.

Total ankle replacements are being used more often to treat end-stage ankle arthritis, but they're also failing sometimes because of PJIs. The infections usually are diagnosed by lab work, imaging, and clinical exams, while management can either consist of limb salvage or amputation. Dr Benjamin D. Umbel and colleagues say a multidisciplinary approach is needed to get rid of the infection, and they take a deep dive into the various management procedures.

Several diagnostic methods usually are needed to help differentiate between an infection and acute Charcot neuroarthropathy in the foot and ankle. Dr Ryan G. Rogero and team discuss the use of radiographs, advanced imaging, scintigraphy, and lab work, along with histopathology if osteomyelitis is suspected.

We thank the authors for their valuable information and hope that readers will find these topics helpful in their practices.

DISCLOSURES

Dr Azar discloses the following outside of this work: 98point6; Pfizer; Zimmer; Elsevier; JSES; *Orthopedic Clinics*; Wolters Kluwer; St. Jude; ABOS; AJSSM.

Frederick M. Azar, MD
Campbell Clinic, Inc
University of Tennessee–Campbell Clinic
Department of Orthopaedic Surgery and
Biomedical Engineering
1211 Union Avenue, Suite 510
Memphis, TN 38104, USA

E-mail address:
fazar@campbellclinic.com

Knee and Hip Reconstruction

Current Concepts on the Clinical and Economic Impact of Periprosthetic Joint Infections

Shaan Sadhwani, DO[a,b], Anthony Kamson, DO[a,b],
Andrew J. Frear, BS[a], Nadine Sadaka, BS, NRP[a],
Kenneth L. Urish, MD, PhD[a,c,d,e,*]

KEYWORDS

- Periprosthetic joint infection • PJI • Total knee arthroplasty • Total hip arthroplasty • TKA • THA
- Revision TKA • Revision THA

KEY POINTS

- Total joint arthroplasty has a high success rate; however, periprosthetic joint infection (PJI) is a costly and devastating complication.
- The cost of PJI is expected to be approximately US$1.85 billion in the United States alone by 2030; however, this may be an underestimation.
- More effective treatment that allows patients to resolve their infection with less operations and higher implant retainment, as well as prevention of PJI is paramount to decrease cost to the health-care system.

INTRODUCTION

Total joint arthroplasty (TJA) is a common procedure performed throughout the entire world to alleviate debilitating hip or knee pain. In the United States alone, it is projected that approximately 1.9 million TJAs will be performed annually by 2030.[1] However, this may even be an underestimation, as SmartTRAK Biomed GPS, a market analytics firm for orthopedics that tracks surgical volume, shows that in 2023 there will be 1.71 million TJAs, growing at 3.8% compound annual growth rate. With this calculation, the yield of TJA in 2030 would actually near 2.2 million. On average, a single TJA can cost upward of US$30,000 when considering the perioperative hospital expenditures as well as the procedural cost.[2,3] Although most TJAs are successful and without complication, periprosthetic joint infection (PJI) remains a potential catastrophic and life-changing complication that adds upward of US$100,000 in direct costs for each additional admission needed to treat the infection.[4] In the United States alone, projected annual hospital costs associated with PJIs of the knee and hip are projected to be approximately US$1.85 billion by 2030.[1] However, this number may actually also be a gross underestimation because many studies estimating these costs do not report the total cost of inpatient or outpatient care involving multiple visits.

---

[a] Arthritis and Arthroplasty Design Group, Department of Orthopaedic Surgery, School of Medicine, University of Pittsburgh, Pittsburgh, PA 15219, USA; [b] Department of Orthopaedic Surgery, UPMC Central PA, Harrisburg, PA 17109, USA; [c] Arthritis and Arthroplasty Design Group, The Bone and Joint Center, Magee Womens Hospital of the University of Pittsburgh Medical Center; [d] Department of Orthopaedic Surgery, Clinical and Translational Science Institute, University of Pittsburgh; [e] Department of Bioengineering, Clinical and Translational Science Institute, University of Pittsburgh
* Corresponding author. Arthritis and Arthroplasty Design Group, Department of Orthopaedic Surgery, School of Medicine, University of Pittsburgh, Pittsburgh, PA 15219.
E-mail address: ken.urish@pitt.edu

Orthop Clin N Am 55 (2024) 151–159
https://doi.org/10.1016/j.ocl.2023.09.001
0030-5898/24/© 2023 Elsevier Inc. All rights reserved.

Because the number of TJAs performed increases globally, the economic burden of a PJI must be understood and respected. Greater understanding of the financial burden created by a PJI on hospitals and patients should serve as one of the many driving factors to minimize its occurrence to allow for optimal patient care and outcomes.

SUMMARY OF THE CLINICAL PROBLEM

TJA of the hip or knee is the most common operative surgery performed in the United States, and it is estimated that in 2030 approximately 5 million new joint replacement procedures will be performed globally.[2,3,5] This increase is attributed to several factors, notably the nation's aging population, obesity, increased access to care, improved technology, and earlier surgical treatment.[6] In addition, the American Academy of Orthopedic Surgeons found that the mean age for primary total hips has declined significantly from 66.3 to 64.9 years and for knees from 68 to 65.9 years.[5] Others have shown that the average age for TJA decreases by 1 year every decade, equating to thousands of new cases per year.

The most common cause of surgical TJA revision is PJI, a life-altering complication with a poor prognosis, high morbidity and mortality, and catastrophic health and socioeconomic outcomes.[7] PJI is attributed to nearly 2.1% of hip and more than 2.3% of knee TJA revision surgeries.[6,8–10] Recent research has suggested that infection rates might be higher than previously reported due to a variety of factors ranging from patient population, variations in how PJI is defined, and length of time until treatment.[6,10–12] A 2019 study by Runner and colleagues[13] showed that infection rates in general university hospitals were significantly higher than rates in orthopedic specialty hospitals, which could skew reported infection rates.[6,9–11] At infection rates of 2.1% and 2.3%, when coupled with projections for a substantial global increase in TJAs by 2030, it is reasonable to estimate that these data equate to more than 150,000 new PJI patients.[8]

PJI revisions are complex, and each of these projected 150,000 patients will require on average 2 to 3 revision surgeries, leading to approximately 300,000 to 450,000 surgeries performed. It has been shown that these patients also average 3.6 hospital readmissions, which can be estimated to correlate to approximately 540,000 hospitalizations.[14] As such, it can be noted that the aforementioned estimation of annual cost of US$1.85 billion is an underestimation of the problem when approximating a cost of US$100,000 per admission.[4] Beyond additional procedures and hospitalizations, readmissions also result in compounding debilitation. The standard of care is a 2-stage revision with removal of the primary implants. Unfortunately, many patients never receive their definitive revision implants and either live with antibiotic spacers or go on to arthrodesis or amputations. Additionally, PJI is associated with frequent and lengthy hospital stays. Kapadia and colleagues compared infected and uninfected total knee arthroplasties and found that patients with PJI had significantly longer hospitalizations (5.3 vs 3 days), more readmissions (3.6 vs 0.1), and more clinic visits (6.5 vs 1.3).[6] In other studies, the mean hospital stay has been found to be longer for patients with hip or knee PJIs than for patients undergoing primary arthroplasty; total hip arthroplasty, 7.6 versus 3.3 days, and total knee arthroplasty, 5.3 versus 3.0 days.[15,16]

Mortality secondary to PJI is also one of great concern. For example, mortality rates for 2-stage hip revisions can be up to 25.8% within 2 years and 45% at 4 to 7 years for recurrent infections.[6,17,18] In another study, it was found that at 5 years postinfection, 1 in 4 total hip arthroplasty patients will die as a direct or indirect result of PJI, whereas nearly 45% will die after 10 years.[10] For 2-stage revisions, 1-year mortality after explantation is 13% for total hip arthroplasties and 9% for total knee arthroplasties.[11] In the literature, it has been cited that comparing the management of PJI to that of cancer is not inaccurate, especially given that the mortality rates associated with 2-stage exchange for PJI 25% to 33% at 5 years postoperatively.[19–22] These mortality rates are higher than many cancers.[23] In fact, PJI is associated with a 5-year mortality rate higher than that of breast cancer, melanoma, Hodgkin's lymphoma, and other malignancies.[1] Additionally, it has been found in the literature that the physical, psychological, and economic influences of PJI recovery process have been compared with the experience of patients undergoing cancer treatment.[22]

What Is Periprosthetic Joint Infection and Why Is It Hard to Treat?

PJI can be caused by the invasion of microorganisms from the skin at the surgical site, the surgical environment or by recurring infection.[10] Although PJI can be caused by a variety of microorganisms (including fungi), the most common pathogens belong to the Staphylococcus species, although one study found that 25% of infections may be caused by multiple microbes.[6,10] When these highly adherent bacteria come in contact with a prosthetic device, they attach to its surface and proliferate to form a biofilm.[10] Biofilms are resilient and difficult to treat with antimicrobial agents because pathogens within it are physically protected, often requiring long periods of time with heavy doses of medication, and potentially leading to antibiotic resistance.[10] One such example can be found in Methicillin-resistant *Staphylococcus aureus*, which accounts for 12% to 23% of all PJIs in the United States.[6]

Despite treating patients with heavy doses of systemic antibiotics, effective therapeutic levels are not reached at the surface of the prosthesis and bio lm. Even with the current standard of care involving surgery and the local use of antiseptics or antibiotics, recurrence rates remain high. In addition, early symptoms of PJI can be vague, presenting a diagnostic challenge that can lead to delayed treatment. Presentation of PJI varies drastically among individuals, which has slowed advances in diagnosis and treatment. Without proper, timely treatment, PJI is progressive and can be life threatening.[22] Although joint pain is the most common symptom, PJI can occur without typical symptoms that indicate an infection, such as redness, swelling, fever, and sinus tract drainage.[10] Careful history and patient examinations looking for satellite infection causes/procedures, combined with diagnostic assessments that involve the evaluation of the surgical site, radiographs, joint fluid, and bloodwork are all required.

The variety of microbes that cause PJI require culture-speci c antibiotics which can also lead to delays in optimal antibiotic treatment due to the time needed to determine the causative pathogen.[6] However, determining the causative organism is crucial and can have a great influence on treatment success. An example of this influence can be demonstrated by treatment success rates, which are as low as 52% in a 2-stage revision for PJI caused by a gram-negative pathogen, as low as 51% for methicillin resistant staphylococcus aureus (MRSA), and as low as 69% for methicillin-sensitive organisms.[10] In addition, up to 45% of PJI, cases are culture negative. These cases require a surgical culture and tissue samples for microbial diagnosis, further complicating and delaying the treatment decision-making process.[10]

Treatment Options and Their Recurrence Rates

The most common, and unfortunately catastrophic, complication of PJI is recurrence of infection, which is complex and challenging to treat. With the current standard of care, morbidity and mortality rates of failed revision are known to be high.[6] Reinfection can lead to amputations and death. In fact, 11% of patients whose DAIR (debridement, antibiotics, implant retention) procedure fails within the first year will require amputation.[24] With repeated surgeries and hospital admissions, mortality rates increase by 20% with each additional major surgery.[8,24] Drain and colleagues found that mortality related to PJI is due to a combination of factors, including frailty and the effects of the infection itself but not the treatment.[23]

Despite an increase in PJI incidence and continued poor outcomes, treatment paradigms for PJI have not changed to address this burden. Infection is still typically a surgical problem, and even combined with both systemic and local antibiotic/antiseptic use, the revisions still often fail.[10] In some patients who are at high risk for surgical complications, long-term antibiotic treatment without surgical intervention can be attempted but is typically not successful in eradicating the infection.[10]

Given the complexity and treatment challenges, there are multiple current treatment options for PJI that include the DAIR procedure, commonly combined with removal and replacement of the mobile components; 1-stage surgical joint removal and revision; and 2-stage surgical joint removal and revision (the current "gold standard" of care).

Many patients require multiple surgeries and high doses of systemic antibiotics for months to years, yet still result in high failure rates and recurrence of infection.[10] DAIR is a more conservative treatment option for acute infection, which allows patients to retain their implant and have a chance at resolution with a single operation. It is used when there is sufficient bone quality with a stable prosthesis, there is no draining sinus, and the soft tissues are not compromised.[10] However, the procedure fails in 1 of 2 patients, and reinfection rates are high.[24] If solutions existed that improved outcomes of this procedure, this option could grow in attractiveness and utilization. One-stage revision for PJI can also be performed but has been a topic of recent debate. Lazic and colleagues reviewed infection eradication in 29 studies with a mean follow-up of 4.9 ± 2.6 years.[25] They found that the mean eradication rate was 87% after 1-stage knee revisions and 83% after 2-stage revisions during the aforementioned mean follow-up time.[25] Two-stage surgical prosthesis removal and revision is the most common treatment of PJI.[6] It is most beneficial in more severe or chronic cases or in the presence of unstable implant, poor bone/ soft tissue quality, and antimicrobial resistant pathogens.[6,10] Outcomes are still challenging and failure with reinfection has been estimated at 23% after a mean follow-up of 94 months.[26] Other studies have estimated that the overall rate of successful completion of 2-stage revisions is less than 50%, with completion rates of 43% for hips and 11% to 48% for knees.[10,11,27,28] It has also been found that in up to 38.4% of 2-stage exchange, patients do not receive the definitive revision prosthesis and either continue with antibiotic spacers and antibiotic suppressive therapy or end up with joints fused or limbs amputated.[29] Of those who do receive new implants, approximately 19% will get reinfected in the first year and restart the treatment process.[29] Furthermore, Kapadia and colleagues found that patients with PJI required significantly more care than patients who required revision surgery without infection (aseptic failure).[10,14] Treatment of aseptic failure can typically be successful after one additional surgery and subsequent hospitalization, whereas septic revisions require longer antibiotic courses, more rehabilitation and clinic and physical therapy visits, and extended hospital stays.[4] As such, septic revisions often drive up the cost of care, which is often underestimated in the literature due to the nature of reporting cost from one hospital admission rather than the full inpatient and outpatient journey that encompasses multiple admissions, skilled nursing facilities, home health care, and so forth.

Depression and Social Issues

PJI recovery is long and arduous and often results in limited mobility, lost wages, social isolation, anxiety, and depression among patients, as well as increased stress on caregivers.[30–33] It was reported that the largest complaints by patients included living with pain, reduced independence, and constant fear of disease progression.[30] In a study by Wildeman, and colleagues, patients with PJI of the hip have a lower quality of life and joint function and are more likely to need assisted living (21% vs 12%) and ambulatory aid (65% vs 42%) when compared with their uncomplicated total hip arthroplasty (THA) counterparts.[10,34]

With such major influences on all facets of a patient's life, the link to depression seems clear. Wilson and colleagues showed that PJI after THA was a significant risk factor for the development of new onset depression (NOD).[31]

Similarly, PJI after total knee arthroplasty (TKA) was also found to be a significant risk factor for NOD.[35] Beyond the diagnosis of a PJI itself, the process of treatment involving the 2-stage revision can also place an enormous strain on patients. The time required between the original and definitive prosthesis is one that has been shown to increase rates of depression as well as other mental health disorders.[30,32,33] When compared with patients who underwent revision for aseptic loosening, patients who underwent 2-stage revision for PJI after TKA were found to have a significantly higher risk of depressive, stress, bipolar, and psychotic disorders within 2 years after surgery.[33]

It is important to remember that when a patient is diagnosed with PJI, the future becomes exactly the opposite of why the patient consulted with an orthopedist initially. Wishes for a pain-free and improved joint are replaced with additional surgeries and treatments, increased burden of care, and lack of symptom resolution.[32] Therefore, the psychological stressor of the patient can be unsurmountable and, in some cases, have an influence on the success of PJI treatment. Prevention, education, and the maintenance of social support, as well as a focus on transparency and communication from the health-care team, have been shown to help patients through the disaster that is a PJI diagnosis.[30]

It is important to note that treating PJI requires significant efforts of health-care teams. When it occurs, it can lead to feelings of guilt and low morale among the surgeons and operative staff, who are aware of the devastating consequences, possibly leading to burnout.[10,36]

SUMMARY OF THE ECONOMIC PROBLEM

Beyond the clinical aspects of a PJI following TJA, understanding the economic burden of this diagnosis is of great importance. Direct costs can be seen due to prolonged hospitalizations, frequent readmissions, laboratory workup, prolonged use of antibiotics and analgesics, extended rehabilitation, and multiple reoperations.[4,8,37] In a 2016 study, the cost of revision procedure per PJI was found to exceed US$566 million in that year and projected to exceed US$1.6 billion by 2020.[37,38] In a 2017 study, the combined cost of TKA and THA PJI was found to be US$1.7 billion in that year and was estimated to be US$1.85 billion by 2030, including US$753.4 million for THA PJI and US$1.1 billion for TKA PJI.[1] Much of this increase can be attributed to the increase in volume of primary TKA and THA, with 1.5 million primary THA and TKA performed in 2014 and an expected 2-fold increase by 2030.[1] In a study by Kapadia and colleagues, in which matched uncomplicated patients with THA were compared with patients with THA diagnosed with PJI, it was found that patients with PJI incurred a 3-fold increase in episode cost, 2-fold increase in length of stay, and had a higher rate of readmission.[37] They reported that the management of these infections, which often requires a 2-stage procedure, has been reported to cost approximately US$60,000 more than revisions for aseptic causes.[37] In another study, costs of PJI procedures were found to be 15% to 28% higher than the cost of a doubled aseptic revision to account for the 2-stage procedure required to treat PJI.[39] In this same study, it was shown that the direct medical costs of irrigation and debridement procedures for PJI compared with partial component exchange for aseptic revisions were also double.[39] When observing hospital costs, it can be seen that operating room services and hospital bed occupation comprised most of the increase in cost.[37,39]

Preoperative Screening

Preoperative screening is paramount in both the diagnosis and successful treatment of PJI. It has been shown that age, comorbidity indices, illicit drug use, sex, and heart failure are all drivers of increased total costs associated to PJI treatment.[1,40–42] Therefore, patient optimization is central to the prevention of PJI, and the benefits of this are widely reported in the literature. Preoperative screening with decolonization protocols have also been implemented for S aureus, given that this bacterium accounts for approximately 30% of surgical site infections. In regards to this intranasal screening, it has been shown that universal screening for all patients and decolonization for bacterial-positive patients has been the most cost-effective method when compared with universal decolonization without screening and screening for high-risk populations only.[43] In many cases, diagnosis can be straightforward with clinical evidence of infection, raised inflammatory markers, and positive culture results from sampling. However, the prevalence of culture-negative PJI ranges from 5% to 42%, which can complicate diagnosis and increase costs of both screening and treatment.[38] In these cases, tests such as alpha-defensin assays, sonication, polymerase chain reaction, mass spectrometry, and next-generation sequencing can help aid in diagnosis but come with the burden of decreased reliability and a large increase in cost.[38] A lower cost alternative to this can be found in leukocyte esterase testing, which allows a specificity of 100% and sensitivity of 80.6%.[37] Although this test will not identify the causative organism, it can be a relatively low-cost alternative to diagnosing the PJI itself.

Perioperative Management

Perioperatively, measures including incorporation of standardized sterilization protocols, shorter operating times, use of laminar ow, body exhaust suits, perioperative antibiotics, antibiotic cement, and antimicrobial adhesive dressings have been implemented to decrease PJI rates; however, the incidence of PJI has remained relatively unchanged.[1] Interestingly, it has been shown in the literature that tranexamic acid is a cost-effective way to reduce infection risk in total shoulder arthroplasty by promoting hemostasis. This benefit was also shown by Kolin, and colleagues, in which use was economically justified in THA and TKA and was shown to prevent at least 1 infection out of 3125 TJAs (ARR = 0.032%).[44]

In terms of antibiotic usage, an increase in PJI can be complicated by an increase in antibiotic resistance, therefore incurring a great cost due to prolonged and more expensive antibiotic use. A 2010 study by Parvizi and colleagues regarding PJI in THA found that the mean in-hospital cost of care was US$110,495 for methicillin-resistant infections and US$65,776 for methicillin-sensitive infections.[9] In the more recent study by Kapadia and colleagues, it was also found that organism type affected hospital stay in THA PJI, in which methicillin-resistant PJI caused a 17-times longer average hospital stay than their methicillin-sensitive counterparts.[37] Although systemic antibiotic use is central to PJI treatment, local antibiotic use to deliver high concentrations to the joint and soft tissues has also been implemented. However, the use of agents such as topical powder, bone cement, and calcium sulfate carriers for local delivery of antibiotics comes with increased costs, and currently no level-1 evidence exists to support their routine use for both prevention of PJI in primary TJA and treatment of PJI in revision TJA.[45] An example of this added cost without substantial clinical evidence can be seen in a study by Yayac and colleagues, which examined antibiotic-loaded bone cement (ALBC) use in primary TKA. In this retrospective review, they found that out of 2511 patients, 1077 patients who underwent TKA with ALBC showed no difference in PJI rates or complications but did have an added cost of US$299 to their episode of care.[29] However, Trentinaglia and colleagues examined antibacterial coatings in primary TJA and found that the use of dual ALBC and antibacterial hydrogel coating can provide an annual direct cost savings by reducing incidence of PJI, whereas silver coating would increase costs.[46] Without a true consensus of local antibiotic use for the prevention of PJI, these methods require further study and larger trials.

Intraoperatively, methodology of revision and implant type and characteristics can play an economic role in treating PJI. Kurtz, and colleagues evaluated the economic burden of 2-stage revision for PJI and found that the mean additional cost for hospitalizations between stages was US$23,582 and US$20,965 per patient for hips and knees, respectively, whereas the likelihood of completing the second stage revision successfully was only 43.1%.[47] In this same study, they found that the overall direct hospital cost of resection and reimplantation was US$63,691 for TKA PJI treatment in 2020, which was similar to the 2018 data published by Yao and colleagues that showed US$50,553 for the treatment of TKA PJI.[39,47] Regarding antibiotic spacer use, Nodzo and colleagues evaluated the success rates and cost of using a prefabricated spacer, homemade mold, or autoclaved femoral component in treating TKA PJI. They found that although there was no difference in success rates, the cost of the surgeon's own intraoperatively created mold had the lowest mean cost per construct, whereas commercial cement molds had the highest mean cost (US$1341 $\pm$ 889.10 vs US$5439.00 $\pm$ 657.80, $P<.0001$).[48] In treatment of THA PJI, it has also been shown that the use of extended trochanteric osteotomy and articulation type regarding the antibiotic spacer are impactful drivers of cost.[41] Charalambous and colleagues showed that in THA PJI management with 2-stage revision, metal-on-poly liners were associated with a 22% decrease in cost at 2-year postoperatively when compared with cement-on-bone articulating spacer and that metal-on-poly constrained liners account for 38% less cost at 1-year postoperatively.[41]

Indirectly, the loss of health team productivity as well as the cost of disability, rehabilitation, and caregivers can be incurred. Given the volume of projected TJAs, the known infection rates, and the challenges of surgical and antibiotic treatments, the associated economic burden, both in direct hospital costs, subacute and long-term care is staggering. In addition, the psychosocial and ﬁnancial burdens on patients, their families, and care teams are signiﬁcant. As the average age of patients undergoing TJA continues to decrease, indirect costs from lost wages (in addition to direct costs) will increase dramatically.[4] This was further extrapolated by Parisi and colleagues in a study that modeled the sum of direct medical costs and indirect costs in the form of lost wages. They found that when the cost of lost productivity is accounted for, the cost of a 55-year old hypothetical patient requiring 2-stage revision approached US$500,000.[4]

Cost of Failure

Periprosthetic joint infections are a complex and difﬁcult problem with a signiﬁcantly high failure of 11% to 35%.[49] In today's world of arthroplasty, PJIs have become the leading cause for revision arthroplasty.[50] It is well known that revision arthroplasty can be a costly expenditure for patients and health-care systems, and when associated with infection, this burden can significantly affect both parties. There are many options for the treatment of PJI that are based on the onset of infection and the specific microorganism. Surgical intervention ranges from DAIR, 1-stage versus 2-stage revision arthroplasty, arthrodesis, and resection arthroplasty.[51] It has been noted that that a main reason for failure when treating PJI is inadequate surgical debridement, which is highly associated with interventions such as DAIR.[52] With inadequate surgical debridement, the likelihood of completely clearing an infection is decreased and the need for secondary procedures is increased. A 2022 study by Mponponsuo and colleagues demonstrated that the 1-year cost of treating a PJI significantly increased based on the procedure performed. They demonstrated a DAIR procedure averaged US$52,124, a 1-stage revision averaged US$148,101, and a 2-stage revision averaged US$111,858 in Calgary, Canada. The cost burden on the hospital system also varied significantly based on the procedure, with 2-stage revision having the highest average cost. A DAIR procedure was found to cost the hospital system US$45,438, 1-stage revision costs US$104,170, and a 2-stage revision costs US$121,793.[53] It is noted that the higher cost seen in 2-stage revisions can most likely be attributed to 2 different operative interventions/hospital admissions and the implantation of revision components once the infection is deemed eradicated.

Unfortunately, it is known that patients who have a revision for PJI on average incur costs approximately 5 times higher than those without a PJI based on hospital cost alone.[54] In treating

PJI, not only the patients ,but also the treatment team is affected. Due to the complex nature of this clinical problem, the treatment team can be significantly influenced emotionally, which can lead to decreased productivity. The patients commonly have extended hospital courses that lead to increased nursing and staffing utilization.[42] Parvizi and colleagues notes that hospital costs were significantly higher in patients with PJI and nearly 2.9 times higher (US$16,999 vs US$5937) when directly compared with patients without a PJI.[9]

Regardless of the procedure performed for PJI, the associated cost is very signi cant. The importance of prevention cannot be stressed enough to avoid this burden on patients and health-care systems. Revision arthroplasty requires longer operative times, expensive prosthesis, extended hospital stays, higher complication rates, higher likelihood of discharge to rehabilitation facilities, and higher incurred cost to patient's and hospitals.[8] It should be noted that the cost of the procedure a patient receives in their care should not be a driving factor. Surgeons should critically analyze every PJI and determine the appropriate treatment of each patient that will optimize the possibility of infection eradication.

SUMMARY

PJIs are a costly and life-changing complication of TJA. As the number of TJAs performed increases, there must be a deliberate focus among surgeons to decrease the occurrence of PJIs and deliver effective surgical and medical treatment. Although health-care systems take on a large economic burden during the treatment of PJI, cost should not be the only determining factor. Surgeons and health-care systems should work in tandem to deliver ef cient care while minimizing the economic burden on patients, surgeons, and the health-care system.

CLINICS CARE POINTS

- TJA is one of the most common surgical procedures and is estimated to exceed 1.9 million cases by 2030.[1]
- PJI is a devastating and common complication of TJA, with occurrence rates between 2.1% and 2.3% for hip and knee TJA, respectively.[6,8–10]
- The overall economic cost of PJI is set to increase due to the increase in TJA with an estimated financial burden of US$1.85 billion in 2030.[1]
- PJI is difficult to eradicate due to the propensity for common microbes to develop a resistant biofilm on prosthetic hardware.[10]
- Revisions and treatments for PJI are often complex and prolonged, resulting in extended hospital stays, multiple procedures, decreased quality of life, and increased monetary burden in relation to those without TJA without PJI.[4,8,10,34]
- The standard of care procedure for PJI is a 2-stage revision; other treatment options, such as a 1-stage revision and DAIR, are also available.[10]
- Even with standard of care, failure rates remain high, with studies producing failure rates ranging from 23% to greater than 50%.[10,11,26–28]

DISCLOSURE

This work is supported in part by NIH NIAMS (R01 AR082167).

REFERENCES

1. Premkumar A, Kolin DA, Farley KX, et al. Projected Economic Burden of Periprosthetic Joint Infection of the Hip and Knee in the United States. J Arthroplasty 2021;36(5):1484–1489 e3.
2. Changjun C, Jingkun L, Yun Y, et al. Enhanced Recovery after Total Joint Arthroplasty (TJA): A Contemporary Systematic Review of Clinical Outcomes and Usage of Key Elements. Orthop Surg 2023;15(5):1228–40.
3. Sloan M, Premkumar A, Sheth NP. Projected Volume of Primary Total Joint Arthroplasty in the U.S., 2014 to 2030. J Bone Joint Surg Am 2018; 100(17):1455–60.
4. Parisi TJ, Konopka JF, Bedair HS. What is the Long-term Economic Societal Effect of Periprosthetic Infections After THA? A Markov Analysis. Clin Orthop Relat Res 2017;475(7):1891–900.
5. Fisher CR, Patel R. Profiling the Immune Response to Periprosthetic Joint Infection and Non-Infectious Arthroplasty Failure. Antibiotics (Basel) 2023;12(2). https://doi.org/10.3390/antibiotics12020296.
6. Kapadia BH, Berg RA, Daley JA, et al. Periprosthetic joint infection. Lancet 2016;387(10016):386–94.
7. Mortazavi SM, Molligan J, Austin MS, et al. Failure following revision total knee arthroplasty: infection is the major cause. Int Orthop 2011;35(8):1157–64.
8. Bozic KJ, Kurtz SM, Lau E, et al. The epidemiology of revision total knee arthroplasty in the United States. Clin Orthop Relat Res 2010;468(1):45–51.

9. Parvizi J, Pawasarat IM, Azzam KA, et al. Periprosthetic joint infection: the economic impact of methicillin-resistant infections. J Arthroplasty 2010;25(6 Suppl):103–7.

10. Patel R. Periprosthetic Joint Infection. N Engl J Med 2023;388(3):251–62.

11. Kurtz S, Ong K, Lau E, et al. Projections of primary and revision hip and knee arthroplasty in the United States from 2005 to 2030. J Bone Joint Surg Am 2007;89(4):780–5.

12. Gundtoft PH, Pedersen AB, Varnum C, et al. Increased Mortality After Prosthetic Joint Infection in Primary THA. Clin Orthop Relat Res 2017; 475(11):2623–31.

13. Runner RP, Mener A, Roberson JR, et al. Prosthetic Joint Infection Trends at a Dedicated Orthopaedics Specialty Hospital. Adv Orthop 2019;2019:4629503.

14. Kapadia BH, McElroy MJ, Issa K, et al. The economic impact of periprosthetic infections following total knee arthroplasty at a specialized tertiary-care center. J Arthroplasty 2014;29(5):929–32.

15. Blanchette CM, Wang PF, Joshi AV, et al. Resource utilization and costs of blood management services associated with knee and hip surgeries in US hospitals. Adv Ther 2006;23(1):54–67.

16. Boettner F, Cross MB, Nam D, et al. Functional and Emotional Results Differ After Aseptic vs Septic Revision Hip Arthroplasty. HSS J 2011;7(3):235–8.

17. Toulson C, Walcott-Sapp S, Hur J, et al. Treatment of infected total hip arthroplasty with a 2-stage reimplantation protocol: update on "our institution's" experience from 1989 to 2003. J Arthroplasty 2009; 24(7):1051–60.

18. Berend KR, Lombardi AV Jr, Morris MJ, et al. Two-stage treatment of hip periprosthetic joint infection is associated with a high rate of infection control but high mortality. Clin Orthop Relat Res 2013; 471(2):510–8.

19. Choi HR, Bedair H. Mortality following revision total knee arthroplasty: a matched cohort study of septic versus aseptic revisions. J Arthroplasty 2014;29(6): 1216–8.

20. Zmistowski B, Karam JA, Durinka JB, et al. Periprosthetic joint infection increases the risk of one-year mortality. J Bone Joint Surg Am 2013; 95(24):2177–84.

21. Choi HR, Beecher B, Bedair H. Mortality after septic versus aseptic revision total hip arthroplasty: a matched-cohort study. J Arthroplasty 2013;28(8 Suppl):56–8.

22. Dietz MJ, Springer BD, Barnes PD, et al. Best practices for centers of excellence in addressing periprosthetic joint infection. J Am Acad Orthop Surg 2015;23(Suppl):S12–7.

23. Drain NP, Bertolini DM, Anthony AW, et al. High Mortality After Total Knee Arthroplasty Periprosthetic Joint Infection is Related to Preoperative Morbidity and the Disease Process but Not Treatment. J Arthroplasty 2022;37(7):1383–9.

24. Urish KL, Bullock AG, Kreger AM, et al. A Multicenter Study of Irrigation and Debridement in Total Knee Arthroplasty Periprosthetic Joint Infection: Treatment Failure Is High. J Arthroplasty 2018;33(4): 1154–9.

25. Lazic I, Scheele C, Pohlig F, et al. Treatment options in PJI - is two-stage still gold standard? J Orthop 2021;23:180–4.

26. Bongers J, Jacobs AME, Smulders K, et al. Reinfection and re-revision rates of 113 two-stage revisions in infected TKA. J Bone Jt Infect 2020;5(3):137–44.

27. Barton CB, Wang DL, An Q, et al. Two-Stage Exchange Arthroplasty for Periprosthetic Joint Infection Following Total Hip or Knee Arthroplasty Is Associated With High Attrition Rate and Mortality. J Arthroplasty 2020;35(5):1384–9.

28. Corona PS, Vicente M, Carrera L, et al. Current actual success rate of the two-stage exchange arthroplasty strategy in chronic hip and knee periprosthetic joint infection. Bone Joint Lett J 2020; 102-B(12):1682–8.

29. Yayac M, Rondon AJ, Tan TL, et al. The Economics of Antibiotic Cement in Total Knee Arthroplasty: Added Cost with No Reduction in Infection Rates. J Arthroplasty 2019;34(9):2096–101.

30. Rowland T, Lindberg-Larsen M, Santy-Tomlinson J, et al. A qualitative study of patients' experiences before, during and after surgical treatment for periprosthetic knee joint infection; "I assumed it had to be like that … ". Int J Orthop Trauma Nurs 2023;48: 100992.

31. Wilson JM, Schwartz AM, Farley KX, et al. Preoperative Patient Factors and Postoperative Complications as Risk Factors for New-Onset Depression Following Total Hip Arthroplasty. J Arthroplasty 2021;36(3):1120–5.

32. Lueck E, Schlaepfer TE, Schildberg FA, et al. The psychological burden of a two-stage exchange of infected total hip and knee arthroplasties. J Health Psychol 2022;27(2):470–80.

33. Das A, Agarwal AR, Gu A, et al. Higher 2-Year Cumulative Incidence of Mental Health Disorders Following Antibiotic Spacer Placement for Chronic Periprosthetic Joint Infection following Total Joint Arthroplasty. J Arthroplasty 2023; 38(7):1349–1355 e1.

34. Wildeman P, Rolfson O, Soderquist B, et al. What Are the Long-term Outcomes of Mortality, Quality of Life, and Hip Function after Prosthetic Joint Infection of the Hip? A 10-year Follow-up from Sweden. Clin Orthop Relat Res 2021;479(10):2203–13.

35. Schwartz AM, Wilson JM, Farley KX, et al. New-Onset Depression After Total Knee Arthroplasty: Consideration of the At-Risk Patient. J Arthroplasty 2021;36(9):3131–6.

36. Mallon CM, Gooberman-Hill R, Moore AJ. Infection after knee replacement: a qualitative study of impact of periprosthetic knee infection. BMC Musculoskelet Disord 2018;19(1):352.

37. Kapadia BH, Banerjee S, Cherian JJ, et al. The Economic Impact of Periprosthetic Infections After Total Hip Arthroplasty at a Specialized Tertiary-Care Center. J Arthroplasty 2016;31(7):1422–6.

38. Palan J, Nolan C, Sarantos K, et al. Culture-negative periprosthetic joint infections. EFORT Open Rev 2019;4(10):585–94.

39. Yao JJ, Hevesi M, Visscher SL, et al. Direct Inpatient Medical Costs of Operative Treatment of Periprosthetic Hip and Knee Infections Are Twofold Higher Than Those of Aseptic Revisions. J Bone Joint Surg Am 2021;103(4):312–8.

40. Rezapoor M, Parvizi J. Prevention of Periprosthetic Joint Infection. J Arthroplasty 2015;30(6):902–7.

41. Charalambous LT, Wixted CM, Kim BI, et al. Cost Drivers in Two-Stage Treatment of Hip Periprosthetic Joint Infection With an Antibiotic Coated Cement Hip Spacer. J Arthroplasty 2023;38(1):6–12.

42. Kurtz SM, Lau E, Watson H, et al. Economic burden of periprosthetic joint infection in the United States. J Arthroplasty 2012;27(8 Suppl):61–65 e1.

43. Tonotsuka H, Sugiyama H, Amagami A, et al. What is the most cost-effective strategy for nasal screening and Staphylococcus aureus decolonization in patients undergoing total hip arthroplasty? BMC Musculoskelet Disord 2021;22(1):129.

44. Kolin DA, Moverman MA, Menendez ME, et al. A break-even analysis of tranexamic acid for prevention of periprosthetic joint infection following total hip and knee arthroplasty. J Orthop 2021;26: 54–7.

45. Bourget-Murray J, Azad M, Gofton W, et al. Is the routine use of local antibiotics in the management of periprosthetic joint infections justified? Hip Int 2023;33(1):4–16.

46. Trentinaglia MT, Van Der Straeten C, Morelli I, et al. Economic Evaluation of Antibacterial Coatings on Healthcare Costs in First Year Following Total Joint Arthroplasty. J Arthroplasty 2018;33(6):1656–62.

47. Kurtz SM, Higgs GB, Lau E, et al. Hospital Costs for Unsuccessful Two-Stage Revisions for Periprosthetic Joint Infection. J Arthroplasty 2022;37(2): 205–12.

48. Nodzo SR, Boyle KK, Spiro S, et al. Success rates, characteristics, and costs of articulating antibiotic spacers for total knee periprosthetic joint infection. Knee 2017;24(5):1175–81.

49. Bernard L, Arvieux C, Brunschweiler B, et al. Antibiotic Therapy for 6 or 12 Weeks for Prosthetic Joint Infection. N Engl J Med 2021;384(21):1991–2001.

50. Tarazi JM, Chen Z, Scuderi GR, et al. The Epidemiology of Revision Total Knee Arthroplasty. J Knee Surg 2021;34(13):1396–401.

51. Miller R, Higuera CA, Wu J, et al. Periprosthetic Joint Infection: A Review of Antibiotic Treatment. JBJS Rev 2020;8(7):e1900224.

52. Pansu N, Hamoui M, Manna F, et al. Implant retention and high rate of treatment failure in hematogenous acute knee and hip prosthetic joint infections. Med Mal Infect 2020;50(8):702–8.

53. Mponponsuo K, Leal J, Puloski S, et al. Economic Burden of Surgical Management of Prosthetic Joint Infections Following Hip and Knee Replacements in Alberta, Canada: An analysis and comparison of two major urban centers. J Hosp Infect 2022. https://doi.org/10.1016/j.jhin.2022.05.002.

54. Garfield K, Noble S, Lenguerrand E, et al. What are the inpatient and day case costs following primary total hip replacement of patients treated for prosthetic joint infection: a matched cohort study using linked data from the National Joint Registry and Hospital Episode Statistics. BMC Med 2020;18(1): 335.

Biofilm and How It Relates to Prosthetic Joint Infection

Ashley E. MacConnell, MD*, Ashley E. Levack, MD, Nicholas M. Brown, MD

KEYWORDS

- Biofilm • Prosthetic joint infection • Total joint arthroplasty • Bacteriophage
- Antimicrobial peptide

KEY POINTS

- Biofilm infections are poorly managed with antibiotics alone given the dormant state of bacteria.
- A combination of surgical and medical intervention is necessary to eradicate a biofilm and thus appropriately treat PJI.
- While active and passive surface modification of an implant can currently be implemented in practice, many alternative infection prevention options require additional study prior to clinical application.

INTRODUCTION

Total knee arthroplasty (TKA) and total hip arthroplasty (THA) are highly effective options for treating end-stage osteoarthritis, resulting in substantial increases in quality of life for patients undergoing these procedures.[1,2] One catastrophic complication is the development of a prosthetic joint infection (PJI), an infection of the joint prosthesis and surrounding soft tissues. The rate of these infections remains fairly low ranging between 0.25% and 2.0% in the literature; a recent registry-based described a rate of 0.92% (0.84–1.01) after THA and 1.41% (1.32–1.51) following TKA.[3–6] Nevertheless, a diagnosis of PJI is associated with increased patient morbidity and mortality, with studies reporting a mortality rate of up to 8% within 1 year of the index procedure and 2 fold increase in in-hospital mortality for every surgical admission.[7–10] It remains imperative that techniques for appropriate prevention, diagnosis, and management of PJI continue to be implemented. However, 1 factor that can complicate the eradication of these infections is the presence of a bacterial biofilm. This review will seek to describe the challenges associated with treating PJI attributed to biofilm in order to better elucidate the best management practices for patients presenting with these infections.

BACKGROUND

Adaptation is critical for the survival of bacteria in a human host. One such survival mechanism is the ability of bacteria to display different phenotypic forms—planktonic versus sessile in biofilm.[11] Bacteria that are independent and free-floating are described as planktonic. Conversely, bacteria can form a biofilm, in which they organize and grow as a surface-associated sessile aggregate, rooted in a self-produced extracellular polymeric substance (EPS).[11–13] Bacteria modify their gene expression and metabolism to accommodate a nutrient-poor and anoxic environment in the dormant biofilm state. This in turn limits the classic targets of antimicrobial agents by minimizing the requirements for cellular function.[14] Mechanisms such as efflux pumps or horizontal gene transfer are used to induce further resistance.[15] Additionally, the extracellular matrix of the biofilm functions as a barrier to the native immune system and charged antimicrobial agents, allowing biofilms to endure antimicrobial concentrations 10 to 1000 times higher than those used to target

---

Department of Orthopaedic Surgery and Rehabilitation, Loyola University Medical Center, 2160 South First Avenue, Suite 1700, Maywood, IL 60153, USA
* Corresponding author.
E-mail address: ashley.macconnell@luhs.org

Orthop Clin N Am 55 (2024) 161–169
https://doi.org/10.1016/j.ocl.2023.10.001

planktonic bacteria.[13] Even at these concentrations, bacteria in biofilms respond inconsistently to treatment.

The process of biofilm formation was elucidated by Sauer and colleagues in 2002 using a number of analytical techniques to examine *Pseudomonas aeruginosa*.[16] The authors found that formation progressed through discrete stages, characterized by differences in gene expression and protein profile. These stages were planktonic, reversible attachment, irreversible attachment, maturation-1, maturation-2, and dispersion. Dispersed cells were able to return to a planktonic form and leave the biofilm, allowing for further dissemination and bacterial colonization.[11] The dispersion process is facilitated by a variety of organism-specific enzymes released in the EPS. Depending on the species and environment, in vitro biofilm formation has been shown to occur in as little as 24 to 48 hours.[17]

Biofilms carry significant relevance for orthopedic surgeons in regards to the potential for colonization of implanted hardware. Surgical site contamination can occur intraoperatively when bacteria from the patient's skin or from the operating room result in direct inoculation of the wound.[15] A "race for the surface," as described by Gristina, subsequently occurs, where the invading bacteria compete with the native host cells for space on the implant.[18] If host tissue establishes itself first, it becomes less likely that the bacteria will be able to successfully colonize the implant.[19] In the event of infection, initial passive surface adhesion via nonspecific interactions between the implant material and bacteria takes place.[20] Combinations of van der Waals, electrostatic, Lewis acid/base, and hydrophobic forces contribute to these interactions.[21] This process is augmented by autolysins, organism-specific proteins that promote binding to abiotic surfaces.[22] Adhesins then enhance the stability of this link, and ultimately facilitate internalization into the host cells through interaction with host extracellular matrix proteins.[20]

Certain bacterial species have a proclivity for orthopedic implants. Specifically, gram-positive staphylococcal species such as *Staphylococcus aureus*, coagulase-negative staphylococci including *Staphylococcus epidermidis*, and enterococci are the most common organisms that cause PJI and account for 75% of biofilm formation.[15,23,24] Infective species vary by geographic location, surgical site, and time since the index procedure, and may be attributed to 1 organism or polymicrobial.[23] Infections can present more acutely, often attributed to contamination with a virulent species such as *S aureus*, or may be chronic and indolent, such as infection with *S epidermidis* or *Cutibacterium acnes*.[15,23]

EVALUATION

The clinical presentation of a patient presenting with PJI varies based on a number of factors, including the pathogen virulence, time of onset, and host immune response.[3] Patients may report continued or progressive joint pain, erythema, delayed wound healing, presence of a sinus tract, or systemic symptoms suggestive of an infection. Parvizi and colleagues developed a scoring system in 2018 that incorporates a number of preoperative and intraoperative factors into criteria for the diagnosis of PJI.[25]

Unfortunately, patients who have biofilm infection may have a subtle clinical presentation, making proper identification challenging. The sessile bacteria in the biofilm are less immunogenic and therefore do not elicit the same inflammatory response that would be appreciated in an infection of planktonic bacteria.[12] Biofilm encapsulation also prevents access to the organism, and the reduced metabolic activity can hinder growth on traditional bacterial media, resulting in falsely negative cultures.[24,26]

Techniques to disrupt biofilm have been implemented in an effort to overcome these diagnostic issues, including chemical and mechanical dislodgement. A reducing agent, dithiothreitol (DTT), functions by reducing the disulfide bonds between neighboring substrates, which allows for the displacement of bacteria from the extracellular polymeric substance matrix.[27] De Vecchi and colleagues demonstrated a high sensitivity (88.0%) and specificity (97.8%) of detecting microbial growth with use of DTT when compared to use of saline in the analysis of periprosthetic tissue samples.[28]

Ultrasound-based sonication is a method of mechanical disruption that has consistently demonstrated promising results. Trampuz and colleagues examined 331 patients using conventional culture of tissue and compared that to samples obtained after sonication.[29] A sensitivity of 78.5% and specificity of 98.8% upon analysis of sonicate fluid were reported, compared to a tissue culture sensitivity and specificity of 60.8% and 99.2%, respectively. These findings were mirrored by Tani and colleagues who noted a sensitivity of 77.04% and specificity of 98.11% when using a sonication method.[30]

Rothenberg and colleagues determined that sensitivity of sonicate fluid culture was found to be statistically significantly higher than that of synovial fluid culture or tissue culture, while specificity was similar between these 3 methods.[31] Additionally, in the setting of recent antibiotic administration (less than 15 days prior to analysis), Scorzolini and colleagues found that sonicate fluid was able to detect pathogens at a rate of 80% compared to 16.6% when standard culture methods were used.[32]

Challenges with sonication include the possibility of damage to micro-organisms, cost of procedural equipment, and potential of sample contamination during the process.[26] Parameters for ultrasound frequency have been studied by Dudek and colleagues to identify a point at which biofilm is disrupted without harming planktonic bacteria.[33] A frequency of 35 kHz and 40 kHz were optimal frequencies when analyzing *S aureus*, *P aeruginosa*, and *Escherichia coli* biofilm cultures, although some planktonic bacteria were shown to be degraded after sonication despite the low-frequency and low-intensity environment. Trampuz and colleagues identified the issue of contamination, noting that several samples for patient with aseptic failure demonstrated sonicate fluid culture growth that did not correspond to tissue cultures; leakage of the ultrasound bath water was ultimately found to be the source.[34]

Multiple studies have been undertaken to compare chemical and mechanical disruption of biofilm on explanted arthroplasty implants. A recent meta-analysis of clinical studies comparing DTT and sonication did not appreciate a statistically significant difference between pooled sensitivity and specificity, suggesting that both are effective methods to obtain diagnostic cultures.[35] Sambri and colleagues reported a sensitivity of 89% for cultures on sonicate fluid and 91% for cultures obtained after using DTT, which were significantly improved from that of 79% for conventional tissue samples.[36] DTT had a greater sensitivity than both sonication and standard tissue culture but similar specificity among patients who did not appear to have a preoperative infection (absence of a fistula, normal *erythrocyte sedimentation rate* [ESR] and *C-reactive protein* [CRP], negative joint aspiration). Finally, a prospective cohort of 187 patients was examined by Karbysheva and colleagues[37] Sonication had a much higher sensitivity compared to DTT at 73.8% versus 43.2%, respectively. Specificity was similar between both methods, at 98% for sonication and 94.6% for DTT. The accuracy of DTT was

posited to be correlated with low pH of a reagent in the system, a finding that had previously been reported as contributing to an increase in false-negative readings.[38]

MANAGEMENT

A combination of operative intervention and systemic treatment is necessary when addressing these complex infections. Different strategies in managing PJI include antibiotic suppression, debridement with retention of hardware, prosthesis resection with reimplantation as a 1-stage or 2-stage exchange, prosthesis resection without reimplantation of hardware, joint fusion, and amputation.[39]

A debridement, antibiotics, and implant retention (DAIR) procedure is an option typically reserved for patients presenting with hematogenous infection or PJI within 30 days of their index procedure.[40] Retaining the original hardware allows for a less invasive or extensive operation, while debridement can serve to reduce the bacterial load and provide a better opportunity for systemic antibiotics to treat the infection.[41] The efficacy of DAIR has not been fully borne out by studies, with rate of successful infection eradication ranging from 11.1% to 100% in the literature.[42] The rationale for selecting this option for early PJI lies in the development of a biofilm. Bacteria causing an infection soon after the index procedure have theoretically not had enough time to form a mature biofilm, and thus may be susceptible to debridement.[43] However, in vitro studies suggest biofilm maturation can occur in a few days[17]; while in vivo data on the timing of biofilm formation is currently lacking, the speed of this process may contribute to the notable inconsistency of successful DAIR treatment.

One-stage and two-stage revision procedures with postoperative antibiotic therapy are alternatives for patients presenting with PJI. One-stage revision occurs with explantation of the implant followed by debridement and direct reimplantation, while 2-stage surgeries allow for interval treatment with antibiotics and stabilization with a spacer followed by delayed reimplantation.[44] Two-stage exchange has been largely considered the "gold standard," but is associated with increased burden on the patient and health care system in the form of reduced function and mobility between surgical procedures, increased expense, and additional risk inherent to multiple operations.[44,45] In a systematic review and meta-analysis, Kunutsor and colleagues found a reinfection rate after 1-stage surgery of 7.6% for TKA and 8.2% for THA, while a rate after 2-stage procedures of 8.8% after TKA and 7.9% for THA patients, prompting the authors to suggest that both techniques may be effective options.[46,47]

Successful 1-stage procedures require vigilance and thorough debridement to remove any tissue or foreign material that could sustain a biofilm infection after implantation of a new prosthesis.[48] Unfortunately, this remains a challenging goal given the inability of the surgeon to see the biofilm and assess the adequacy of their debridement. Methods of enhancing intraoperative visualization of the biofilm include the use of methylene blue, a cationic dye under investigation as a biofilm-disclosing agent.[49] In vitro studies have demonstrated the efficacy of this compound in staining different implant materials to identify the location of S aureus and P aeruginosa biofilms[50] and established that use of methylene blue does not preclude the acquisition of adequate bacterial culture.[51] Shaw and colleagues performed a small study trialing dilute methylene blue in patients with PJI after TKA.[49] Tissue stained with methylene blue demonstrated a statistically significant difference compared to unstained tissue, with greater bacterial bioburden on culture, quantitative polymerase chain reaction, and tissue pathology.

Arthroplasty resection and antibiotic spacer placement without prosthesis reimplantation, known as the 1.5-stage treatment, has gained popularity as a surgical option. While use of functional spacers can potentially allow a patient to forgo a second surgery, concerns about implant survivorship have been raised, as the prosthesis and implantation techniques may not be as robust compared to a traditional 1-stage approach.[52] Studies have demonstrated that despite this theoretic disadvantage, 1.5-stage revision is an excellent option in a lower demand patient.[53,54] Amputation is the last resort for patients who have either failed alternative treatments or who require emergent source control of their infection. Fortunately, this is not often necessary, with approximately 0.1% of patients who underwent TKA at 1 institution over 30 years requiring an above-knee amputation for persistent infection.[55]

Antibiotic therapy alone is not recommended, as it does not serve to directly reduce the bacterial burden by removing the hardware that serves as an ongoing source of infection and cannot reach intra-articular concentrations that would be bactericidal. This strategy is typically reserved for patients who are not surgical candidates given other comorbidities or who have failed multiple attempts at surgical eradication of infection.[39] Leijtens and colleagues completed a retrospective study of patients treated with antibiotic suppression given increased complication risk with revision surgery; 43.5% of patients ultimately required further operation or succumbed to PJI-related causes of death.[56] However, the rate of failure increased to 80% for patients diagnosed with PJI caused by S aureus. Burr and colleagues examined chronic antibiotic suppression and reported a success rate of 67% in their patient cohort.[57] This strategy was more successful in patients diagnosed with infections of the hip or gram-positive infections.

Given the metabolic inactivity of biofilms, investigation into different irrigation solutions that do not target cellular processes has been undertaken. Oxidizing agents such as hydrogen peroxide or sodium hypochlorite have been trialed as irrigants.[58] While in vitro studies have demonstrated the efficacy of these agents against bacterial biofilms,[59] cytotoxicity upon exposure of healthy tissue to these chemicals remains a limitation.[60] Similarly, cationic synthetic biguanides such as chlorhexidine are widely used antiseptics in the operating room, but have cytotoxic effects at concentrations necessary to disrupt biofilms.[61] Premkumar and colleagues examined the impact of different antimicrobial solutions on biofilm grown for 24 hours and for 72 hours on biomaterials including titanium, cement, and plastic 48-well plates.[62] Efficacy of the different irrigants varied significantly, with only povidone-iodine 10% and a 1:1 mixture of povidone-iodine 10% and 4% hydrogen peroxide successfully diminishing biofilm bacterial counts by ten-thousand-fold at both time points. Commonly used solutions such as Irrisept (0.05% chlorhexidine gluconate in water) and Bactisure (acetic acid, water, sodium acetate, ethanol, and benzalkonium chloride) were highly effective on planktonic bacteria but did not consistently eradicate biofilm infection. However, the authors cautioned that these findings need to be translated to clinical application before drawing conclusions on use in the human body.

PREVENTION

The addition of antibiotics to polymethylmethacrylate (PMMA) when cementing components in total joint arthroplasty has been a common practice for over 50 years.[19] Beyond the disadvantage of increased cost, risks with routine use of antibiotic cement include toxicity locally and systemically, inhibition of bony healing and osseointegration, and the development of antibiotic resistance.[63,64] Further, there are concerns regarding the biodistribution of the antimicrobial agent, and thus their effectiveness on a biofilm, as well as potential for colonization of the PMMA or development of resistance after antibiotic concentration becomes subtherapeutic.[63,65] Studies have sought to address these issues by examining procedural or material changes that may affect the elution properties of the antibiotics. Use of a mechanical device such as a mixing drill piece when preparing the cement, reduction in the ratio of liquid: powder components, increase in the proportion of radiopacifier (barium sulfate), and formation of intracement tunnels (specifically when making cement beads) have been found to improve porosity and thus antibiotic elution.[66–68] These strategies unfortunately also serve to diminish the mechanical properties of the cement. Consequently, the use of antibiotic-impregnated cement as both a prophylactic measure and in addressing biofilm infection in PJI remains an ongoing topic of discussion and investigation.

One opportunity to inhibit the formation of a biofilm would be to alter the surface characteristics of the implant itself. The surface characteristics of a metal implant, such as hydrophilicity and roughness profile, can serve to promote or inhibit bacterial colonization.[19,23] Smooth, hydrophilic surfaces reduce the surface area available for adhesion and present less optimal environments for the proliferation of microorganisms.[19,21] Sorrentino and colleagues compared common arthroplasty materials and found that bioceramics were superior to metals and polymers in their ability to resist bacterial adhesion and thus biofilm formation.[69] Coatings can also be applied to confer adhesion-resistant or bacteria-repellent properties to hardware, with the goal of efficacy without compromising the integrity of the implant.[23,24] These coatings can be either passive or active. Passive coatings function by preventing adhesion to the surface of the implant.[70] Examples include polyethylene oxide or polyethylene glycol added to the implant surface, ultraviolet irradiation of titanium dioxide to enhance wettability and decrease adhesion, and incorporation of zinc into titanium surfaces.[23,70] Active coatings work by releasing bactericidal substances into the surrounding tissue.[70] Modification with a silver coating results in the release of metal cations which possess multiple mechanisms of action, triggering the formation of reactive oxygen species, targeting

bacterial cell metabolism, and destroying membrane proteins.[71] Antibiotic-hydroxyapatite coatings are another option, although likely only function on microorganisms adjacent to the hardware and present an opportunity for antibiotic resistance.[23] In vivo studies utilizing active and passive coatings are currently lacking, and concerns of osteoblast impairment, inhibition of osseointegration, and decreased wear properties have been raised.

FUTURE DIRECTIONS

The literature suggests that, despite our best efforts, the rate of PJI has not changed significantly over the past few years.[72] The key as we progress into the future may very well be the advancement of new technologies or techniques for addressing these infections.

Nanotube arrays and nanoparticles offer an alternative method of prolonged local delivery of antimicrobial agents to the surface of an implant. Nanotubes have demonstrated an ability to bind to different antibiotics and, when anchored to the surface of an implant, may prevent the formation of a biofilm through continuous release of these agents.[73] Hirshfeld and colleagues examined multi-walled carbon nanotubes that were impregnated with varied concentrations of rifampicin and found that S epidermidis biofilm formation was significantly inhibited for up to 5 days.[73] Nanoparticles can also be used in antibiotic delivery. One example is that of a liposome, a phospholipid vesicle can transport and protect antimicrobial agents from degradation.[74,75] Liposomes have demonstrated the ability to fuse with the outer membrane of bacteria to allow for targeted release of the enclosed antimicrobial into the cell, thus reducing the systemic effects of medical therapies in the treatment of biofilm infection.[58] Limitations of liposomal nanoparticles include the expense and potential for inconsistent drug delivery.[76]

Antimicrobial peptides (AMP) are a category of molecules that are either produced by various organisms or created synthetically and possess certain antimicrobial properties.[77] Hundreds of AMPs have been described in the human body as contributing to the innate immune system.[78] Depending on the length, charge, and structure, AMP can demonstrate mechanisms of action such as translocation across the cell membrane to disrupt DNA, RNA, or proteins synthesis, and formation of pores in the cellular membrane.[74] Kang and colleagues evaluated LL-37, a cathelicidin-derived AMP with known antimicrobial efficacy against multiple gram-positive and gram-negative organisms, against *S aureus* biofilms and found that LL-37 was more effective in eradicating these biofilms than conventional antibiotics.[78] Historically, these organic peptides have not been utilized as therapeutic options, as they have demonstrated toxicity when delivered systemically and are vulnerable to environmental factors such as ion concentration and pH.[79] Huang and colleagues tested an engineered AMP PLG0206, which was designed to minimize the adverse effects of natural AMP and enhancing the antibacterial properties.[79] In vitro studies suggested PLG0206 was highly effective against planktonic and biofilm *S aureus*, and an acceptable safety profile was demonstrated in a Phase 1 trial of healthy volunteers. Studies assessing different AMPs and combination strategies for addressing biofilm infections remain ongoing.

Bacteriophages, or viruses that specifically target and kill bacteria, are another technique under investigation. Lytic phages identify certain surface proteins on the bacteria. The phages then infect the cell, replicate their genomic material, and ultimately lyse the cell to release new phages that seek out additional bacterial targets.[74,80] The specificity with which bacteriophages identify bacterial cells allows for the preservation of host cells, thus reducing adverse reactions to this modality.[80] Further, this cycle of viral infection and lysis perpetuates for the duration of time that a bacterial infection is present, which is in contrast to the time-dependent nature of conventional antibiotics. Totten and colleagues performed an in vitro study of multiple phages against dozens of *S aureus* isolates, demonstrating statistically significant reductions in biofilm growth in 96% to 100% of the cultures.[81] Morris and colleagues mirrored these findings with a similar in vitro study evaluating a combination of 5 different bacteriophages against *S aureus* isolates.[80] Statistically significant reductions in viable bacteria within isolates that demonstrated strong biofilm growth after 48 hours incubation were noted following phage exposure, a finding that was not appreciated when exposing biofilm to cefazolin alone. Independent case reports of bacteriophage therapy in patients with chronic PJI have demonstrated generally positive results, with authors describing eradication of the infection after treatment.[82,83] Unfortunately, the specificity of the phage and uncertainty on the best method of administration present challenges to the widespread clinical implementation of this modality.

SUMMARY

PJI is an uncommon but challenging condition to address, in part due to the development of a bacterial biofilm on the orthopedic hardware. The authors present the nuances of PJI in the context of biofilm formation and how it relates to diagnosis, treatment, and prevention of this complex problem. Bacteria in biofilms demonstrate multiple protective mechanisms, including envelopment in an extracellular polymeric substance, diminished metabolic activity, physical sequestration from the host immune system, and antibiotic resistance. Prevention, diagnosis, and treatment are all impaired and eradication often involves implant removal. Investigation into new techniques including implant surface coating, nanotechnology, antimicrobial peptides, and bacteriophages are of the utmost importance as we seek to minimize the harm associated with PJI.

CLINICS CARE POINTS

- Conventional antibiotic regimens are ineffective against biofilm infections due to the reduced metabolic activity and relatively dormant state of bacteria.

- Diagnosis typically requires chemical or mechanical disruption of the biofilm.

- Debridement or implant removal is necessary in combination with targeted antibiotic therapy to eradicate a biofilm.

- Various methods of prevention and treatment of biofilm infections are currently under investigation.

DISCLOSURE

The authors have nothing to disclose.

REFERENCES

1. Konopka JF, Lee YY, Su EP, et al. Quality-adjusted life years after hip and knee arthroplasty: health-related quality of life after 12,782 Joint replacements. JB JS Open Access 2018;3(3):e0007.

2. Ethgen O, Bruyère O, Richy F, et al. Health-related quality of life in total hip and total knee arthroplasty. A qualitative and systematic review of the literature. J Bone Joint Surg Am 2004;86(5):963–74.

3. Gomez-Urena EO, Tande AJ, Osmon DR, et al. Diagnosis of Prosthetic Joint Infection: Cultures,

Biomarker and Criteria. Infect Dis Clin North Am 2017;31(2):219–35.

4. Matar WY, Jafari SM, Restrepo C, et al. Preventing infection in total joint arthroplasty. J Bone Joint Surg Am 2010;92(Suppl 2):36–46.

5. Ren X, Ling L, Qi L, et al. Patients' risk factors for periprosthetic joint infection in primary total hip arthroplasty: a meta-analysis of 40 studies. BMC Muscoskel Disord 2021;22(1):776.

6. Huotari K, Peltola M, Jämsen E. The incidence of late prosthetic joint infections: a registry-based study of 112,708 primary hip and knee replacements. Acta Orthop 2015 Jun;86(3):321–5.

7. Gundtoft PH, Pedersen AB, Varnum C, et al. Increased Mortality After Prosthetic Joint Infection in Primary THA. Clin Orthop Relat Res 2017; 475(11):2623–31.

8. Fischbacher A, Borens O. Prosthetic-joint Infections: Mortality Over The Last 10 Years. J Bone Jt Infect 2019;4(4):198–202.

9. Shahi A, Tan TL, Chen AF, et al. In-Hospital Mortality in Patients with Periprosthetic Joint Infection. J Arthroplasty 2017;32(3):948–52.e1.

10. Drain NP, Bertolini DM, Anthony AW, et al. High Mortality After Total Knee Arthroplasty Periprosthetic Joint Infection is Related to Preoperative Morbidity and the Disease Process but Not Treatment. J Arthroplasty 2022;37(7):1383–9.

11. Sauer K, Stoodley P, Goeres DM, et al. The biofilm life cycle: expanding the conceptual model of biofilm formation. Nat Rev Microbiol 2022;20(10):608–20.

12. Zoubos AB, Galanakos SP, Soucacos PN. Orthopedics and biofilm—what do we know? A review. Med Sci Mon Int Med J Exp Clin Res 2012;18(6):RA89–96. https://doi.org/10.12659/msm.882893.

13. Jefferson KK. What drives bacteria to produce a biofilm? FEMS Microbiol Lett 2004;236(2):163–73.

14. Vestby LK, Grønseth T, Simm R, et al. Bacterial Biofilm and its Role in the Pathogenesis of Disease. Antibiotics (Basel) 2020;9(2):59.

15. Rodríguez-Merchán EC, Davidson DJ, Liddle AD. Recent Strategies to Combat Infections from Biofilm-Forming Bacteria on Orthopaedic Implants. Int J Mol Sci 2021;22(19):10243.

16. Sauer K, Camper AK, Ehrlich GD, et al. Pseudomonas aeruginosa displays multiple phenotypes during development as a biofilm. J Bacteriol 2002;184(4):1140–54.

17. Staats A, Li D, Sullivan AC, et al. Biofilm formation in periprosthetic joint infections. Ann Jt 2021;6:43.

18. Gristina AG. Biomaterial-centered infection: microbial adhesion versus tissue integration. Science 1987;237(4822):1588–95.

19. Levack AE, Cyphert EL, Bostrom MP, et al. Current Options and Emerging Biomaterials for Periprosthetic Joint Infection. Curr Rheumatol Rep 2018; 20(6):33.

20. Arciola CR, Campoccia D, Ehrlich GD, et al. Biofilm-based implant infections in orthopaedics. Adv Exp Med Biol 2015;830:29–46.

21. Getzlaf MA, Lewallen EA, Kremers HM, et al. Multi-disciplinary antimicrobial strategies for improving orthopaedic implants to prevent prosthetic joint infections in hip and knee. J Orthop Res 2016;34(2): 177–86.

22. Heilmann C, Hussain M, Peters G, et al. Evidence for autolysin-mediated primary attachment of Staphylococcus epidermidis to a polystyrene surface. Mol Microbiol 1997;24(5):1013–24.

23. Davidson DJ, Spratt D, Liddle AD. Implant materials and prosthetic joint infection: the battle with the biofilm. EFORT Open Rev 2019;4(11):633–9.

24. Arciola CR, Campoccia D, Montanaro L. Implant infections: adhesion, biofilm formation and immune evasion. Nat Rev Microbiol 2018;16(7):397–409.

25. Parvizi J, Tan TL, Goswami K, et al. The 2018 Definition of Periprosthetic Hip and Knee Infection: An Evidence-Based and Validated Criteria. J Arthroplasty 2018;33(5):1309–14.e2.

26. Goh GS, Parvizi J. Diagnosis and Treatment of Culture-Negative Periprosthetic Joint Infection. J Arthroplasty 2022;37(8):1488–93.

27. Drago L, Signori V, De Vecchi E, et al. Use of dithiothreitol to improve the diagnosis of prosthetic joint infections. J Orthop Res 2013;31(11):1694–9.

28. De Vecchi E, Bortolin M, Signori V, et al. Treatment With Dithiothreitol Improves Bacterial Recovery From Tissue Samples in Osteoarticular and Joint Infections. J Arthroplasty 2016;31(12):2867–70.

29. Trampuz A, Piper KE, Jacobson MJ, et al. Sonication of removed hip and knee prostheses for diagnosis of infection. N Engl J Med 2007;357(7): 654–63.

30. Tani S, Lepetsos P, Stylianakis A, et al. Superiority of the sonication method against conventional periprosthetic tissue cultures for diagnosis of prosthetic joint infections. Eur J Orthop Surg Traumatol 2018;28(1):61–5.

31. Rothenberg AC, Wilson AE, Hayes JP, et al. Sonication of Arthroplasty Implants Improves Accuracy of Periprosthetic Joint Infection Cultures. Clin Orthop Relat Res 2017;475(7):1827–36.

32. Scorzolini L, Lichtner M, Iannetta M, et al. Sonication technique improves microbiological diagnosis in patients treated with antibiotics before surgery for prosthetic joint infections. New Microbiol 2014;37(3):321–8.

33. Dudek P, Grajek A, Kowalczewski J, et al. Ultrasound frequency of sonication applied in microbiological diagnostics has a major impact on viability of bacteria causing PJI. Int J Infect Dis 2020;100: 158–63.

34. Trampuz A, Piper KE, Hanssen AD, et al. Sonication of explanted prosthetic components in bags for

diagnosis of prosthetic joint infection is associated with risk of contamination. J Clin Microbiol 2006; 44(2):628–31.

35. Tsikopoulos K, Christofilos SI, Kitridis D, et al. Is sonication superior to dithiothreitol in diagnosis of periprosthetic joint infections? Int Orthop 2022; 46(6):1215–24.

36. Sambri A, Cadossi M, Giannini S, et al. Is Treatment With Dithiothreitol More Effective Than Sonication for the Diagnosis of Prosthetic Joint Infection? Clin Orthop Relat Res 2018;476(1):137–45.

37. Karbysheva S, Cabric S, Koliszak A, et al. Clinical evaluation of dithiothreitol in comparison with sonication for biofilm dislodgement in the microbiological diagnosis of periprosthetic joint infection. Diagn Microbiol Infect Dis 2022;103(2): 115679.

38. Randau TM, Molitor E, Fröschen FS, et al. The Performance of a Dithiothreitol-Based Diagnostic System in Diagnosing Periprosthetic Joint Infection Compared to Sonication Fluid Cultures and Tissue Biopsies. Z Orthop Unfall 2021;159(4):447–53.

39. Tande AJ, Patel R. Prosthetic joint infection. Clin Microbiol Rev 2014;27(2):302–45.

40. Veerman K, Raessens J, Telgt D, et al. Debridement, antibiotics, and implant retention after revision arthroplasty: antibiotic mismatch, timing, and repeated DAIR associated with poor outcome. Bone Joint Lett J 2022;104-B(4):464–71.

41. Qasim SN, Swann A, Ashford R. The DAIR (debridement, antibiotics and implant retention) procedure for infected total knee replacement - a literature review. SICOT J 2017;3:2.

42. Kunutsor SK, Beswick AD, Whitehouse MR, et al. Debridement, antibiotics and implant retention for periprosthetic joint infections: A systematic review and meta-analysis of treatment outcomes. J Infect 2018;77(6):479–88.

43. Xu Y, Wang L, Xu W. Risk factors affect success rate of debridement, antibiotics and implant retention (DAIR) in periprosthetic joint infection. Arthroplasty 2020;2(1):37.

44. Goud AL, Harlianto NI, Ezzafzafi S, et al. Reinfection rates after one- and two-stage revision surgery for hip and knee arthroplasty: a systematic review and meta-analysis. Arch Orthop Trauma Surg 2023;143(2):829–38.

45. van den Kieboom J, Tirumala V, Box H, et al. One-stage revision is as effective as two-stage revision for chronic culture-negative periprosthetic joint infection after total hip and knee arthroplasty. Bone Joint Lett J 2021;103-B(3):515–21.

46. Kunutsor SK, Whitehouse MR, Blom AW, et al, INFORM Team. Re-Infection Outcomes following One- and Two-Stage Surgical Revision of Infected Hip Prosthesis: A Systematic Review and Meta-Analysis. PLoS One 2015;10(9):e0139166.

47. Kunutsor SK, Whitehouse MR, Lenguerrand E, et al, INFORM Team. Re-Infection Outcomes Following One- And Two-Stage Surgical Revision of Infected Knee Prosthesis: A Systematic Review and Meta-Analysis. PLoS One 2016;11(3):e0151537.

48. Maale GE, Eager JJ, Srinivasaraghavan A, et al. The evolution from the two stage to the one stage procedure for biofilm based periprosthetic joint infections (PJI). Biofilm 2020;2:100033.

49. Shaw JD, Miller S, Plourde A, et al. Methylene Blue-Guided Debridement as an Intraoperative Adjunct for the Surgical Treatment of Periprosthetic Joint Infection. J Arthroplasty 2017;32(12):3718–23.

50. Shaw JD, Brodke DS, Williams DL, et al. Methylene Blue Is an Effective Disclosing Agent for Identifying Bacterial Biofilms on Orthopaedic Implants. J Bone Joint Surg Am 2020;102(20):1784–91.

51. Parry JA, Karau MJ, Kakar S, et al. Disclosing Agents for the Intraoperative Identification of Biofilms on Orthopedic Implants. J Arthroplasty 2017; 32(8):2501–4.

52. Hernandez NM, Buchanan MW, Seyler TM, et al. 1.5-Stage Exchange Arthroplasty for Total Knee Arthroplasty Periprosthetic Joint Infections. J Arthroplasty 2021;36(3):1114–9.

53. Siddiqi A, Mahmoud Y, Forte SA, et al. One and a Half-Stage Revision With Prosthetic Articulating Spacer for Definitive Management of Knee Periprosthetic Joint Infection. Arthroplast Today 2022; 19:100993.

54. Nabet A, Sax OC, Shanoada R, et al. Survival and Outcomes of 1.5-Stage vs 2-Stage Exchange Total Knee Arthroplasty Following Prosthetic Joint Infection. J Arthroplasty 2022;37(5):936–41.

55. Sierra RJ, Trousdale RT, Pagnano MW. Above-the-knee amputation after a total knee replacement: prevalence, etiology, and functional outcome. J Bone Joint Surg Am 2003;85(6):1000–4.

56. Leijtens B, Weerwag L, Schreurs BW, et al. Clinical Outcome of Antibiotic Suppressive Therapy in Patients with a Prosthetic Joint Infection after Hip Replacement. J Bone Jt Infect 2019;4(6):268–76.

57. Burr RG, Eikani CK, Adams WH, et al. Predictors of Success With Chronic Antibiotic Suppression for Prosthetic Joint Infections. J Arthroplasty 2022; 37(8S):S983–8.

58. Koo H, Allan RN, Howlin RP, et al. Targeting microbial biofilms: current and prospective therapeutic strategies. Nat Rev Microbiol 2017;15(12):740–55.

59. Röhner E, Jacob B, Böhle S, et al. Sodium hypochlorite is more effective than chlorhexidine for eradication of bacterial biofilm of staphylococci and Pseudomonas aeruginosa. Knee Surg Sports Traumatol Arthrosc 2020;28(12):3912–8.

60. Böhle S, Röhner E, Zippelius T, et al. Cytotoxic effect of sodium hypochlorite (Lavanox 0.08%) and chlorhexidine gluconate (Irrisept 0.05%) on human

osteoblasts. Eur J Orthop Surg Traumatol 2022 Jan; 32(1):81–9.

61. George J, Klika AK, Higuera CA. Use of Chlorhexidine Preparations in Total Joint Arthroplasty. J Bone Jt Infect 2017;2(1):15–22.

62. Premkumar A, Nishtala SN, Nguyen JT, et al. Comparing the Efficacy of Irrigation Solutions on Staphylococcal Biofilm Formed on Arthroplasty Surfaces. J Arthroplasty 2021;36(7S):S26–32.

63. Schwarz EM, McLaren AC, Sculco TP, et al. Adjuvant antibiotic-loaded bone cement: Concerns with current use and research to make it work. J Orthop Res 2021;39(2):227–39.

64. Antoci V Jr, Adams CS, Hickok NJ, et al. Antibiotics for local delivery systems cause skeletal cell toxicity in vitro. Clin Orthop Relat Res 2007;462:200–6.

65. van Vugt TAG, Arts JJ, Geurts JAP. Antibiotic-Loaded Polymethylmethacrylate Beads and Spacers in Treatment of Orthopedic Infections and the Role of Biofilm Formation. Front Microbiol 2019;10:1626.

66. Shiramizu K, Lovric V, Leung A, et al. How do porosity-inducing techniques affect antibiotic elution from bone cement? An in vitro comparison between hydrogen peroxide and a mechanical mixer. J Orthop Traumatol 2008;9(1):17–22.

67. Chen IC, Su CY, Nien WH, et al. Influence of Antibiotic-Loaded Acrylic Bone Cement Composition on Drug Release Behavior and Mechanism. Polymers (Basel) 2021;13(14):2240.

68. Tseng TH, Chang CH, Chen CL, et al. A simple method to improve the antibiotic elution profiles from polymethylmethacrylate bone cement spacers by using rapid absorbable sutures. BMC Muscoskel Disord 2022;23(1):916.

69. Sorrentino R, Cochis A, Azzimonti B, et al. Reduced bacterial adhesion on ceramics used for arthroplasty applications. J Eur Ceram 2018;38(3):963–70.

70. Gbejuade HO, Lovering AM, Webb JC. The role of microbial biofilms in prosthetic joint infections. Acta Orthop 2015;86(2):147–58.

71. Diez-Escudero A, Hailer NP. The role of silver coating for arthroplasty components. Bone Joint Lett J 2021;103-B(3):423–9.

72. Murphy MP, MacConnell AE, Killen CJ, et al. Prevention Techniques Have Had Minimal Impact on the Population Rate of Prosthetic Joint Infection for Primary Total Hip and Knee Arthroplasty: A National Database Study. J Arthroplasty 2023. S0883-S5403(23)00190-0.

73. Hirschfeld J, Akinoglu EM, Wirtz DC, et al. Long-term release of antibiotics by carbon nanotube-coated titanium alloy surfaces diminish biofilm formation by Staphylococcus epidermidis. Nanomedicine 2017;13(4):1587–93.

74. Taha M, Abdelbary H, Ross FP, et al. New Innovations in the Treatment of PJI and Biofilms-Clinical and Preclinical Topics. Curr Rev Musculoskelet Med 2018;11(3):380–8.

75. Zaidi S, Misba L, Khan AU. Nano-therapeutics: A revolution in infection control in post antibiotic era. Nanomedicine 2017;13(7):2281–301.

76. Indelli PF, Ghirardelli S, Iannotti F, et al. Nanotechnology as an Anti-Infection Strategy in Periprosthetic Joint Infections (PJI). Trav Med Infect Dis 2021;6(2):91.

77. Visperas A, Santana D, Klika AK, et al. Current treatments for biofilm-associated periprosthetic joint infection and new potential strategies. J Orthop Res 2022;40(7):1477.

78. Kang J, Dietz MJ, Li B. Antimicrobial peptide LL-37 is bactericidal against Staphylococcus aureus biofilms. PLoS One 2019;14(6):e0216676.

79. Huang D, Pachuda N, Sauer JM, et al. The Engineered Antibiotic Peptide PLG0206 Eliminates Biofilms and Is a Potential Treatment for Periprosthetic Joint Infections. Antibiotics (Basel) 2021;11(1):41.

80. Morris J, Kelly N, Elliott L, et al. Evaluation of Bacteriophage Anti-Biofilm Activity for Potential Control of Orthopedic Implant-Related Infections Caused by Staphylococcus aureus. Surg Infect 2019;20(1):16–24.

81. Totten KMC, Patel R. Phage Activity against Planktonic and Biofilm Staphylococcus aureus Periprosthetic Joint Infection Isolates. Antimicrob Agents Chemother 2022;66(1):e0187921.

82. Neuts AS, Berkhout HJ, Hartog A, et al. Bacteriophage therapy cures a recurrent Enterococcus faecalis infected total hip arthroplasty? A case report. Acta Orthop 2021;92(6):678–80.

83. Ramirez-Sanchez C, Gonzales F, Buckley M, et al. Successful Treatment of Staphylococcus aureus Prosthetic Joint Infection with Bacteriophage Therapy. Viruses 2021;13(6):1182.

Innovations in the Isolation and Treatment of Biofilms in Periprosthetic Joint Infection

A Comprehensive Review of Current and Emerging Therapies in Bone and Joint Infection Management

Spencer A. Ward, BS, Akram A. Habibi, MD,
Itay Ashkenazi, MD, Armin Arshi, MD,
Morteza Meftah, MD, Ran Schwarzkopf, MD, MSc*

KEYWORDS

• Periprosthetic joint infection • Biofilm • Management • Review

KEY POINTS

- The formation of biofilms occurs in a two-step process: rapid bacterial adherence phase and accumulation phase.
- *Staphylococcus aureus* plays a major role in the pathogenesis of periprosthetic joint infection-associated biofilms, representing 30% to 35% of all orthopedic implant-related infections.
- Surgical management with debridement, antibiotics, and implant retention and one- and two-stage revisions remains the mainstay of treatment.
- Emerging therapies such as combination and conjugated antibiotics, antimicrobial peptides, bacteriophages, and advancements in bearing surfaces offer alternatives for biofilm management.

INTRODUCTION

Total joint arthroplasty (TJA) has been one of the most successful orthopedic surgeries following its introduction in the 1960s, demonstrating both impressive survivorship and meaningful improvements in pain, physical function, and overall quality of life.[1–4] Although modern TJA is associated with a relatively low risk of adverse events, approximately 0.5% to 1.4% of all patients who undergo TJA suffer from infection of the implanted joint at 10 years, and this metric approaches 20% in revision TJA.[5,6] More importantly, periprosthetic joint infection (PJI) is one of the most common causes of implant failure

in TJA patients, with around 2% of these patients undergoing revision for PJI at 15 years following surgery, representing both a significant financial risk and clinical challenge.[5,6] Morcos and colleagues found that patients who undergo two-stage revision in the management of PJI following total knee arthroplasty (TKA) on average had overall costs of $35,429 versus $6809 on average associated with the costs from primary TKA patients.[7] Clinically, PJI remains one of the most feared and deleterious complications following TJA and is associated with increased morbidity, mortality, and worse functional outcomes.[4,8] This represents a substantial source of both health care utilization

NYU Langone Orthopedic Hospital, NYU Langone Health, 301 East 17th Street, Room 1402, New York, NY 10003, USA
* Corresponding author. Department of Orthopedic Surgery, NYU Langone Health, 301 East 17th Street, New York, NY 10003.
E-mail address: Ran.Schwarzkopf@nyulangone.org

Orthop Clin N Am 55 (2024) 171–180
https://doi.org/10.1016/j.ocl.2023.10.002
0030-5898/24/© 2023 Elsevier Inc. All rights reserved.

and financial burden placed on patients, and it is critical to understand current and emerging treatments to reduce costs and improve clinical outcomes for this patient population. In recent years, the role of biofilm in PJI has received increased interest due to its ability to prevent PJI eradication.[9–11] Therefore, in this review, we aim to identify the current understanding of PJI related to TJA and to discuss both the current and emerging technologies in the identification and management of biofilms and PJIs.

Biofilms and Biofilm-Associated Bacteria

Biofilms can be defined broadly as a structured aggregation of one or several organisms within a self-forming matrix of extracellular matrix components adherent to an organic or inorganic surface.[11,12] The formation of biofilms occurs in a two-step process. The first step involves rapid bacterial adherence to a polymer or device surface. In vitro, this process involves direct interaction with host matrix proteins such as fibronectin, fibrinogen, and von Willebrand factor that rapidly coat orthopedic devices following implantation.[13–15] This is then followed by an accumulation phase during which bacteria proliferate to form thick clusters of cells within the extracellular space on the device surface via intercellular adhesion, thus forming a dense matrix of polysaccharides, proteins, glycoproteins, and extracellular DNA[16] (Fig. 1). This process typically takes between 4 and 6 weeks before a mature biofilm is fully formed.[17,18] Once formed, this interwoven matrix of polymers and organisms is referred to as a glycocalyx, which confers resistance to local environmental factors.[19] The role of biofilms is critically important to the management of PJI as they shield bacteria from antibiotic treatment, and once this interconnected ecosystem is established bacteria demonstrate substantially increased resistance to antiseptic treatment.[20] This is critical since several bacteria responsible for PJI are known to acquire the ability to create a biofilm.[12,21]

The common bacterial organisms associated with biofilm production in PJI include the gram-negative organism *Pseudomonas aeruginosa* and the gram-positive *Staphylococcus epidermidis* and *S aureus* species. Including orthopedic devices, *these organisms account* for 75% of all identified biofilms detected on medical devices such as catheters, shunts, and pacemakers.[10,22] *S epidermidis* and more broadly coagulase-negative staphylococcal species are one of the most commonly isolated biofilm-producing organisms in medicine and, in the case of PJI, have been reported to be associated with treatment failure rates between 46.7% and 60%.[23,24] Koch and colleagues demonstrated that *S epidermidis*-associated biofilms have a high resistance to many commonly used antibiotics, with only rifampin and doxycycline demonstrating a quantifiable minimum biofilm bactericidal concentration.[25] In the case of *P aeruginosa*, bacterial biofilms may confer up to a 1000-fold increase in antibacterial resistance.[26]

S aureus represents one of the most common pathogens causing musculoskeletal infections and plays a major role in the pathogenesis of PJI-associated biofilms, representing 30% to 35% of all orthopedic implant-related infections.[27,28] There are several virulence factors associated with *S aureus* that allow it to not only produce a favorable environment for adherence to implant surfaces but also allow for invasion into native bone and joint tissue via evasion of host immunity and conferring a high resistance to antibiotics.[29–31] *S aureus* possesses several microbial surface components for recognizing adhesive matrix molecules and plasma proteins that allow it to recognize and interact with host extracellular matrix.[32,33] In addition, molecules such as protein A, coagulase, enterotoxins, exfoliatins, toxic shock syndrome toxins, and hemolysins have been shown to increase the pathogenicity of this organism.[32,33]

Identification and Isolation of Biofilm-Forming Bacteria

The diagnosis of PJI and the identification of bacteria that form biofilms have been critical for providing the appropriate treatment for patients with PJI after TJA. Currently, laboratory methods for the diagnosis of biofilm-forming bacteria PJI depend on pathogen isolation through cultural incubation. However, the use of cultures to identify pathogens has not provided the necessary sensitivity and specificity to reliably diagnose these infections preoperatively, with culture negativity rates as high as 15%, especially for biofilm-producing bacteria.[34,35] Most commonly, the diagnostic process for PJI following TJA involves a combination of clinical presentation, laboratory results, and radiographic evaluation. Currently, the gold standard for the diagnosis of PJI remains the guidelines put forth by the Musculoskeletal Infection Society, most recently updated in 2018.[36] Despite the effectiveness in the usage of this tool in the diagnosis of PJI, it remains an imperfect method of detection as the usage of inflammatory markers have been shown to be unreliable method of diagnosis, with a sensitivity as low as 45%.[36,37]

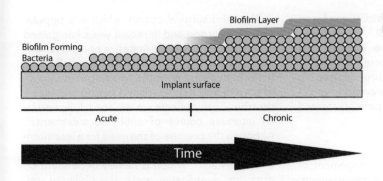

Fig. 1. Visualization of biofilm layering as time progresses.

Critical to the detection and diagnosis of biofilm-associated PJI is the understanding of the timing of the infection. Generally, it is accepted that acute PJIs present within 4 to 6 weeks postoperatively or 4 to 6 weeks from initiation of signs and symptoms of infection.[17,18,38] These infections are more often associated with bacteria in active growth phases and are less likely to be associated with biofilm production. In contrast, following formation of a biofilm, bacteria are notoriously difficult to detect. Hall-Stoodley and colleagues only detected biofilms on culture 30% of the time compared with 80% to 90% when using histology and microscopy, demonstrating the difficulties of identifying the insulting organism in a clinical setting once a biofilm has formed.[26] Multiple methods have been used as previously there were no known methods for the detection of biofilms clinically. Congo Red Agar was an early method studied for the detection of biofilm, although its poor sensitivity proved it to be far inferior to traditional tissue culture.[39]

A promising new development in the detection of biofilm-associated bacteria involves sonication, which incorporates long-wave ultrasound implementation before obtaining a culture, which aims to dislodge bacteria growing within the biofilm.[40,41] Following removal of infected implants during revision arthroplasty, implants are placed in sterile solution and undergo a series of vortexing in combination with sonication, from which cultures are obtained and incubated.[42] Kobayashi and colleagues found that the usage of sonication before obtaining cultures produced consistently higher quantitative yields of biofilm forming Staphylococcal species.[43] Recent literature has suggested a potential role for sonication cultures in the presence of inconclusive MSIS criteria, as 93% (76/82) patients diagnosed with PJI using clinical criteria had positive sonication cultures, compared with only 57% (47/82) of traditional tissue cultures.[44] Likewise, Merchan and colleagues

reported a sensitivity of 75% for sonicate cultures in comparison to only 57% for tissue cultures in the diagnosis PJI following TKA.[42] The consistent positive results for sonication suggest a role for this technique as a dependable test for the diagnosis of PJI, especially in the potential presence of biofilm (ie, chronic infections). Next-generation sequencing (NGS) has been identified as a potential future diagnostic method for biofilm detection due to decreasing costs and increasing availability.[45,46] NGS typically involves the extraction and sequencing of all nucleic acid material in a fluid sample to identify organisms without the need of traditional cultures.[45,46]

Current and Emergent Methodologies in the Management of Periprosthetic Joint Infection-Associated Biofilms

Prevention of periprosthetic joint infection

The most effective treatment of biofilm-associated PJI remains prevention of infection through the management of chronic medical conditions and thorough preoperative management before surgery. It has been shown that rigorous management of chronic medical conditions before TJA reduces morbidity, costs, and mortality.[47] Risk factors for PJI include rheumatoid arthritis, an American Society of Anesthesiologists Score of 2 or above, and uncontrolled diabetes, especially in conjunction with other comorbidities.[48–50] Among the risk factors for PJI following TJA, factors such as anemia, injection drug use, malnutrition, tobacco usage, obesity, and diabetes are modifiable targets for optimization before surgery.[51,52] Marchant and colleagues found that diabetic patients with increased preoperative hemoglobin A1c levels were at increased risk for PJI with an odds ratio of 2.31, and Mraovic and colleagues demonstrated that elevated postoperative glucose levels likewise predisposed patients to increased risk for PJI.[53,54] Preoperative testing and decolonization of Staphylococcus with intranasal mupirocin and chlorhexidine can be an effective method for reducing PJI.[55–57] Recently, preoperative interventions have incorporated the usage of prophylactic interosseous regional antibiotics, with recent literature suggesting either comparable or superior prevention of PJI in TJA patients in comparison to patients treated with systemic antibiotics.[58]

Surgical management

The mainstay treatment in the management of PJI-associated biofilms is surgical management, with debridement, antibiotics, and implant retention (DAIR) and both one- and two-stage revision procedures being the most used methods due to the insufficiency of PJI management with antibiotics in isolation. DAIR involves a combination of a thorough irrigation and debridement with aggressive antibiotic treatment and the exchange of modular components (ie, polyethylene liner exchange). Irrigation solutions can involve a combination of several agents, including normal saline, povidone-iodine, chlorhexidine, hydrogen peroxide, bacitracin, and hypochlorite.[59] Generally, DAIR is more commonly used in the acute phase of a PJI, when bacteria are more commonly still in growth phases and a biofilm has either not formed or is in the very early stages of formation, typically within 4 to 6 weeks after implantation.[60] The lack of a stable biofilm allows for the treatment of acute PJI with DAIR while rendering it less effective for more chronic infections with robust biofilms that confer resistance.[61] Intraosseous antibiotics have been reported to have a role intraoperatively, showing significantly reduced rates of PJI following TKA in comparison to intravenous administration when given following tourniquet inflation.[62]

In chronic PJI, two-stage revision is a more comprehensive approach to the treatment of biofilms in PJI and has established itself as the gold standard treatment of PJIs in the United States. Two-stage revision involves an initial stage for the removal of all joint prostheses with diligent resection of infected tissue and implantation of a temporary antibiotic-coated cement spacer, in conjunction with several months of antibiotic treatment.[63–65] A complete removal of all infected foreign material is mandatory due to robust biofilm formation that may harbor residual infection. This is then followed by the second stage, in which the spacer is removed and a new prosthesis is implanted. Although this is the gold standard treatment for PJI, failure is still not uncommon and chronic infections can be notoriously difficult to eradicate, ranging from 8% to 20%[66,67] (Fig. 2).

The third surgical option, which is a popular choice in Europe and in recent years has gained popularity in the United States, is one-stage revision surgery.[66–68] This procedure essentially combines both elements of the two-stage revision, in which a radical debridement is performed and all prosthetic components are replaced, followed by an intensive course of antibiotic treatment.[68] Although the premise of the need for a less intensive operative experience is enticing, the success of a one-stage revision is heavily dependent on organism identification and susceptibility of antibiotics.[64] Failure rates of one-stage revision are comparable to two-stage, ranging from 6% to 17%.[66,67] Both one- and two-stage revisions provide effective revision solutions particularly for biofilm-forming organisms in chronic infections. The investigators have argued for the selective use of single-stage exchange in patients who are healthy with an identified, antibiotic-susceptible organism, good bone stock and soft tissue coverage, and the use of antibiotic-loaded cement.[69]

The role of implant material of biofilm production

In recent years, there has been increasing research studying the role of implant surface material and the risk of biofilm formation following TJA. There have been several studies that suggest that implant designs incorporating ceramic material may decrease the formation of biofilms in PJI following total hip arthroplasty (THA).[70–72] Despite evidence supporting the potential benefits of ceramic surfaces in reducing the risk of biofilm-associated PJI, a systematic review by Hexter and colleagues found no difference in the choice of bearing material influencing the risk of PJI following THA.[73] Other studies have focused on the enhancement of existing metallic surfaces with various coating treatments to reduce the risk of biofilm formation. Pilz and colleagues observed decreased S epidermidis biofilm formation on zirconium nitride-coated cobalt–chromium–molybdenum alloy surfaces when compared with other common prosthetic surface materials.[74] Norambuena and colleagues found an 80% reduction in biofilm cell density on materials coated with titanium-copper oxide in comparison to other tested materials.[75]

Antibiotic management

In addition to surgical intervention, combination antibiotic therapy has been an essential component in the treatment of biofilms in PJI. An antibiotic that has been established within the literature as a consistently effective choice in the

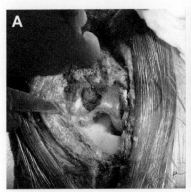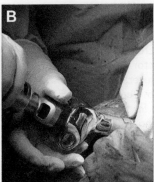

Fig. 2. Intraoperative image of a total knee arthroplasty with (A) prior implants from a chronic infection and (B) newly implanted distal femur replacement.

treatment of PJI-associated biofilms is rifampin, an inhibitor of bacterial DNA-dependent RNA synthesis that has demonstrated the ability to penetrate biofilms, especially from *Staphylococcal* infections.[76–78] A randomized, double-blind, placebo-controlled trial conducted by Zimmerli and colleagues observed a cure rate of 100% from the 12 patients who were infected with *Staphylococcal spp* treated with rifampin in combination ciprofloxacin when compared with placebo, which saw a cure rate of only 58%.[78] Similarly, O'Reily and colleagues reported the highest rate of bone sterilization when rifampin was given in combination with either azithromycin or clindamycin, in comparison to independent treatment.[79] Other antibiotic alternatives that have been shown to be effective in the treatment of biofilm-producing bacteria, especially *staphylococcal* infections, are moxifloxacin and flucloxacillin. Greimel and colleagues found that both moxifloxacin and flucloxacillin demonstrated comparable and effective treatment for *S aureus*-related PJI in when given in combination with rifampin.[77]

In recent years, there have been new developments in the available antibiotics and the formulations of commonly available antibiotics that have shown promising results in the treatment of biofilm-producing bacterial organisms that incorporate intracellular colonization to evade the host response. Surewaard and colleagues demonstrated vancomycin-loaded liposomes to be superior to conventional vancomycin therapy (100% vs 50% survival) in mouse models infected with methicillin-resistant *S. aureus* (MRSA).[80] In addition to lipophilic formulations of commonly used antibiotics, nanoparticles have recently been shown to be effective in enhancing penetration of the bacterial biofilm.[81] Primarily these studies have focused on enhancing the antibiofilm activity of rifampin, which can penetrate biofilms produced by but has limited efficacy

against biofilm cells.[82,83] Bazzaz and colleagues reported that solid lipid nanoparticles loaded with rifampin was superior in the treatment of *S epidermidis* when comparing biofilm count in vitro.[81]

Antimicrobial peptides

Owing to the increasing prevalence of highly antibiotic-resistant biofilm-producing organisms, recent research has been focused on the role of antimicrobial peptides (AMPs) in the treatment of biofilm-producing organisms in PJI.[84] Owing to the inherent toxicity of these charged particles and high sensitivity to pH, research has been focused on engineering a potential solution to mitigate this problem.[85,86] An example of an AMP generating interest within the literature is PLG0206, which is an engineered cationic AMP. PLG0206 has shown promising effectiveness against biofilm-producing bacteria, demonstrating dose-dependent reductions in biofilm formation in multiple physiologic environments.[87,88] With regard to its application to PJI, PLG0206 achieved 99.9% reductions in biofilm mass on infected implant surfaces at high concentrations in a lactated ringer's and diphosphate buffered saline irrigation solution at higher pH levels and achieved complete inhibition of growth at physiologic pH on blood agar.[89]

Phage therapy

In addition to the usage of AMPs as a potential solution to the increasing resistance of biofilm-producing bacteria, there has been increasing research into the usage of bacteriophages in both the treatment of biofilm-associated PJI and in enhancing the delivery of existing antibiotic regimens. Bacteriophages are viruses that preferentially infect bacterial cells and in the case of PJI can be engineered to deliver antibiotics or aid in the prevention of biofilms in

PJI.[90] An experimental study by Samokhin and colleagues demonstrated effective phage delivery via implantation into polymethyl methacrylate, although an effective antimicrobial titer was lost after 1 to 2 weeks.[91] As a vector for antibiotic delivery, there have been several case studies demonstrating responses to treatment following a course of phage therapy for biofilm-producing bacteria, either eliminating all signs of PJI or avoiding the need for further surgical intervention.[54,91] With regard to prevention, a mouse model study by Kaur and colleagues using phage and anti-*S aureus* antibody coated Kirschner wire following TJA in combination with linezolid led to a reduction of bacterial implant adhesion, reduced inflammation, and more rapid improvements in function and ambulation.[92] When considering the obvious potential benefits of phage therapy, there is a clear need for further investment into studies to better understand this treatment.

SUMMARY

The management of biofilms in PJIs continues to be a significant challenge for clinicians. Current treatment strategies, including surgical approaches and antibiotic treatment, have limitations and may not always be effective in eradicating biofilms. However, emerging therapies such as combination and conjugated antibiotics, AMPs, bacteriophages, and advancements in bearing surfaces offer promising alternatives in biofilm management. Future research should focus on developing innovative and targeted therapies to combat biofilms in PJI and improve clinical outcomes for patients. Overall, a multidisciplinary approach and continued research efforts are necessary to overcome the challenges of biofilm-associated infections and improve the management of PJI.

CLINICS CARE POINTS

- Bacterial biofilms may result in a 1000-fold increase in antibacterial resistance.

- Preoperative optimization can reduce the risk of periprosthetic joint infection (PJI).

- Debridement, antibiotics, and implant retention procedures have limited success in chronic infections with robust biofilms.

- Antimicrobial peptides and bacteriophages offer promising results for the treatment of PJI with biofilm-forming bacteria.

DISCLOSURE

S Ward, A Habibi, and I Ashkenazi have nothing to disclose. A Arshi is on the editorial or governing board at The Journal of Arthroplasty. M Meftah is a paid consultant for Conformis and Intellijoint and has stock or stock options in CAIRA surgical and Constance. R Schwarzkopf is a paid consultant for Intellijoint and Smith & Nephew and holds stock options in Gauss Surgical.

REFERENCES

1. Ritter MA, Albohm MJ, Keating EM, et al. Comparative outcomes of total joint arthroplasty. J Arthroplasty 1995;10:737–41.

2. Ethgen O, Bruyère O, Richy F, et al. Health-Related Quality of Life in Total Hip and Total Knee Arthroplasty. J Bone Joint Surg 2004;86:963–74.

3. Learmonth ID, Young C, Rorabeck C. The operation of the century: total hip replacement. Lancet 2007;370.

4. Rissanen P, Aro S, Slätis P, et al. Health and quality of life before and after hip or knee arthroplasty. J Arthroplasty 1995;10:169–75.

5. Beam E, Osmon D. Prosthetic Joint Infection Update. Infect Dis Clin 2018;32:843–59.

6. Huotari K, Peltola M, Jämsen E. The incidence of late prosthetic joint infections. Acta Orthop 2015; 86:321–5.

7. Morcos MW, Kooner P, Marsh J, et al. The economic impact of periprosthetic infection in total knee arthroplasty. Can J Surg 2021;64. https://doi.org/10.1503/cjs.012519.

8. Blom AW, Lenguerrand E, Strange S, et al. Clinical and cost effectiveness of single stage compared with two stage revision for hip prosthetic joint infection (INFORM): pragmatic, parallel group, open label, randomised controlled trial. BMJ 2022;e071281. https://doi.org/10.1136/bmj-2022-071281.

9. Arciola CR, Campoccia D, Ehrlich GD, et al. Biofilm-based implant infections in orthopaedics. Adv Exp Med Biol 2015;830. https://doi.org/10.1007/978-3-319-11038-7_2.

10. McConoughey SJ, Howlin R, Granger JF, et al. Biofilms in periprosthetic orthopedic infections. Future Microbiol 2014;9:987–1007.

11. Gbejuade HO, Lovering AM, Webb JC. The role of microbial biofilms in prosthetic joint infections. Acta Orthop 2015;86:147–58.

12. Staats A, Li D, Sullivan AC, et al. Biofilm formation in periprosthetic joint infections. Ann Jt 2021;6.

13. Dickinson GM, Bisno AL. Infections associated with indwelling devices: Concepts of pathogenesis; Infections associated with intravascular devices. Antimicrob Agents Chemother 1989;33. https://doi.org/10.1128/AAC.33.5.597.

14. Kochwa S, Litwak RS, Rosenfield RE, et al. Blood elements at foreign surfaces: a biochemical approach to the study of the adsorption of plasma proteins. Ann N Y Acad Sci 1977;283. https://doi.org/10.1111/j.1749-6632.1977.tb41751.x.

15. Cottonaro CN, Roohk HV, Shimizu G, et al. Quantitation and characterization of competitive protein binding to polymers. Trans Am Soc Artif Intern Organs 1981;27.

16. Flemming H-C, Neu TR, Wozniak DJ. The EPS Matrix: The "House of Biofilm Cells". J Bacteriol 2007; 189:7945–7.

17. Della Valle C, Parvizi J, Bauer TW, et al. American Academy of Orthopaedic Surgeons clinical practice guideline on: the diagnosis of periprosthetic joint infections of the hip and knee. J Bone Joint Surg Am 2011;93:1355–7.

18. Parvizi J, Della Valle CJ. AAOS Clinical Practice Guideline: diagnosis and treatment of periprosthetic joint infections of the hip and knee. J Am Acad Orthop Surg 2010;18:771–2.

19. Costerton JW, Geesey GG, Cheng KJ. How bacteria stick. Sci Am 1978;238. https://doi.org/10.1038/scientificamerican0178-86.

20. Ceri H, Olson ME, Stremick C, et al. The Calgary Biofilm Device: New technology for rapid determination of antibiotic susceptibilities of bacterial biofilms. J Clin Microbiol 1999;37. https://doi.org/10.1128/jcm.37.6.1771-1776.1999.

21. Gbejuade HO, Lovering AM, Webb JC. The role of microbial biofilms in prosthetic joint infections: A review. Acta Orthop 2015;86. https://doi.org/10.3109/17453674.2014.966290.

22. Fakhro A, Jalalabadi F, Brown R, et al. Treatment of Infected Cardiac Implantable Electronic Devices. Semin Plast Surg 2016. https://doi.org/10.1055/s-0036-1580733.

23. Charalambous LT, Kim BI, Schwartz AM, et al. Prosthetic Knee Infection With Coagulase-Negative Staphylococcus: A Harbinger of Poor Outcomes. J Arthroplasty 2022;37:S313–20.

24. von Eiff C, Peters G, Heilmann C. Pathogenesis of infections due to coagulase-negative staphylococci. Lancet Infect Dis 2002;2:677–85.

25. Koch JA, Pust TM, Cappellini AJ, et al. Staphylococcus epidermidis biofilms have a high tolerance to antibiotics in periprosthetic joint infection. Life 2020;10. https://doi.org/10.3390/life10110253.

26. Hall-Stoodley L, Hu FZ, Gieseke A, et al. Direct detection of bacterial biofilms on the middle-ear mucosa of children with chronic otitis media. JAMA 2006;296. https://doi.org/10.1001/jama.296.2.202.

27. Montanaro L, Speziale P, Campoccia D, et al. Scenery of Staphylococcus implant infections in orthopedics. Future Microbiol 2011;6. https://doi.org/10.2217/fmb.11.117.

28. Arciola CR, An YH, Campoccia D, et al. Etiology of Implant Orthopedic Infections: A Survey on 1027 Clinical Isolates. Int J Artif Organs 2005;28:1091–100.

29. Ricciardi BF, Muthukrishnan G, Masters E, et al. Staphylococcus aureus Evasion of Host Immunity in the Setting of Prosthetic Joint Infection: Biofilm and Beyond. Curr Rev Musculoskelet Med 2018; 11. https://doi.org/10.1007/s12178-018-9501-4.

30. Hofstee MI, Riool M, Terjajevs I, et al. Three-dimensional in vitro staphylococcus aureus abscess communities display antibiotic tolerance and protection from neutrophil clearance. Infect Immun 2020;88. https://doi.org/10.1128/IAI.00293-20.

31. Alder KD, Lee I, Munger AM, et al. Intracellular Staphylococcus aureus in bone and joint infections: A mechanism of disease recurrence, inflammation, and bone and cartilage destruction. Bone 2020; 141. https://doi.org/10.1016/j.bone.2020.115568.

32. Darouiche RO, Landon GC, Patti JM, et al. Role of Staphylococcus aureus surface adhesins in orthopaedic device infections: Are results model-dependent? J Med Microbiol 1997;46. https://doi.org/10.1099/00222615-46-1-75.

33. Elasri MO, Thomas JR, Skinner RA, et al. Staphylococcus aureus collagen adhesin contributes to the pathogenesis of osteomyelitis. Bone 2002;30. https://doi.org/10.1016/S8756-3282(01)00632-9.

34. Vasoo S. Improving the diagnosis of orthopedic implant-associated infections: Optimizing the use of tools already in the box. J Clin Microbiol 2018; 56. https://doi.org/10.1128/JCM.01379-18.

35. Stoodley P, Nistico L, Johnson S, et al. Direct demonstration of viable Staphylococcus aureus biofilms in an infected total joint arthroplasty: A case report. J Bone Joint Surg 2008;90. https://doi.org/10.2106/JBJS.G.00838.

36. Parvizi J, Tan TL, Goswami K, et al. The 2018 Definition of Periprosthetic Hip and Knee Infection: An Evidence-Based and Validated Criteria. J Arthroplasty 2018;33:1309–14.e2.

37. Berbari E, Mabry T, Tsaras G, et al. Inflammatory blood laboratory levels as markers of prosthetic joint infection: A systematic review and meta-analysis. J Bone Joint Surg 2010;92. https://doi.org/10.2106/JBJS.I.01199.

38. Widmer AF. New developments in diagnosis and treatment of infection in orthopedic implants. Clin Infect Dis 2001;33. https://doi.org/10.1086/321863.

39. Knobloch JKM, Horstkotte MA, Rohde H, et al. Evaluation of different detection methods of biofilm formation in Staphylococcus aureus. Med Microbiol Immunol 2002;191. https://doi.org/10.1007/s00430-002-0124-3.

40. Liu H, Zhang Y, Li L, et al. The application of sonication in diagnosis of periprosthetic joint infection. Eur J Clin Microbiol Infect Dis 2017;36. https://doi.org/10.1007/s10096-016-2778-6.

41. Carmen JC, Roeder BL, Nelson JL, et al. Treatment of biofilm infections on implants with low-frequency ultrasound and antibiotics. Am J Infect Control 2005;33. https://doi.org/10.1016/j.ajic.2004.08.002.

42. Rodriguez-Merchan EC. The Function of Sonication in the Diagnosis of Periprosthetic Joint Infection After Total Knee Arthroplasty. Arch Bone Jt Surg 2022;10:735–40.

43. Kobayashi H, Oethinger M, Tuohy MJ, et al. Improved detection of biofilm-formative bacteria by vortexing and sonication: A pilot study. Clin Orthop Relat Res 2009;467. https://doi.org/10.1007/s11999-008-0609-5.

44. Ribeiro TC, Honda EK, Daniachi D, et al. The impact of sonication cultures when the diagnosis of prosthetic joint infection is inconclusive. PLoS One 2021;16. https://doi.org/10.1371/journal.pone.0252322.

45. Thoendel MJ, Jeraldo PR, Greenwood-Quaintance KE, et al. Identification of prosthetic joint infection pathogens using a shotgun metagenomics approach. Clin Infect Dis 2018;67. https://doi.org/10.1093/cid/ciy303.

46. Street TL, Sanderson ND, Atkins BL, et al. Molecular diagnosis of orthopedic-device-related infection directly from sonication fluid by metagenomic sequencing. J Clin Microbiol 2017;55. https://doi.org/10.1128/JCM.00462-17.

47. Kamal T, Conway RM, Littlejohn I, et al. The role of a multidisciplinary pre-assessment clinic in reducing mortality after complex orthopaedic surgery. Ann R Coll Surg Engl 2011;93. https://doi.org/10.1308/003588411X561026.

48. Buller LT, Sabry FY, Easton RW, et al. The Preoperative Prediction of Success Following Irrigation and Debridement With Polyethylene Exchange for Hip and Knee Prosthetic Joint Infections. J Arthroplasty 2012;27. https://doi.org/10.1016/j.arth.2012.01.003.

49. Bozic KJ, Lau E, Kurtz S, et al. Patient-related risk factors for postoperative mortality and periprosthetic joint infection in Medicare patients undergoing TKA. Clin Orthop Relat Res 2012;470. https://doi.org/10.1007/s11999-011-2043-3.

50. Pulido L, Ghanem E, Joshi A, et al. Periprosthetic joint infection: The incidence, timing, and predisposing factors. Clin Orthop Relat Res 2008;466. https://doi.org/10.1007/s11999-008-0209-4.

51. Patel R. Periprosthetic Joint Infection. N Engl J Med 2023;388:251–62.

52. American Academy of Orthopaedic Surgeons. Diagnosis and prevention of periprosthetic joint infections: evidencebased clinical practice guideline. Available at:Https://WwwAaosOrg/Globalassets/Quality-and-Practice-Resources/Pji/Diagnosis And-preventionofperiprosthetic Jointinfections-7-24-19 Pdf 2019.

53. Mraovic B, Suh D, Jacovides C, et al. Perioperative hyperglycemia and postoperative infection after lower limb arthroplasty. J Diabetes Sci Technol 2011;5. https://doi.org/10.1177/193229681100500231.

54. Marchant MH, Viens NA, Cook C, et al. The impact of glycemic control and diabetes mellitus on perioperative outcomes after total joint arthroplasty. J Bone Joint Surg 2009;91. https://doi.org/10.2106/JBJS.H.00116.

55. Ashkenazi I, Thomas J, Lawrence KW, et al. Positive Preoperative Colonization With Methicillin Resistant Staphylococcus Aureus Is Associated With Inferior Postoperative Outcomes in Patients Undergoing Total Joint Arthroplasty. J Arthroplasty 2023. https://doi.org/10.1016/j.arth.2023.02.065.

56. Moroski NM, Woolwine S, Schwarzkopf R. Is preoperative staphylococcal decolonization efficient in total joint arthroplasty. J Arthroplasty 2015;30:444–6.

57. Chen AF, Heyl AE, Xu PZ, et al. Preoperative decolonization effective at reducing staphylococcal colonization in total joint arthroplasty patients. J Arthroplasty 2013;28:18–20.

58. Wells Z, Zhu M, Young SW. Intraosseous Regional Administration of Prophylactic Antibiotics in Total Knee Arthroplasty. Antibiotics 2022;11. https://doi.org/10.3390/antibiotics11050634.

59. Siddiqi A, Abdo ZE, Springer BD, et al. Pursuit of the ideal antiseptic irrigation solution in the management of periprosthetic joint infections. J Bone Jt Infect 2021;6. https://doi.org/10.5194/jbji-6-189-2021.

60. Sousa R, Abreu MA. Treatment of Prosthetic Joint Infection with Debridement, Antibiotics and Irrigation with Implant Retention - A Narrative Review. J Bone Jt Infect 2018;3. https://doi.org/10.7150/jbji.24285.

61. Visperas A, Santana D, Klika AK, et al. Current treatments for biofilm-associated periprosthetic joint infection and new potential strategies. J Orthop Res 2022;40:1477–91.

62. Kildow BJ, Patel SP, Otero JE, et al. Results of debridement, antibiotics, and implant retention for periprosthetic knee joint infection supplemented with the use of intraosseous antibiotics. Bone Joint Lett J 2021;103. B:185–90.

63. Silva M, Tharani R, Schmalzried TP. Results of direct exchange or debridement of the infected total knee arthroplasty. Clin Orthop Relat Res 2002;404. https://doi.org/10.1097/00003086-200211000-00022.

64. Jackson WO, Schmalzried TP. Limited role of direct exchange arthroplasty in the treatment of infected total hip replacements. Clin Orthop Relat Res 2000;381. https://doi.org/10.1097/00003086-200012000-00012.

65. Charette RS, Melnic CM. Two-Stage Revision Arthroplasty for the Treatment of Prosthetic Joint Infection. Curr Rev Musculoskelet Med 2018;11. https://doi.org/10.1007/s12178-018-9495-y.

66. Goud AL, Harlianto NI, Ezzafzafi S, et al. Reinfection rates after one- and two-stage revision surgery for hip and knee arthroplasty: a systematic review and meta-analysis. Arch Orthop Trauma Surg 2023;143. https://doi.org/10.1007/s00402-021-04190-7.

67. Van Den Kieboom J, Tirumala V, Box H, et al. One-stage revision is as effective as twostage revision for chronic culture-negative periprosthetic joint infection after total hip and knee arthroplasty a retrospective cohort study. Bone and Joint Journal 2021. https://doi.org/10.1302/0301-620X.103B.BJJ-2020-1480.R2. 103-B.

68. Wroblewski BM. One-stage revision of infected cemented total hip arthroplasty. Clin Orthop Relat Res 1986;211. https://doi.org/10.1097/00003086-198610000-00014.

69. Dersch G, Winkler H. Periprosthetic Joint Infection (PJI)—Results of One-Stage Revision with Antibiotic-Impregnated Cancellous Allograft Bone—A Retrospective Cohort Study. Antibiotics 2022;11. https://doi.org/10.3390/antibiotics11030310.

70. Chisari E, Magnuson JA, Ong CB, et al. Ceramic-on-polyethylene hip arthroplasty reduces the risk of postoperative periprosthetic joint infection. J Orthop Res 2022;40. https://doi.org/10.1002/jor.25230.

71. Madanat R, Laaksonen I, Graves SE, et al. Ceramic bearings for total hip arthroplasty are associated with a reduced risk of revision for infection. HIP Int 2018;28. https://doi.org/10.1177/1120700018776464.

72. Pitto RP, Sedel L. Periprosthetic Joint Infection in Hip Arthroplasty: Is There an Association Between Infection and Bearing Surface Type? Clin Orthop Relat Res 2016;474. https://doi.org/10.1007/s11999-016-4916-y.

73. Hexter AT, Hislop SM, Blunn GW, et al. The effect of bearing surface on risk of periprosthetic joint infection in total hip arthroplasty: A systematic review and meta-analysis. Bone and Joint Journal 2018. https://doi.org/10.1302/0301-620X.100B2.BJJ-2017-0575.R1. 100B.

74. Pilz M, Staats K, Tobudic S, et al. Zirconium Nitride Coating Reduced Staphylococcus epidermidis Biofilm Formation on Orthopaedic Implant Surfaces: An in Vitro Study. Clin Orthop Relat Res 2019; 477. https://doi.org/10.1097/CORR.0000000000000568.

75. Norambuena GA, Patel R, Karau M, et al. Antibacterial and Biocompatible Titanium-Copper Oxide Coating May Be a Potential Strategy to Reduce Periprosthetic Infection: An In Vitro Study. Clin Orthop Relat Res 2017;475. https://doi.org/10.1007/s11999-016-4713-7.

76. Albano M, Karau MJ, Greenwood-Quaintance KE, et al. In Vitro Activity of Rifampin, Rifabutin, and Rifapentine against Enterococci and Streptococci from Periprosthetic Joint Infection. Microbiol Spectr 2021;9:e0007121.

77. Greimel F, Scheuerer C, Gessner A, et al. Efficacy of antibiotic treatment of implant-associated Staphylococcus aureus infections with moxifloxacin, flucloxacillin, rifampin, and combination therapy: An animal study. Drug Des Dev Ther 2017;11. https://doi.org/10.2147/DDDT.S138888.

78. Zimmerli W, Sendi P. Role of Rifampin against Staphylococcal Biofilm Infections In Vitro, in Animal Models, and in Orthopedic-Device-Related Infections. Antimicrob Agents Chemother 2019;63. https://doi.org/10.1128/AAC.01746-18.

79. O'Reilly T, Kunz S, Sande E, et al. Relationship between antibiotic concentration in bone and efficacy of treatment of staphylococcal osteomyelitis in rats: Azithromycin compared with clindamycin and rifampin. Antimicrob Agents Chemother 1992;36. https://doi.org/10.1128/AAC.36.12.2693.

80. Surewaard BGJ, Deniset JF, Zemp FJ, et al. Identification and treatment of the Staphylococcus aureus reservoir in vivo. J Exp Med 2016;213. https://doi.org/10.1084/jem.20160334.

81. Fazly Bazzaz BS, Khameneh B, Zarei H, et al. Antibacterial efficacy of rifampin loaded solid lipid nanoparticles against Staphylococcus epidermidis biofilm. Microb Pathog 2016;93. https://doi.org/10.1016/j.micpath.2015.11.031.

82. Peck KR, Kim SW, Jung SI, et al. Antimicrobials as potential adjunctive agents in the treatment of biofilm infection with Staphylococcus epidermidis. Chemotherapy 2003;49. https://doi.org/10.1159/000071143.

83. Szczuka E, Kaznowski A. Antimicrobial activity of tigecycline alone or in combination with rifampin against Staphylococcus epidermidis in biofilm. Folia Microbiol (Praha) 2014;59. https://doi.org/10.1007/s12223-013-0296-9.

84. Chen CH, Lu TK. Development and challenges of antimicrobial peptides for therapeutic applications. Antibiotics 2020;9. https://doi.org/10.3390/antibiotics9010024.

85. Deslouches B, Di YP. Antimicrobial Peptides: A Potential Therapeutic Option for Surgical Site Infections. Clin Surg 2017;2.

86. Deslouches B, Islam K, Craigo JK, et al. Activity of the de novo engineered antimicrobial peptide WLBU2 against Pseudomonas aeruginosa in human serum and whole blood: Implications for systemic applications. Antimicrob Agents Chemother 2005;49. https://doi.org/10.1128/AAC.49.8.3208-3216.

87. Melvin JA, Lashua LP, Kiedrowski MR, et al. Simultaneous Antibiofilm and Antiviral Activities of an Engineered Antimicrobial Peptide during Virus-Bacterium Coinfection. mSphere 2016;1. https://doi.org/10.1128/msphere.00083-16.

88. Lashua LP, Melvin JA, Deslouches B, et al. Engineered cationic antimicrobial peptide (eCAP) prevents Pseudomonas aeruginosa biofilm growth on airway epithelial cells. J Antimicrob Chemother 2016;71. https://doi.org/10.1093/jac/dkw143.

89. Mandell JB, Koch J A, Deslouches B, et al. Direct antimicrobial activity of cationic amphipathic peptide WLBU2 against Staphylococcus aureus biofilms is enhanced in physiologic buffered saline. J Orthop Res 2020;38. https://doi.org/10.1002/jor.24765.

90. Azeredo J, Sutherland I. The Use of Phages for the Removal of Infectious Biofilms. Curr Pharmaceut Biotechnol 2008;9. https://doi.org/10.2174/13892 0108785161604.

91. Samokhin AG, Kozlova YN, Korneev DV, et al. Experimental study of the antibacterial activity of the lytic staphylococcus aureus bacteriophage Ph20 and lytic pseudomonas aeruginosa bacteriophage Ph57 when modelling impregnation into poly (methylmetacrylate) orthopedic implants (bone cement). Vestn Ross Akad Med Nauk 2018;73. https://doi.org/10.15690/vramn905.

92. Kaur S, Harjai K, Chhibber S. In Vivo Assessment of Phage and Linezolid Based Implant Coatings for Treatment of Methicillin Resistant S. aureus (MRSA) mediated orthopaedic device related infections. PLoS One 2016;11. https://doi.org/10.1371/journal.pone.0157626.

Articulating Spacers in Total Hip Arthroplasty
Surgical Technique and Outcomes

Babar Kayani, MBBS, BSc, FRCS (Tr & Orth), PhD[a,b,*],
Francisco Bengoa, MD[a,b],
Lisa C. Howard, MD, MHSc, FRCSC[a,b],
Michael E. Neufeld, MD, MSc, FRCSC[a,b],
Bassam A. Masri, MD, FRCSC[a,b]

KEYWORDS

• Arthroplasty • Hip: infection • Outcomes • Spacer • Technique

KEY POINTS

- Periprosthetic joint infection remains a leading cause of revision surgery following total hip arthroplasty and is associated with high morbidity and mortality.
- Two-stage exchange arthroplasty continues to be the gold-standard treatment for chronic periprosthetic joint infections but is associated with increased hospitalization and increased cost compared with one-stage exchange arthroplasty.
- The surgical technique for the first-stage procedure must ensure meticulous debridement of all infected tissue and removal of all foreign material, obtaining tissue samples for microbiological analysis, and grading the degree of bone and soft tissue compromise to aid with planning for the second stage.
- Articulating spacers effectively maintain the joint space, permit hip motion, and enable controlled weight-bearing. In combination, these features help to reduce hip joint contractures and maintain bone stock before the second stage, and maintain patient comfort and function between stages.
- Patients and surgeons need to be cognizant of the risks of fractures and dislocations associated with articulating spacers. In patients with significant bone loss and/or abductor muscle weakness, static spacers should be considered to minimize these risks during the interstage interval.

INTRODUCTION

Periprosthetic joint infection (PJI) is a devastating complication that occurs in 1.0% to 3.0% of patients following primary total hip arthroplasty (THA) and 3% to 10% of patients following revision THA.[1,2] Despite advances in preoperative screening, optimization of patient-specific risk factors, skin preparation agents, antibiotic prophylaxis, laminar theater flow systems, and antibiotic-impregnated cement, the overall prevalence of PJI following THA continues to increase worldwide.[1] This has been attributed to increasing life expectancy, rising prevalence of comorbidities, and increasing numbers of implanted prosthetic joints. Within the United States alone, it is estimated that the number of PJIs will increase by 10,000 cases per year by 2030.[1] PJIs are associated with increased morbidity in physical health and psychological well-being, with a substantial mortality at 5 years.[3,4] Importantly, PJIs also place a significant

[a] Division of Lower Limb Reconstruction & Oncology, Vancouver General Hospital, Vancouver, British Columbia V5Z 1M9, Canada; [b] Department of Orthopaedics, University of British Columbia, Vancouver, British Columbia V6T 1Z4, Canada
* Corresponding author. Division of Lower Limb Reconstruction & Oncology, Vancouver General Hospital, 899 West 12th Avenue, Vancouver, British Columbia V5Z 1M9, Canada.
E-mail address: babar.kayani@gmail.com

Orthop Clin N Am 55 (2024) 181–192
https://doi.org/10.1016/j.ocl.2023.06.002

financial burden on the health care institution, with costs of treating a PJI being almost 5 times greater than a primary THA.[2] Early diagnosis and appropriate surgical treatment are essential for optimizing patient outcomes and limiting the financial burden of this complication to the health care institution.

The overall objective of treating a PJI following THA is to eradicate infection, reduce pain, and improve function; however, there is no uniform consensus on the optimal treatment strategy to achieve this.[3,5–9] Surgical management of these patients is often guided by local surgical experience, expert opinions, and consensus statements. The treatment algorithm is often influenced by the duration of symptoms, time from surgery, health status of the host, soft tissue status, and infecting organism.[3,5–9] Debridement and irrigation with change of modular components may be used for acute infections, but single-stage or two-stage exchange arthroplasties are indicated for chronic infections. Single-stage exchange arthroplasty involves a comprehensive debridement of the infected bone and soft tissue, removal of the infected components, and implantation of the new prostheses at a single setting. Conceptually, this helps to eradicate the infection with less morbidity of surgery to the patient and less cost to the health care institution.[6] Two-stage revision procedures involve 2 separate procedures for the debridement and definitive implantation, with an interval period using an antibiotic spacer and intravenous antibiotic treatment. Two-stage exchange arthroplasty with an antibiotic-eluting interstage spacer remains the gold standard for treating PJIs.[1,10]

This review describes the surgical technique for undertaking a first-stage exchange arthroplasty using an articulating spacer and discusses the pertinent literature on key concepts relating to PJIs in THA to guide effective surgical decision making in these patients.

Periprosthetic Joint Infection Diagnosis

The diagnosis of a PJI continues to be a challenge. Several attempts have been made to organize and unify criteria for diagnosis and management. The 2018 International Consensus Meeting (ICM) on Musculoskeletal Infections proposed the most accepted criteria for diagnosis of a PJI. These criteria include major criteria (2 positive cultures of the same organism and/or sinus tract with evidence of communication to the joint) and minor criteria. The presence of one minor criterion or 6 or more minor criteria is diagnostic of PJI (Tables 1 and 2).

Recently, the European Bone and Joint Infection Society (EBJIS) proposed a new diagnostic criteria, supported by the Musculoskeletal Infection Society and the European Society of Clinical Microbiology and Infectious Diseases.[11] They proposed a three-level approach to diagnosis: infection unlikely, infection likely, and infection confirmed (Table 3), This may, however, overcall infections relative to the ICM criteria, resulting in unnecessary treatment and patient morbidity.

Regardless of the used criteria, a PJI should be suspected in any patient with a painful arthroplasty. In order to diagnose and classify patients, the workup can include clinical and blood investigations, synovial fluid analysis and biomarkers, microbiology, history, and nuclear imaging. Inflammatory markers, such as C-reactive protein (CRP) and erythrocyte sedimentation rate (ESR), should be obtained as a screening tool, as they are inexpensive and have a high sensitivity. If they are elevated, an aspiration of the joint should be performed. However, even in patients with normal inflammatory markers, an aspiration should be obtained if the index of suspicion for infection is high, given that 10% to 15% of PJI associated with low virulence microorganisms will have normal inflammatory markers. After aspiration, synovial fluid should be sent for cytologic analysis, including leukocyte count and differential, synovial biomarkers if available, alpha-defensin (if available), and 10- to 14-day aerobic and anaerobic cultures. Multiple values have been used as a diagnostic threshold for leukocyte counts and polymorphonuclear leukocyte (PMN)%, but both the EBSIS criteria and the 2018 ICM criteria agree that a threshold of 3000 leukocytes should be used for chronic PJI,[9,11,12] and the authors prefer a threshold of 80% for PMN% in keeping with both sets of criteria. Consideration should be

Table 1 2018 International Consensus Meeting periprosthetic joint infection diagnostic major criteria	
Major Criteria (at Least One of the Following)	**Decision**
Two positive growths of the same organism using standard culture methods	Infected
Sinus tract with evidence of communication to the joint or visualization of the prosthesis	

Table 2
2018 International Consensus Meeting periprosthetic joint infection diagnostic minor criteria

Minor Criteria	Threshold (Acute PJI)	Threshold (Chronic PJI)	Score	Decision
Serum CRP (mg/L) Or	100	10	2	Combined preoperative and postoperative score: ≥6 infected 3–5 inconclusive <3 not infected
D-dimer (µg/L)	Unknown	860		
Elevated serum ESR (mm/h)	No role	30	1	
Elevated synovial white blood cell (WBC; cells/µL) Or	10,000	3000	3	
Leukocyte esterase Or	++	++		
Positive alpha-defensin (signal/cutoff)	1.0	1.0		
Elevated synovial PMN (%)	90	70	2	
Single positive culture			2	
Positive histology			3	
Positive intraoperative purulence[a]			3	

[a] No role in suspected adverse local tissue reaction.
The strip that tests for leukocyte esterase shows ++ signs.

given for manual cell counts in the presence of metal debris to improve diagnostic accuracy.

Given the lack of consensus on diagnostic criteria and threshold values, there has been a significant interest in developing alternative testing to accurately identify infected patients. Leukocyte esterase strip testing, using bedside urinalysis strips, is an inexpensive and quick test that has been used as a proxy for leukocyte counts[13] and can be used as a screening test at the time of aspiration, as long as the specimen is not bloody. Leukocyte esterase strip testing may also serve as a valuable diagnostic tool intraoperatively in the setting of a failed aspiration, with excellent specificity. The use of a combination of synovial alpha-defensin and synovial CRP has been reported to have high sensitivity and high specificity.[14] D-dimer has been a controversial criterion and has not been included in the EBJIS definition, as there are conflicting reports regarding its accuracy. Recently, Tarabichi and colleagues[15] demonstrated D-dimer (using a cutoff of 471 ng/mL) had a high sensitivity for the diagnosis of PJI by indolent organisms, and that it was noninferior to CRP and ESR. As such, the authors of that article suggested it might be useful as a screening tool, although the authors of this review do not believe that it adds value to ESR and CRP and may lead to confusion regarding thrombosis in emergency departments.

Indications and Contraindications for Articulating Spacers

The main functions of antibiotic-loaded cement spacers are to safely deliver antibiotics to the surrounding bone and soft tissue to eradicate infection; maintain soft tissue tension before definitive component implantation at the second-stage procedure; and minimize any dead space for potential fluid collections.[16] Two main systems used for these spacers in the interval period are articulating (dynamic) spacers or static spacers. The main advantage of using an articulating spacer is that it allows hip joint motion, which limits contractures, stiffness, and leg shortening before the second-stage procedure. Furthermore, controlled weight-bearing may help to preserve bone stock and maintain lower-limb and core muscle function.[17] Articulating spacers may be handmade spacers, molded around a metal endoskeleton for strength, or facsimiles of real components coated with high-dose antibiotic-impregnated cement.[18]

The absolute contraindication for the use of articulating spacers in the treatment of PJI following THA is the inability to have a stable construct at the end of the procedure. Among all types of articulating spacers designs, the overall reinfection rate is between 1.7% and 10.7%; dislocation rate is between 3.4% and 4.4%, and fracture rate is between 1.5%

Table 3
2021 European Bone and Joint Infection Society periprosthetic joint infection diagnostic criteria

	Infection Unlikely (All Findings Negative)	Infection Likely (Two Positive Findings)	Infection Confirmed (Any Positive Finding)
Clinical and blood workup			
Clinical features	Clear alternative reason for implant dysfunction	1. Radiologic signs of loosening within the first 5 years after implantation 2. Previous wound healing problems 3. History of recent fever or bacteremia 4. Purulence around the prosthesis	Sinus tract with evidence of communication to the joint or visualization of the prosthesis
CRP		>10 mg/L (1 mg/dL)	
Synovial fluid cytologic analysis			
Synovial WBC (cells/μL)	≤1500	>1500	>3000
Synovial PMN (%)	≤65	>65	>80
Synovial fluid biomarkers			
Alpha-defensin			Positive immunoassay or lateral-flow assay
Microbiology			
Aspiration fluid		Positive culture	
Intraoperative (fluid and tissue)	All cultures negative	Single positive culture	≥2 positive samples with the same microorganism
Sonication (CFU/mL)	No growth	>1 CFU/mL of any organism	>50 CFU/mL of any organism
Histology			
High-power field (HPF; 400× magnification)	Negative	Presence of ≥5 neutrophils in a single HPF	Presence of ≥5 neutrophils in ≥5 HPF Presence of visible microorganisms
Others			
Nuclear imaging	Negative three-phase isotope bone scan	Positive WBC scintigraphy	

and 3.4%.[19–22] To minimize the risk of these complications, articulating spacers are relatively contraindicated in patients with significant acetabular bone loss and/or abductor muscle deficiency, unless the spacer includes a cemented polyethylene liner with a snap-fit configuration.[16,21,23] In instances of acetabular bone loss, investigators have published techniques using cement, screws, and various constructs, including dual-mobility articulations, to try to maintain a stable spacer and avoid acetabular failure.[24,25] Static spacers are usually manually molded using the antibiotic-impregnated cement and inserted by hand into the acetabulum and femoral canal. If structural support is required with a static spacer, antibiotic-impregnated cement may be coated around a supportive endoskeleton, such as a Steinman pin or intramedullary nail.[18] As static spacers have limited sizes and the shapes are poorly matched to the native hip anatomy, there remains a risk of pain and acetabular erosion.[18]

Surgical Technique

At the authors' center, preparation for the first-stage exchange arthroplasty begins with preoperative assessment of up-to-date anteroposterior, lateral, and Judet view radiographs, or possibly a computed tomographic scan to assess the degree of bone loss. These images should be assessed for component positioning, integrity of the anterior and posterior acetabular columns, bone loss, osteomyelitis, and any cement mantles, plugs, or additional hardware that needs to be removed. Significant bone loss, particularly of the anterior and posterior column or migration of the acetabular component medial to Kohler line, or pelvic discontinuity may necessitate the insertion of a nonarticulating spacer to preserve as much residual pelvic bone stock ahead of the second-stage reimplantation. With full-length ingrowth/ongrowth uncemented prostheses or cemented prostheses without evidence of lucency at the cement-bone interface, an extended trochanteric osteotomy is required for safe removal of implants.

Preoperative templating is essential for establishing the depth of acetabular reaming, positioning of any femoral osteotomies, and planning component sizes and positions for achieving the desired hip biomechanics. In addition, the operative report from the index procedure and implant stickers should be obtained before the first-stage procedure. Specialized implant and extraction instruments are often required in readiness for the first-stage procedure. As often as

possible, antibiotics should be withheld in the period leading up to the first-stage procedure, especially when the diagnosis is in doubt and preoperative cultures were negative. An integrated management strategy encompassing the surgeon, a pathologist, and an infectious diseases specialist, preferably with an interest in PJIs, is mandatory to the successful treatment of PJI of the hip, and involvement early in the treatment is recommended. As such, centralizing these procedures at specialist centers, whenever possible, is desired for the best outcomes.

The previous incision should be extended to healthy tissue to allow adequate exposure, excising any sinuses and excising the tract down to the prosthesis, provided it is compatible with the proposed surgical approach. The approach must provide adequate exposure to the prosthesis and periarticular soft tissue region to allow a complete debridement of the infected tissue. The authors' preference is to start with a posterior approach owing to its versatility and optional extensile nature. The initial dissection should be performed sequentially in layers using cautery or sharp dissection. Several Kocher clamps may be placed along the fascia lata and used to lift the fascial layer up, while cautery or sharp dissection and finger dissection are used to carefully release any subfascial adhesions and scar tissue. A modified Charnley retractor is then used to expose the posterior aspect of the hip joint, which is entered by detaching the short rotators and capsule and tagging them with sutures for later repair. The inside of the capsule is often inflamed and is excised leaving the thin outer layer of the posterior capsule for repair. Further extensile releases may be required to gain further exposure of any infected tissue and reduce excessive tension on the femur during dislocation. This typically includes the scar tissue along the anterior aspect of the femur after dislocation and internal rotation of the femur. Samples of representative inflamed tissue from both the acetabular and femoral regions should be sent for microbiological assessment. Antibiotics may be administered after the culture samples are obtained. The authors obtain at least 5 samples, but often more. The samples are sent immediately to the laboratory with instructions for aerobic, anaerobic, fungal, and mycobacterial cultures with a minimum 14-day bacterial incubation protocol. Although some investigators advocate sonication of the extracted implants, the authors do not sonicate the extracted implants.

Further extensile maneuvers include releasing the gluteus maximus at its femoral insertion, which often helps to further reduce the tension on the femur, but this is not always needed. The cautery is used to perform an anterior release; resect any thickened capsule, synovium, and scar tissue anterosuperiorly around the trunnion; and develop an anterior acetabular pocket. The hip is carefully dislocated with the aid of a bone hook around the trunnion, and the femoral head is removed using an osteotome and mallet. A cobra retractor is then inserted under the trunnion and gently positioned over the anterior acetabular wall to help retract this anteriorly and expose the acetabular cup. An osteotome and cautery are then used to remove any overhanging bone and soft tissue from the acetabular cup-bone interface.

Extraction of the femoral component requires clearance of the shoulder of the prosthesis using a rongeur or high-powered burr to prevent fracture on stem extraction. Shorter, proximally coated stems can often be removed from within the femoral canal without a femoral osteotomy using a combination of flexible osteotomes, saws, and pencil-tip high-speed burrs. On the other hand, well-fixed protheses with good bony ingrowth/ongrowth, and well-fixed cement mantles necessitate an extended trochanteric osteotomy. The residual cement mantle may need to be removed using high-speed burrs, specialized cement removal osteotomes, and rongeurs. Any distal cement plug is removed using a drill and a tap, or sequentially larger drills and flexible reamers with a reverse hook to remove any residual cement. All cement and residual hardware from previous procedures should be removed. The extent of femoral and acetabular bone loss should be carefully assessed and documented in preparation for the second-stage procedure.

An uncemented acetabular component may be removed in a bone-conserving manner using a size-specific acetabular cup removal system device, such as the explant system (Zimmer, Warsaw, IN, USA), or similar systems from other manufacturers. The central head component is anchored into the polyethylene liner, and the stiff truncated curved blades are penetrated into dense peripheral bone around the cup. The handles are then rotated to create channels around the acetabular shell to loosen the implant and facilitate its removal while preserving the underlying bone stock. The full-radius osteotomes are then used, and once the implant is debonded circumferentially, it can be removed. If screws are present, the polyethylene liner will need to be removed using an osteotome; the screws can be removed, and then the acetabular cup removal system can be positioned into the acetabular shell with a trial liner. In the case of a cemented acetabular component, the polyethylene liner should be removed first (reamer or osteotomes); curved osteotomes should then be used to disrupt the cup-cement interface, and then the residual cement base can be removed using a combination of osteotomes and rongeurs.

The thick fibrous membrane often present at the bone-implant interface must be removed from the femoral canal and the acetabulum and sent for cultures. This may be done using the Cobb elevator, curved curette, and reverse cutting hooks. The debrided acetabular bone and femoral canal are then washed with 6 L of normal saline using pulsed lavage and irrigated with 0.5% aqueous betadine solution, with the solution resting for 5 minutes before suctioning. This is followed by a further 3 L of wash with normal saline via pulsed lavage. The operative site is then packed with gauze. While in one-stage exchange, the surgeons should then change into fresh gowns and gloves; surgical instruments should be replaced, and new surgical drapes applied around the operative field. When preparing for an articulated spacer, the authors tend to size the implant before irrigation, and a temporary spacer is manufactured on the back table while the authors are irrigating to save time. Before implantation of the spacer, new drapes are applied, and a new suction, new gowns, and new gloves are used.

The PROSTALAC (Prosthesis of antibiotic loaded acrylic cement; DePuy Orthopedics, Warsaw, IN, USA) hip system provides an articulating spacer for two-stage exchange arthroplasty with a reported infection eradication rate of 82% to 96%.[19,22,26] This is a facsimile of a femoral stem where antibiotic-loaded cement is molded around a metal endoskeleton with a femoral neck and morse taper in a size-specific mold. The femoral component is available in 4 lengths: 120 mm, 150 mm, 200 mm, and 240 mm. The 120-mm stems are available in 5 sizes and 2 offsets to allow for an excellent press-fit and immediate weight-bearing when appropriate. These stems are sized using size-specific broaches, which allows for the exact size mold to be used for the preparation of the spacer. The 3 larger stems are only available in the standard offset option and a single size. The appropriate length and offset are selected on the basis of femoral bone loss and integrity, and soft tissue tension. In cases whereby the femur has been weakened by osteotomy or osteolysis, or in the case of segmental bone loss, a longer stem with an anterior bow may be used.

Following judicious broaching of the femur for the 120-mm length or reaming for the longer stems up to 13 mm, the spacer is prepared using polymethyl methacrylate cement and augmented with heat-stable antibiotics. For each 40-g pack of cement, 3.6 g of tobramycin and 1.5 g of vancomycin are added, although the exact antibiotic regimen should be based on any cultures and sensitivities before spacer construction. Alternatively, ceftazidime at a dose of 3 g per package may be used instead of tobramycin if powdered tobramycin is not available.[27] For fungal infections, amphotericin B doses of 185.5 mg or 1200 mg or fluconazole dose of 200 mg per 40 g pack of cement may be used.[28] The spacer is prepared by inserting the antibiotic cement into an open mold. The endoskeleton is then inserted in the cement mantle and covered with more antibiotic-loaded cement, and the mold is then closed. In general, the authors use 2 packages of Palacos-R cement. Once the cement has hardened, the mold is dissembled, and the PROSTALAC implant is removed. The rongeur is used to clear any excess cement around the femoral stem before implantation. One technical tip is that the tip of the cement at the end of the stem should be broken off before stem insertion so that it does not break on insertion, making it more difficult to remove it at the second stage. The femoral spacer can then be inserted, and a press fit is achieved to allow rotational stability. In instances whereby there is deficiency of the proximal femur, a cuff or collar of cement can be applied to the proximal spacer to maintain torsional and vertical stability.

The acetabular component is a 45 mm × 32 mm ultrahigh-molecular-weight polyethylene cup with a snap-fit constrained configuration. A rongeur is used to make a small rent in the acetabular liner. This allows any fluid collecting within the cup to escape and reduces the hydrostatic pressures to decrease the risk of dislocation. Antibiotic cement is inserted into the acetabular cavity, without making fixation holes, and the acetabular cup is then cemented and held in position (20° of anteversion and 40° inclination) until the cement sets. Great care should be taken to avoid overmedialization of the cup. A cup impactor with a 28-mm femoral head is used to position the cup, as a 32-mm inserter will get stuck because of the snap-fit configuration of the cup. A trial reduction is then performed with the PROSTALAC femoral head trials, which is 2 mm less than the actual 32-mm head to prevent snapping of the trial head into the cup. Hip stability, range of motion, leg lengths, and soft tissue tension are assessed, before definitive femoral 32-mm head size selection. The final femoral head is impacted onto the trunnion and then positioned on the mouth of the acetabular cup, and gentle abduction pressure is applied to engage the snap-fit configuration.

In all cases, the wound should be closed in layers where possible, and drains should not be used to maximize the local concentration of antibiotic eluted from the cement. The application of negative pressure dressing for the first 5 days after surgery should be considered around a water-tight deep seal to help drain any residual fluid collections and to aid wound healing. The articulating spacer design often lends itself to weight-bearing as tolerated, although this should be within the context of any osteotomy required during the first stage as well as the remaining bone stock. Antibiotics should be based on the organism identified from the preoperative or intraoperative workup or on the basis of the probable infecting organism. A peripherally inserted central catheter (PICC) line should be obtained as soon as possible for long-term intravenous antibiotic administration.

Static Versus Dynamic Spacers Outcomes

The use of antibiotic-impregnated articulating spacers for two-stage exchange arthroplasties for PJIs in THAs have demonstrated infection eradication rates in excess of 80%.[10,20–23,26,29–31] Hofmann and colleagues[10] reviewed outcomes in 42 patients undergoing two-stage revisions with an articulating spacer formed using a cemented, sterilized, explanted femoral component with an all-polyethylene cup and reported 94% of patients remained infection-free at 74 months after surgery. Infection eradication was achieved in 100% of patients in culture-positive patients. Similarly, Younger and colleagues[26] reviewed outcomes in 48 patients undergoing two-stage revisions with the aforementioned PROSTALAC system and reported an infection eradication rate of 94% at a mean of 43 months' follow-up. Quayle and colleagues[32] reviewed outcomes in 53 patients undergoing two-stage revisions with custom-made articulating spacers and reported an infection eradication rate of 88.7% at 46.8 months' follow-up. The overall reported reinfection rate with articulating spacers remains between 1.7% and 10.7%, which is comparable with static spacers that have a reported reinfection rate between 1.4% and 8%in two-stage exchange arthroplasties in THA.[10,22,26,29,30,32–37]

Proponents of articulating spacers cite that retaining range of motion and controlled weight-bearing may help to maintain some function and mobility in preparation for the second-stage procedure. In the above study by Younger and colleagues,[26] articulating spacers were associated with improved interstage patient comfort levels compared with static spacers for Girdlestone excision arthroplasty. Other investigators also anecdotally noted that articulating spacers were associated with improved interstage comfort levels and reduced interstage inpatient hospitalization compared with static spacers.[31,35] D'Angelo and colleagues[29] reviewed outcomes in 28 patients undergoing two-stage exchange arthroplasty with an articulating spacer formed using a cement-coated hemiarthroplasty and reported improvements in the Harris hip score from 43 points preoperatively to 82 points at a mean of 53 months follow-up. Similarly, Masri and colleagues[22] reviewed outcomes in 29 patients undergoing two-stage revisions with the PROSTALAC hip system and reported the Harris hip score improved from 38 points before surgery to 70 points at 47 months' follow-up. Tsung and colleagues[37] followed 76 patients and reported improvements in the Charnley–D'Aubigne–Postel pain and function scores, Harris hip score, and Oxford hip score at 80.4 months' follow-up.

Some studies have shown that articulating spacers may help to reduce the duration of the inpatient hospital admission or operative times for the second-stage procedure compared with static spacers.[38,39] Nahhas and colleagues[39] conducted a prospective randomized controlled trial comparing static versus articulating spacers for the treatment of 40 patients with PJIs following THA. The study reported no differences in the primary outcome measure of operative time between the 2 treatment groups, although patients with static spacers had longer inpatient admissions compared with articulating spacers. Both groups had comparable secondary outcomes relating to the Harris hip scores, failure secondary to infection, dislocation rates, and reoperation for any reason at a mean of 3.2 years' follow-up. Warwick and colleagues[38] retrospectively reviewed outcomes in 99 patients undergoing static versus articulating spacers for PJI following THAs. The study found that articulating spacers were associated with reduced operative times for the second-stage procedure compared with static spacers, but there were no differences between the groups in relation to the need for second-stage extensile procedures, reimplantation rates, or overall mortality at a minimum of 1-year follow-up.

SINGLE-STAGE VERSUS TWO-STAGE OUTCOMES

Single-stage revision has been reported to be as effective at eradicating infection as two-stage revision, although trials comparing both strategies are lacking.[40–43] Leonard and colleagues[42] performed a systematic review including 9 studies and found that single-stage revision allows comparable reinfection rates and a trend toward better functional outcomes, when compared with a two-stage revision. Unfortunately, the quality of the included studies was poor, and no randomized controlled trials were identified. Choi and colleagues[43] reported infection control rates of 82% with single-stage revisions, versus 75% using two-stage revisions for PJI after THA. Similarly, Kunutsor and colleagues[41] performed a systematic review and meta-analysis, identifying reinfection rates from 38 one-stage studies and 60 two-stage studies. They found no differences in reinfection rates, with an 8.2% reinfection rate in single-stage revisions versus 7.9% in two-stage revisions. Recently, van den Kieboom and colleagues[40] retrospectively compared 105 consecutive patients with culture-negative PJI, a factor that has been considered to be a contraindication to a single-stage revision. Interestingly, they found no differences between one-stage and two-stage revisions for 30-, 60-, and 90-day readmissions, 1-year mortality, and amputation.

To the authors' knowledge, the only trial comparing one-stage versus two-stage revisions in PJI is the recently published INFORM trial.[44] This was a multicentric, pragmatic, parallel group, open-label, randomized controlled trial that compared the effectiveness and cost-effectiveness of single-stage versus two-stage revisions in PJI of the hip. One hundred forty patients were randomized to undergo single-stage revision or two-stage revision. They found no differences in infection control at 18 months' follow-up (14% of the single-stage revision group had at least one marker of possible infection vs 11% in the two-stage group). Patients undergoing single-stage revisions had higher functional scores at 3 months, but not from 6 months onward. Although there were no differences in terms of infection control or functional scores, single-stage revisions were cost-effective when compared with two-stage revisions.

Although the evidence does not show superiority of one approach over the other, it is important to interpret these findings with caution. First, to the authors' knowledge there is only one published level I study, and most studies are level IV retrospective series, some of them of poor quality. Therefore, most meta-analyses replicate these findings and limitations. Second, patients with more complex presentations, aggressive organisms, and difficult technical factors are likely to undergo two-stage revisions and as such are overrepresented in this group in retrospective series. The inherent limitations of retrospective studies are likely to replicate these selection biases and therefore obscure true differences between single- and two-stage procedures. Last, the lack of a consensus in diagnosis and management means there is a marked heterogeneity in hospital-specific protocols, including differences in surgical indications for either procedure, surgical technique, timing of surgeries, and antibiotic treatment, among other factors. This makes studies different to compare and the external validation of their findings somewhat limited.

Postoperative Management, Including Antibiotic Duration

After surgery, patients must continue antibiotic treatment. Antibiotics should be targeted to the identified agent in the preoperative or intraoperative cultures, or based on the probable infecting organism if none has been identified. A multidisciplinary approach, including infectious diseases specialists, is paramount to obtaining optimal outcomes.[45] Patients should be mobilized as much as possible, and thromboprophylaxis should be ensured. Although PJI is known to increase venous thromboembolism risk, there is no evidence to support maintaining different thromboprophylaxis practices in this population of patients.[46] Rehabilitation should be tailored to the intraoperative findings and postoperative results. Articulating spacers allow for weight-bearing and maintaining a relatively preserved length of the extremity.

There is mounting evidence supporting the use of oral antibiotics to treat bone or joint infections, as an alternative to intravenous antibiotics. The Oral versus Intravenous Antibiotic (OVIVA) trial included 1054 participants with bone or joint infection, including PJI, at 26 United Kingdom hospitals.[47] Within 7 days of surgery, they randomized patients to receive oral or intravenous antibiotics to complete the first 6 weeks of treatment. Oral antibiotic therapy was noninferior to intravenous antibiotics when comparing treatment failure at 1 year. Unfortunately, there was no subanalysis comparing osteomyelitis, fracture-related infections, and PJI outcomes. Given the difficulties, cost, and

complications associated with intravenous antibiotics, the current recommendation is to use oral antibiotics after achieving organism and susceptibility identification, if possible. If intravenous antibiotics need to be used, long-term peripheral venous access should be obtained. With reference to intravenous versus oral antibiotics, the authors defer to the infectious diseases consultant, and if they feel that oral bioavailability is sufficient, then oral antibiotics are given.

Antibiotic duration has not been stablished, although most studies have used 4- to 6-week antibiotic regimens. As such, the 2018 ICM has also recommended 4 to 6 weeks of antibiotics after single-stage revisions, and 2 to 6 weeks after the first stage of a two-stage revision.[48,49] However, emerging evidence suggests longer treatment periods may be necessary for some patients. Bernard and colleagues[50] performed an open-label, randomized, controlled, noninferiority trial in 28 French hospitals, comparing 6 weeks of antibiotic therapy versus 12 weeks, in patients with PJI. They found 6 weeks of antibiotics were not shown to be noninferior and resulted in a higher number of patients with persistent infection at 2 years. Of note, they included patients undergoing debridement, antibiotics, and implant retention (DAIR), single-stage revisions, and two-stage revisions. Only in DAIR procedures was 12 weeks of antibiotics clearly superior, as the study was not powered to demonstrate differences between different surgeries.

There is no consensus on when to reimplant. Some centers perform reimplantation after finishing antibiotic treatment, whereas others maintain an antibiotic holiday period between finishing antibiotic treatment and reimplantation. Patients should have completed their antibiotic treatment, and the medical team should be satisfied the infection has resolved. Timing of reimplantation should consider the resolution of the signs of infection and inflammatory markers trending downward. However, no marker has been identified as a predictor of a successful reimplantation. Also, it is unclear whether the PJI diagnostic criteria have any role in deciding reimplantation.[51] In the presence of any clinical signs of infection or active inflammatory markers, a repeat first-stage procedure should be considered.

COMPLICATIONS

Mechanical complications are a significant concern after an articulating spacer has been implanted. Complications are more frequent in handmade dynamic spacers and in spacers that articulate with host bone.[52] The most common ones are dislocation, spacer fracture, and femoral fracture.

Dislocation has been reported to occur in about 8% to 16% of patients.[36,52,53] Several factors influence the risk of instability, including limited head sizes and offset alternatives. Handmade spacers are prone to dislocate, as obtaining an adequate head-to-neck ratio is difficult, and femoral fixation can be compromised.[54] The use of dynamic spacers, such as the PROSTALAC system, or other custom-made versions using cemented cups or liners has improved the stability of the constructs, as they allow for adequate sizing, increased femoral head and offset, as well as varying degrees of constraint.

Spacer fracture is associated with the use of handmade or injection-molded dynamic spacers, and it can occur in up to 3% to 6% of patients.[55] Of note, the mechanical stability of the cement is not affected the addition of antibiotics up to a proportional ratio of approximately 5%.[56] If the antibiotic ratio increases more than 20%, however, the ease of manufacture of the cement will be affected.[20]

Similarly, femoral fractures can occur, particularly in patients with a spacer that has not obtained adequate fixation and in patients with increasing bone loss.[31] The lack of proper cement interdigitation may result in motion of the femoral implant, which may increase the risk of sustaining a fracture.

SUMMARY

PJI following THA is a devastating complication associated with high morbidity and mortality. Two-stage revision surgery remains the gold standard treatment for eradication of infection. The surgical technique for the first-stage procedure must ensure meticulous debridement of all infected tissue and removal of metalwork, obtain tissue samples for microbiological analysis, and grade the degree of bone and soft tissue compromise. Articulating spacers effectively maintain the joint space, permit hip motion, and enable controlled weight-bearing. In combination, these features help to reduce hip joint contractures and maintain bone stock before the second stage. Articulating spacers are associated with improvements in functional outcomes, and infection eradication rates remain greater than 80%. The main complications with articulating spacers are fractures and dislocations.

CLINICS CARE POINTS

- Periprosthetic joint infection remains a leading cause of revision surgery following total hip arthroplasty and is associated with high morbidity and mortality.

- Two-stage exchange arthroplasty continues to be the gold-standard treatment for chronic periprosthetic joint infections but is associated with increased hospitalization and increased cost compared with one-stage exchange arthroplasty.

- The surgical technique for the first-stage procedure must ensure meticulous debridement of all infected tissue and removal of metalwork, obtain tissue samples for microbiological analysis, and grade the degree of bone and soft tissue compromise.

- Static or articulating spacers may be used for localized antibiotic-elution before the definitive second-stage procedure.

- Articulating spacers effectively maintain the joint space, permit hip motion, and enable controlled weight-bearing. In combination, these features help to reduce hip joint contractures and maintain bone stock before the second stage.

- Two-stage exchange arthroplasty with articulating spacers is associated with improvements in functional outcomes and infection eradication rates greater than 80%.

- Patients and surgeons need to be cognizant of the risks of fractures and dislocations associated with articulating spacers. In patients with significant bone loss and/or abductor muscle weakness, static spacers should be considered to minimize these risks during the interstage interval.

DISCLOSURE

The authors have nothing to disclose.

REFERENCES

1. Kurtz S, Ong K, Lau E, et al. Projections of primary and revision hip and knee arthroplasty in the United States from 2005 to 2030. J Bone Joint Surg Am 2007;89:780–5.

2. Kurtz SM, et al. Future clinical and economic impact of revision total hip and knee arthroplasty. J Bone Joint Surg Am 2007;89(Suppl 3): 144–51.

3. Berend KR, et al. Two-stage treatment of hip periprosthetic joint infection is associated with a high

rate of infection control but high mortality. Clin Orthop Relat Res 2013;471:510–8.

4. Bozic KJ, Ries MD. The impact of infection after total hip arthroplasty on hospital and surgeon resource utilization. J Bone Joint Surg Am 2005; 87:1746–51.

5. Matthews PC, Berendt AR, McNally MA, et al. Diagnosis and management of prosthetic joint infection. Bmj 2009;338:b1773.

6. Gehrke T, Kendoff D. Peri-prosthetic hip infections: in favour of one-stage. Hip Int 2012;22(Suppl 8): S40–5.

7. Zimmerli W, Trampuz A, Ochsner PE. Prosthetic-joint infections. N Engl J Med 2004;351:1645–54.

8. Klouche S, Sariali E, Mamoudy P. Total hip arthroplasty revision due to infection: a cost analysis approach. Orthop Traumatol Surg Res 2010;96: 124–32.

9. Parvizi J, Tan TL, Goswami K, et al. The 2018 Definition of Periprosthetic Hip and Knee Infection: An Evidence-Based and Validated Criteria. J Arthroplasty 2018;33(5):1309–14.e2.

10. Hofmann AA, Goldberg TD, Tanner AM, et al. Ten-year experience using an articulating antibiotic cement hip spacer for the treatment of chronically infected total hip. J Arthroplasty 2005;20:874–9.

11. McNally M, et al. The EBJIS definition of periprosthetic joint infection. Bone Joint Lett J 2021;103-b:18–25.

12. Shohat N, et al. Hip and Knee Section, What is the Definition of a Periprosthetic Joint Infection (PJI) of the Knee and the Hip? Can the Same Criteria be Used for Both Joints?: Proceedings of International Consensus on Orthopedic Infections. J Arthroplasty 2019;34:S325–7.

13. Parvizi J, Jacovides C, Antoci V, et al. Diagnosis of periprosthetic joint infection: the utility of a simple yet unappreciated enzyme. J Bone Joint Surg Am 2011;93:2242–8.

14. Deirmengian C, et al. Combined measurement of synovial fluid α-Defensin and C-reactive protein levels: highly accurate for diagnosing periprosthetic joint infection. J Bone Joint Surg Am 2014; 96:1439–45.

15. Tarabichi M, et al. Diagnosis of Periprosthetic Joint Infection: The Potential of Next-Generation Sequencing. J Bone Joint Surg Am 2018;100:147–54.

16. Younger AS, Duncan CP, Masri BA. Treatment of infection associated with segmental bone loss in the proximal part of the femur in two stages with use of an antibiotic-loaded interval prosthesis. J Bone Joint Surg Am 1998;80:60–9.

17. Chalmers BP, et al. Two-Stage Revision Total Hip Arthroplasty With a Specific Articulating Antibiotic Spacer Design: Reliable Periprosthetic Joint Infection Eradication and Functional Improvement. J Arthroplasty 2018;33:3746–53.

18. Kildow BJ, Della-Valle CJ, Springer BD. Single vs 2-Stage Revision for the Treatment of Periprosthetic Joint Infection. J Arthroplasty 2020;35:S24–30.

19. Wentworth SJ, Masri BA, Duncan CP, et al. Hip prosthesis of antibiotic-loaded acrylic cement for the treatment of infections following total hip arthroplasty. J Bone Joint Surg Am 2002;84-A-(Suppl 2):123–8.

20. Hsieh PH, et al. Two-stage revision hip arthroplasty for infection: comparison between the interim use of antibiotic-loaded cement beads and a spacer prosthesis. J Bone Joint Surg Am 2004;86:1989–97.

21. Masri BA, Duncan CP, Beauchamp CP. Long-term elution of antibiotics from bone-cement: an in vivo study using the prosthesis of antibiotic-loaded acrylic cement (PROSTALAC) system. J Arthroplasty 1998;13:331–8.

22. Masri BA, Panagiotopoulos KP, Greidanus NV, et al. Cementless two-stage exchange arthroplasty for infection after total hip arthroplasty. J Arthroplasty 2007;22:72–8.

23. Romanò CL, Romanò D, Albisetti A, et al. Preformed antibiotic-loaded cement spacers for two-stage revision of infected total hip arthroplasty. Long-term results. Hip Int 2012;22(Suppl 8):S46–53.

24. Lausmann C, et al. Preliminary results of a novel spacer technique in the management of septic revision hip arthroplasty. Arch Orthop Trauma Surg 2018;138:1617–22.

25. Patel JN, Pizzo RA, Yoon RS, et al. Addressing Antibiotic Hip Spacer Instability via Hybrid Screw-cement Fixation of a Constrained Liner and Cement-rebar Interface Techniques: A Technical Narrative. J Am Acad Orthop Surg 2020;28:166–70.

26. Younger AS, Duncan CP, Masri BA, et al. The outcome of two-stage arthroplasty using a custom-made interval spacer to treat the infected hip. J Arthroplasty 1997;12:615–23.

27. Iarikov D, Demian H, Rubin D, et al. Choice and doses of antibacterial agents for cement spacers in treatment of prosthetic joint infections: review of published studies. Clin Infect Dis 2012;55:1474–80.

28. Kuiper JW, van den Bekerom MP, van der Stappen J, et al. 2-stage revision recommended for treatment of fungal hip and knee prosthetic joint infections. Acta Orthop 2013;84:517–23.

29. D'Angelo F, Negri L, Binda T, et al. The use of a preformed spacer in two-stage revision of infected hip arthroplasties. Musculoskelet Surg 2011;95: 115–20.

30. Hsieh PH, Huang KC, Lee PC, et al. Two-stage revision of infected hip arthroplasty using an antibiotic-loaded spacer: retrospective comparison between short-term and prolonged antibiotic therapy. J Antimicrob Chemother 2009;64:392–7.

31. Pattyn C, De Geest T, Ackerman P, et al. Preformed gentamicin spacers in two-stage revision hip

arthroplasty: functional results and complications. Int Orthop 2011;35:1471–6.

32. Quayle J, Barakat A, Klasan A, et al. External validation study of hip peri-prosthetic joint infection with cemented custom-made articulating spacer (CUMARS). Hip Int 2022;32:379–85.

33. Haddad FS, Muirhead-Allwood SK, Manktelow AR, et al. Two-stage uncemented revision hip arthroplasty for infection. J Bone Joint Surg Br 2000;82: 689–94.

34. Charlton WP, Hozack WJ, Teloken MA, et al. Complications associated with reimplantation after girdlestone arthroplasty. Clin Orthop Relat Res 2003; 407:119–26.

35. Jacobs C, Christensen CP, Berend ME. Static and mobile antibiotic-impregnated cement spacers for the management of prosthetic joint infection. J Am Acad Orthop Surg 2009;17:356–68.

36. Romanò CL, Romanò D, Logoluso N, et al. Long-stem versus short-stem preformed antibiotic-loaded cement spacers for two-stage revision of infected total hip arthroplasty. Hip Int 2010;20:26–33.

37. Tsung JD, Rohrsheim JA, Whitehouse SL, et al. Management of periprosthetic joint infection after total hip arthroplasty using a custom made articulating spacer (CUMARS); the Exeter experience. J Arthroplasty 2014;29:1813–8.

38. Warwick HS, et al. Comparison of Static and Articulating Spacers After Periprosthetic Joint Infection. J Am Acad Orthop Surg Glob Res Rev 2023;7. https://doi.org/10.5435/JAAOSGlobal-D-22-00284.

39. Nahhas CR, et al. Randomized Trial of Static and Articulating Spacers for Treatment of the Infected Total Hip Arthroplasty. J Arthroplasty 2021;36: 2171–7.

40. van den Kieboom J, et al. One-stage revision is as effective as two-stage revision for chronic culture-negative periprosthetic joint infection after total hip and knee arthroplasty. Bone Joint Lett J 2021; 103-b:515–21.

41. Kunutsor SK, Whitehouse MR, Blom AW, et al. Re-Infection Outcomes following One- and Two-Stage Surgical Revision of Infected Hip Prosthesis: A Systematic Review and Meta-Analysis. PLoS One 2015; 10:e0139166.

42. Leonard HA, Liddle AD, Burke O, et al. Single- or two-stage revision for infected total hip arthroplasty? A systematic review of the literature. Clin Orthop Relat Res 2014;472:1036–42.

43. Choi HR, Kwon YM, Freiberg AA, et al. Comparison of one-stage revision with antibiotic cement versus two-stage revision results for infected total hip arthroplasty. J Arthroplasty 2013;28:66–70.

44. Blom AW, et al. Clinical and cost effectiveness of single stage compared with two stage revision for hip prosthetic joint infection (INFORM): pragmatic, parallel group, open label, randomised controlled trial. Bmj 2022;379:e071281.

45. Abblitt WP, et al. Hip and Knee Section, Outcomes: Proceedings of International Consensus on Orthopedic Infections. J Arthroplasty 2019;34:S487–95.

46. Recommendations from the ICM-VTE: Hip & Knee. J Bone Joint Surg Am 2022;104:180–231.

47. Li HK, et al. Oral versus Intravenous Antibiotics for Bone and Joint Infection. N Engl J Med 2019;380: 425–36.

48. de Beaubien B, et al. Hip and Knee Section, Treatment, Antimicrobials: Proceedings of International Consensus on Orthopedic Infections. J Arthroplasty 2019;34:S477–82.

49. Bialecki J, et al. Hip and Knee Section, Treatment, One Stage Exchange: Proceedings of International Consensus on Orthopedic Infections. J Arthroplasty 2019;34:S421–6.

50. Bernard L, et al. Antibiotic Therapy for 6 or 12 Weeks for Prosthetic Joint Infection. N Engl J Med 2021;384:1991–2001.

51. Aalirezaie A, et al. Hip and Knee Section, Diagnosis, Reimplantation: Proceedings of International Consensus on Orthopedic Infections. J Arthroplasty 2019;34:S369–79.

52. D'Angelo F, Negri L, Zatti G, et al. Two-stage revision surgery to treat an infected hip implant. A comparison between a custom-made spacer and a pre-formed one. Chir Organi Mov 2005;90:271–9.

53. Rava A, Bruzzone M, Cottino U, et al. Hip Spacers in Two-Stage Revision for Periprosthetic Joint Infection: A Review of Literature. Joints 2019;7:56–63.

54. Leunig M, Chosa E, Speck M, et al. A cement spacer for two-stage revision of infected implants of the hip joint. Int Orthop 1998;22:209–14.

55. Citak M, Masri BA, Springer B, et al. Are Preformed Articulating Spacers Superior To Surgeon-Made Articulating Spacers in the Treatment Of PJI in THA? A Literature Review. Open Orthop J 2015;9: 255–61.

56. Murray WR. Use of antibiotic-containing bone cement. Clin Orthop Relat Res 1984;190:89–95.

Recurrent Periprosthetic Joint Infections

Diagnosis, Management, and Outcomes

Christopher F. Deans, MD*, Beau J. Kildow, MD,
Kevin L. Garvin, MD

KEYWORDS

- Arthroplasty • Prosthetic joint infection • Infected total joint arthroplasty • Persistant infection
- Recurrent infection

KEY POINTS

- Recurrent prosthetic joint infections are associated with significant patient morbidity and mortality and are a financial burden to the health care system.
- Multiple joint and limb salvage surgical options exist and require careful patient counseling and patient participation in management decision-making for this challenging problem.
- A multidisciplinary approach with providers who are experienced in the management of prosthetic joint infection optimizes patients' treatment.
- Novel pathogen identification techniques, surgical protocols, and medical treatment modalities are under investigation, with promising early results in difficult-to-treat cases.

INTRODUCTION/BACKGROUND/PREVALENCE

Periprosthetic joint infection (PJI) remains one of the most devastating and challenging complications after primary total joint arthroplasty (TJA). It has been associated with signi cant morbidity and mortality and has shown to be costly for the health care system.[1–4] Two-stage revision has been established as the standard of care for treating chronic PJI in North America with early infection eradication success rates reported from 73% to 94%[5–17] (Table 1).

Failure following 2-stage revisions for chronic PJI is thought to be secondary to either an entirely new infection with a different pathogen or recurrent infection due to failed index treatment. Recent studies have demonstrated dichotomous results, with reinfection rates by the same organism ranging from 5% to 55%[9,10] (see Table 1). The majority of studies would suggest that most failures are due to a new infection rather than

the persistence of previous infection, using modern 2-stage management protocols.[5,6,9,18] An alternative to this theory was explored in a recent report by Della Valle and colleagues.[19] They postulated that reinfections with a different organism could be the persistence of an organism at index 2-stage revision that was not identified via conventional culture methods; however, their report did not support this hypothesis.

Recurrent PJI rates after index 2-stage revision have been reported to increase with greater length of follow-up (Table 2). One recent study by Petis and colleagues reported failure rates of 4% at 1-year, 14% at 5-year, 16% at 10-year, and 17% at 15-year follow-up.[7] Another recent study reported 9% reinfection at 2-year and 14.8% at 10-year follow-up.[12] Other studies with at least 7.5-year follow-up concur, with reinfection rates ranging from 9% to 33%.[6–9,11,12,15] Reports suggesting that the majority of reinfections are secondary to new pathogens and higher reinfection rate with longer-term follow-up support

---

Department of Orthopaedic Surgery and Rehabilitation, University of Nebraska Medical Center, 985640 Nebraska Medical Center, Omaha, NE 68198, USA
* Corresponding author.
E-mail address: christopher.deans@unmc.edu

Orthop Clin N Am 55 (2024) 193–206
https://doi.org/10.1016/j.ocl.2023.09.002
0030-5898/24/Published by Elsevier Inc.

Table 1
Selected comparative outcomes of 2-stage revision total joint arthroplasty for chronic periprosthetic joint infection with length of follow-up and reported pathogens

Author, Year	N (hips, knees)	Reinfection After 2-Stage Revision, N (%)	Follow-up Term (Mean)	Same Organism	Different Organism	Resistant Pathogens
Hartman et al,[5] 2022	158 (hips, knees)	31(19.6%)	3.35 y	22.5%	77.5%	MRSA 14 (45%) MDR 1(3.2%)
Petis et al,[7] 2019	245 (knees)	10(4%) @ 1 y 34(14%) @5 y 39(16%) @10 y 42 (17%) @15 y	14 y	—	—	MRSA 6(2%)
Stambough et al,[15] 2019	291(hips, knees)	48(16%)	2 y	—	—	—
Garvin et al,[9] 2018	97 (hips, knees)	12 (12.3%)	11 y	5%	95%	MRSA 1(8.3%) MRSE 2 (16.6%)
Ma et al,[12] 2018	108(knees)	16(14.8%)	5.6 y	—	—	—
Sabry et al,[8] 2014	314 (knees)	105 (33%)	3.3 y	—	—	MRSA 35 (33.3%) MRSE 2 (1.9%) VRE 5 (4.8%)
Kubista et al,[6] 2012	368 (knees)	58(15.8%)	7.8 y	—	—	MRSA 21(36%)
Mortazavi et al,[14] 2011	117 (knees)	33(28%)	3.4 y	—	—	MRSA 11(33%)
Kurd et al,[10] 2010	96 (knees)	26(27%)	2.1 y	54%	46%	MRSA 4 (15.4%) MRSE 2 (7.7%)
Haleem et al,[11] 2004	96 (knees)	9(9%)	7.2 y	44%	56%	MRSA 2 (22%)
McPherson et al,[13] 2002	50 (hips)	21(42%)	1.9 y	—	—	—

Abbreviations: MDR, multiple drug-resistant; MRSA, methicillin-resistant *Staphylococcus aureus*; MRSE, methicillin-resistant *Staphylococcus epidermidis*; N, number; VRE, vancomycin-resistant *Enterococcus*.

Table 2
Selected comparative outcomes of repeat 2-stage revision total joint arthroplasty for recurrent periprosthetic joint infection, reported pathogens, and final management

Author, Year	N (Hips, Knees)	Reinfection After Second 2-Stage Revision	Follow-up Term (Mean)	Same Organism	Different Organism	Final Management
Steinicke et al,[16] 2021	43 (hips, knees)	14 (33%) @1 y 27 (62%) @ 5 y	2.9 y	21%	79%	Amputation 14%
Gathen et al,[60] 2018	45(knees)	9(20%)	2.9 y	—	—	—
Bejon et al,[17] 2010	152 (hips. knees)	41(27%)	5.75 y	4%	6%	Amputation 12%
Maheshwari et al,[32] 2010	35(knees)	11(31.4%)	4.9 y	—	—	Amputation 45% Retained spacer 27% Arthrodesis 18% Resection arthroplasty 9%
Azzam et al,[59] 2009	18 (knees)	4 (22%)	3.83 y	75%	25%	Third 2-stage 50% Resection arthroplasty 25% I&D with suppressive abx 25%
Haleem et al,[11] 2004	9 (knees)	4 (44%)	7.2 y	—	—	Amputation 50% Arthrodesis 50%
Hanssen et al,[53] 1995	24 (knees)	—	—	—	—	Arthrodesis 54% I&D with suppressive abx 21% Amputation 17% Resection arthroplasty 4.2%

Abbreviations: abx, antibiotics; I&D, incision and drainage; N, number.

the theory of altered local immune function in certain individuals with various comorbidities and risk factors. Heim and colleagues explored this hypothesis in 2017, finding high levels of myeloid-derived suppressor cells (MDSCs) in PJI tissues, which inhibit T-cell proliferation and blunt immune response in the affected joint.[20]

Greater volume of primary TJAs being performed annually will result in an increase in chronic PJIs in the near future. It is crucial to expand our understanding of the etiologies and contributing factors of 2-stage revision failure, the management options after a failed 2-stage revision and outcomes related to these options, new diagnostic and therapeutic developments, and deficits in our understanding that future research efforts may address. The purpose of this study is to review current literature and expert opinions on such topics.

PATIENT EVALUATION OVERVIEW

Careful assessment of each patient's unique presentation—surgical history, medical conditions, soft tissue/limb integrity, virulence of infecting pathogen, patient compliance with therapeutic management, and other risk factors—empowers the surgeon and treating team to recommend the best medical and surgical options for treatment of recurrent PJI. A thorough understanding of patient, pathogen, and surgical risk factors for failure of 2-stage revision may improve risk assessment, lead to more aggressive or patient-specific management, and allow for consideration of alternative surgical or medical therapies.

DIAGNOSIS OF RECURRENT PERIPROSTHETIC JOINT INFECTION

The diagnosis of recurrent hip and knee PJI requires a combination of clinical findings, laboratory results from peripheral blood and synovial fluid, and microbiological cultures, with potential utilization of intraoperative findings and histologic evaluation of periprosthetic tissues. In patients who have had previous PJI, presentation with a painful total joint is infected until proven otherwise. Other common clinical findings include effusion, warmth, erythematous skin, sinus tract or draining wound, and low-grade fever. Special consideration should be given on the presence of other active infections, recent surgeries or potential for skin tissue penetration (colonoscopy, dental work, cosmetic interventions, other joint injections, and so forth), and patient comorbidities including immunosuppressed state, uncontrolled

diabetes, smoking status, obesity, alcohol consumption, intravenous (IV) drug use, and oral hygiene, among many others. Timing since symptom onset should be identified, if possible. Any patient being evaluated for a painful total joint should be sent for standard roentgenographic imaging, serum erythrocyte sedimentation rate (ESR), and C-reactive protein (CRP), with aspiration in the setting of effusion or elevated inflammatory markers. Consideration of serum D-dimer may be performed at provider discretion. Synovial analysis with cell count and routine culture should be performed, with specimens held at least 14 days. Advanced diagnostic modalities that may be considered include alpha-defensin, synovial leukocyte esterase, or molecular methods including rapid polymerase chain reaction (PCR) diagnostics, 16s sequencing, and/or shotgun/targeted whole genome sequencing. The authors prescribe to the 2018 diagnostic criteria for PJI.[21] Preoperative consultation of an infectious disease specialist is a valuable addition to help guide advanced diagnostic modalities, patient counseling on expectations, and postoperative antibiotic selection and duration.

PATIENT-RELATED OUTCOME PREDICTORS

Many studies have reported clinical and patient-related factors that predict treatment failure (Table 3). Consistent patient-related factors include chronic lymphedema, immunocompromised state, diabetes, anemia, age greater than 70, obesity and morbid obesity, tobacco use, inflammatory arthritis, coagulopathies, peripheral vascular disease, chronic disease of major organ systems, recurrent urinary tract infections, and malnutrition.[5–8,10,12,16,22–26] As more generalized markers of the preceding patient risk factors, several have noted the American Society of Anesthesiologists (ASA) score and the Charlson Comorbidity Index as representative of the risk of reinfection.[8,16,24]

Other historical findings and laboratory markers have also been found predictive of treatment failure. Elevated CRP (12.65 g/dL vs 5.0 g/dL) at index PJI 2-stage revision may indicate host immune system under assault by a more virulent pathogen or a compromised immune response struggling to control an infection.[5,8] A longer duration of symptoms prior to surgical management and gross purulence at time of surgery are both associated with increased failure rates. It has been suggested that purulence is a marker of a more virulent pathogen and established infection, with tissue

Table 3
Predictors of treatment failure in 2-stage management of periprosthetic joint infection

Author, Year	N (Hips, Knees)	Predictors of Treatment Failure
Hartman et al,[5] 2022	158 (hips, knees}	MSSA CRP>12.65 g/dL ESR>69 Time to reimplantation (>101 days)
Kubista et al,[6] 2012	368 (knees)	Chronic lymphedema Repeat surgery between resection and reimplantation Time to reimplantation (>66 d)
Petis et al,[7] 2019	245 (knees)	BMI≥30 kg/m Previous revision surgery McPherson host grade C
Sabry et al,[8] 2014	314 (knees)	Longer duration of symptoms Increased time from index TKA Greater number of previous surgeries Time to reimplantation (>96 d) Gram-negative pathogen
Cancienne et al,[85] 2017	7146 (hips)	Age>85 y Obesity Inflammatory arthritis Depression Hyperlipidemia Chronic kidney disease Chronic liver disease
Cancienne et al,[26] 2018	18,533 (knees)	Male gender Age 70–74 y Obesity, morbid obesity Tobacco use Inflammatory arthritis Depression Hypercoagulable disorder Hypertension Peripheral vascular disease Hyperlipidemia Chronic liver disease Chronic kidney disease
Houdek et al,[25] 2015	653 (hips)	Obesity
Watts et al,[23] 2014	2423 (knees)	Obesity Diabetes
Kurd et al,[10] 2010	96 (knees)	Age>65 y Obesity, morbid obesity Thyroid disease Methicillin-resistant pathogen
Ma et al,[12] 2018	108 (knees)	Obesity Operative time at reimplantation>4 h Gout *Enteroroccus* species
Steinicke e et al,[16] 2021	55 (hips, knees)	Higher Charlson Comorbidity Index Obesity Diabetes
Zhang et al,[22] 2022	241 (hips, knees)	Lower serum albumin
Kilgus et al,[30] 2022	70 (hips, knees)	Antibiotic-resistant pathogens

(continued on next page)

Author, Year	N (Hips, Knees)	Predictors of Treatment Failure
Klemt et a1,[31] 2021	256 (hips, knees)	Higher Charlson Comorbidity Index Requiring interim spacer exchange *Enterococcus* species
Maheshwari et a1,[32] 2010	35 (knees)	Antibiotic-resistant pathogens
Mortazavi et a1,[14] 2011	117 (knees)	Culture-negative pathogen Methicillin-resistant pathogen
George et al,[37] 2018	347 (hips, knees)	Higher Charlson Comorbidity Index Longer time to reimplantation Requiring interim spacer exchange Antibiotic-resistant pathogens
Puetzler et al,[36] 2023	Meta-analysis	Longer time to reimplantation
Tan et al,[35] 2018	785 (hips, knees)	Longer time to reimplantation (>88 d)
Rajagopal et a1,[38] 2018	184 (knees)	Prior failed DAIR Methicillin-resistant pathogens *Pseudomonas* species

Abbreviations: BMI, body mass index; CRP, C-reactive protein; DAIR, debridement, antibiotics, and implant retention; ESR, erythrocyte sedimentation rate; MSSA, methicillin-susceptible *Staphylococcus aureus*; N, number.

devitalization and higher likelihood of extension into the periprosthetic bone.[14] Some bacteria, such as *Staphylococcus aureus*, produce virulence factors such as adhesions which allow the bacteria to penetrate and remain within periarticular soft tissues and potentially alter local immune function.[8,12,14,27,28] It has also been posed that more subjectively necrotic-appearing tissues at the time of surgery suggest penetration of bacteria into the soft tissues, associated with bacterial quiescence that is resistant to antibiotic penetration and efficacy, much in the way of biofilm.[27–29]

PATHOGEN-RELATED OUTCOME PREDICTORS

Specific pathogens have been noted consistently in the literature as predictors of treatment failure. These pathogens include methicillin-resistant *S aureus* (MRSA), *Enterococcus*, and culture-negative (CN) and gram-negative bacteria.[8,10,12,14,30–33] Kilgus and team demonstrated this in 2002, finding treatment success at 2.5-year follow-up after 2-stage revision of hips to be 81% for methicillin-susceptible *S aureus* (MSSA) and 48% for MRSA, and of knees to be 89% and 18%, respectively.[30] Kurd and team reported 3.37 times greater failure rate if index infection was MRSA.[10] Klemt in 2021 found *Enterococcus* as an independent risk factor for requiring spacer exchange during 2-stage management.[31] Mortazavi noted a 42% failure of

2-stage at a mean 3.4-year follow-up if CN or methicillin-resistant pathogens, compared to 15% without.[14]

It seems that the pathogen profile with recurrent infection shifts based on time to recurrence. Early failure, defined variably as within 1 to 3 years of index 2-stage, has been found more commonly to be the same organism.[9,11,16] Late failure, in contrast, has been more often reported as a different organism or polymicrobial.[9,11,16] Haleem and colleagues recently reported 60% of failures within 1 year with same microorganism, and 75% of failures at greater than 1 year with a different microorganism.[11] Steinicke reported only 21% of failures with same organism at median approximately 3-year follow-up.[16] At the authors' own institution with a mean 11-year follow-up, the authors found only 5% of reinfections with same microorganism.[9]

A recent report by Egbulefu and colleagues addressed the likelihood that recurrent infections were persistent or new infections.[19] In their retrospective study looking at 30 patients with recurrent PJI that failed 2-stage management, cultures and sensitivities at the first PJI were compared to cultures and sensitivities at the recurrent PJI. If there was a new organism, they sought to determine if the new organism was susceptible to previous antibiotic therapy. Of the recurrent infections, 83.3% were new organisms, and 64% of those were susceptible to the index antibiotics. This suggests that most failures were new infections entirely, rather than persistent infections not previously detected by culture data on index PJI.

Potentially most impactful on the future of treatment failure are pathogen-related factors, particularly with the evolution of multiple drug-resistant (MDR) microorganisms (see Table 2). Recent reports have demonstrated the increase in MDR pathogens in the United States relative to other countries. In the United States, 48.1% of *S aureus* infections are MRSA and 26.7% of enterococcus infections are vancomycin-resistant *Enterococcus* (VRE) compared to 12.8% and 0% in Europe, respectively.[34] As stated earlier, MDR organisms have been demonstrated repeatedly as independent risk factors for failure of 2-stage management.[8,10,12,14,30–33]

SURGERY-RELATED OUTCOME PREDICTORS

The time to reimplantation (TTR), duration of surgery at reimplantation, prior failed surgical interventions, and repeated spacer exchange mid-therapy have been demonstrated to affect outcomes after initial 2-stage management of PJI.

TTR, de ned as time duration from explant and antibiotic spacer placement until the second stage revision, is important. Hartman and colleagues reported an increased failure rate at a mean of 141 days to reimplantation compared to 101 days.[5] Others have reported correlative findings, including increased failure rates at 66 days compared to 61 days, 124 days compared to 96 days, and 112 days to 87.9 days.[6,8,35] Puetzler recently reported a meta-analysis of 11 studies reporting on TTR, finding significant variation in what is regarded as "long" TTR. No study observed benefit for long TTR; however, similar or better infection control was observed in "short" TTR in all studies.[36] Several reasons for this finding have been posed. This may be a demonstration of the potential benefit of a second debridement within a short timeframe prior to reimplantation. It also may be indicative of the dangers of prolonged periods without antibiotic coverage prior to reimplantation, assuming patients are receiving 6 to 8 weeks of oral or IV antibiotics per most widely accepted 2-stage revision practices.

Need for interim spacer exchange has been shown detrimental to 2-stage management success. In a study of 347 TJA PJIs undergoing 2-stage exchange, George and colleagues found that 17% required mid-treatment spacer exchange due to persistent infection. Five-year failure rates were greater for the interim exchange group than the non-exchange group (37% vs 22%).[37] In agreement, Klemt and team in 2021 required spacer exchange in 19% of 256 two-stage TJA PJI patients. With minimum 2-year follow-up, they reported 24% failure in exchange group and 15% failure in non-exchange group.[31] Requiring exchange mid-therapy would suggest particularly virulent pathogen, unidentified organism not covered by antibiotic therapy, or incomplete debridement of persistent infectious agent.

Previous failed PJI management with any technique other than a 2-stage treatment is variably associated with failure of subsequent 2-stage management. Rajgopal and colleagues reported on 184 consecutive knees that underwent 2-stage revision for PJI with an average follow-up of 5.3 years, nding prior debridement and irrigation with implant retention is associated with nearly twice the risk of failure of subsequent 2-stage management when compared to direct 2-stage revision, 23.9% versus 15.6%, respectively.[38] In contrast, Brimmo and colleagues reported on 750 patients who underwent 2-stage management, among which 57 had prior incision and drainage (I&D).[39] The I&D preceding 2-stage group had a significantly lower failure rate than the direct 2-stage revision group, 8.7% versus 17.5%, respectively. Nodzo and colleagues reported equivalent success amongst patients undergoing I&D prior to 2-stage revision compared to direct 2-stage revision, 82.2% versus 82.5%, respectively.[40] While further study is needed, it may be that more timely intervention at diagnosis of PJI, whether direct to 2-stage revision or temporizing debridement and irrigation with implant retention, is preventative against bacterial penetration into soft tissues and bone and the establishment of local immune-modulating effects of pathogens.

Intraoperative time has also been demonstrated to be important at the time of reimplantation. Mortazavi and colleagues in a study including 117 patients who underwent 2-stage management noted increased operative time, 174 minutes compared to 165 minutes, as a risk factor for failure.[14] This is a finding that is supported in the primary total joint literature, with several reports noting increased risk of postoperative complications, including wound complications and PJI, related to longer surgical time.[41–44]

STAGING SYSTEMS AND PREDICTIVE TOOLS FOR 2-STAGE PERIPROSTHETIC JOINT INFECTION MANAGEMENT

These patient and pathogen-related risk factors have been organized in attempts at staging systems and predictive models for success in the management of PJI. While grouping orthopedic-related infections was not novel, McPherson and colleagues were among the first to propose a clinical staging system and apply this to knee and hip PJI.[13,45–49] This system was devised based on the investigators' subjective experience with patients with systemic comorbidities that predispose a patient to infection, making infection more difficult to manage. Their 1999 paper retrospectively applied the staging system to 70 total knee arthroplasty (TKA) PJIs, and subsequently, their 2002 paper retrospectively applied it to 50 total hip arthroplasty (THA) PJIs. After applying their staging system, they found that patients who were healthier at baseline, with fewer local findings of severe infection and better soft tissue status and healing ability, were more likely to have success after the second stage reimplantation.[13,49] Although widely used, the McPherson staging system has not been validated with intra-observer and inter-observer studies.[50] This system addresses 3 parameters of host grading—infection type, host status, and soft tissue quality.[13,49] However, it has been proposed that the system does not account for multiple other parameters that affect outcome prediction, including infecting organism and resistance profiles, bone loss, and multiple additional host comorbidities.[50,51] Despite this, the International Consensus Group on Orthopedic Infections has advocated the use, development, and further research into the system.[50,52]

A tool to predict the probability of failure of 2-stage revision has more recently been proposed. Sabry and colleagues retrospectively reviewed 3809 TKAs, with 314 undergoing 2-stage revision for chronic PJI and 105 (33.4%) treatment failures.[8] Using univariate analyses, factors associated with failure were determined, and a nomogram was developed to preoperatively predict a patient's probability of failure. Independently associated variables included in the 2-stage revision nomogram were assigned a weight and score, correlating with the probability of treatment failure. Organisms were grouped to provide clinical utility for the nomogram, including group 1 (MRSA, VRE, methicillin-resistant S epidermidis [MRSE], or acid-fast bacteria [AFB]), group 2 (MSSA, methicillin-sensitive coagulase-negative Staphylococcus species), group 3 (other gram-positive bacteria or fungus), and group 4 (gram-negative bacteria). Factors included body mass index, time from index surgery to surgical intervention, duration of symptoms prior to surgical intervention, number of previous surgeries, hemoglobin, soft tissue coverage requirements,

previous infection of the same joint, previous 2-stage revision, group 1 through 4 organism, diabetes, immunocompromised state, and heart disease. This tool has yet to be externally validated.

The authors concur with the calls for a validated, comprehensive staging system with the potential to assist surgeons in the decision-making process and accurately counseling patients, understanding rates of success in eradication of infection, or considering alternative treatments to decrease surgical complications and costs. This may be an area where machine-learning or artificial intelligence could be utilized.

TREATMENT OPTIONS FOR RECURRENT PERIPROSTHETIC JOINT INFECTION

Multiple management options exist for medical and surgical management of recurrent PJI, but the ultimate goal persists—infection eradication. Treatments described in the literature include repeat 2-stage revision, arthrodesis, resection arthroplasty or girdlestone, and amputation.

Current management trends after recurrent PJI in the United States demonstrate patients are most commonly offered debridement, antibiotics, and implant retention (DAIR) with variable antibiotic suppressive regimens, repeat 2-stage revision, arthrodesis, or amputation. Hanssen and colleagues in 1995 described the management of recurrent PJIs after 2-stage knee revision. Of 24 patients, 10 patients underwent successful knee arthrodesis, 5 repeat surgical debridement with prolonged suppressive antibiotics, 4 above-knee amputations (AKAs), 3 knees with attempted arthrodesis and persistent pseudoarthrosis, 1 resection arthroplasty, and 1 repeat 2-stage management.[53] McPherson and team reported 34% girdlestone and 8% hip disarticulation after failed 2-stage THA PJI.[13] More recently, a large Medicare database review described rates of alternative management options after index 2-stage management failure, finding only 4.5% knee arthrodesis and 3.1% amputation rates.[26] This agrees with another Medicare database review including patients older than 65 with failed 2-stage revision, which noted a declining trend in the number of both arthrodesis and AKAs, suggesting clinicians are more aggressively attempting to preserve the joint with repeat 2-stage revision.[54] Limited data exist on the rates of girdlestone or hip disarticulation.

DAIR is typically indicated in patients with acute perioperative or hematogenous PJI, or patients who may not be candidates for 2-stage revision due to medical comorbidities or difficult-to-remove components. Eradication success for DAIR varies quite widely in reports, ranging from 18% to 87% success after primary TJA.[55–57] Reports of outcomes after DAIR for recurrent PJI are less common. Vahedi and team reported on DAIR for recurrent PJI in 24 patients with minimum 2-year follow-up, reporting 71% success.[58] Of 7 failed DAIRs, 3 underwent a repeat DAIR with 66% success at 2 years; the remainder underwent a second 2-stage revision. Treatment of DAIR after primary TJA has a failure rate of 57% and 84% in patients infected with S aureus and MRSA, respectively.[18,55,57] Surgeons should be aware of and counsel patients accordingly in regard to outcomes for DAIR, attempt to identify organisms prior to consideration of DAIR, and keep in mind the higher failure rates of 2-stage revisions in the setting of prior attempted DAIR.[38]

Infection eradication success of repeat 2-stage revision is poorer than that of index 2-stage revision, with failure rates reported from 23% to 62% at 5 years.[16,17,59,60] Steinicke and colleagues in a cohort of 55 patients with repeat 2-stage revision TKA or THA after failed index 2-stage management reported 23% failure at 1 year and 62% failure at 5 years.[16] Bejon and team, with a 152-patient cohort, reported 27% failure of the second 2-stage revision at a mean of 5.75 years.[17]

Gathen and colleagues reported 20% failure at a mean 2.5-year follow-up in a group of 45 repeat 2-stage knee PJIs.[60] In a smaller cohort of 18 patients, Azzam and colleagues reported 22% failure after the second 2-stage revision, and 50% failure after a third 2-stage revision attempt.[59] While there is significant variation amongst these reports in postoperative antibiotic therapy, including prolonged IV antibiotics, prolonged oral antibiotics, and lifelong antibiotic suppression, it is clear that subsequent attempts at infection eradication are less successful.

Outcomes of salvage operations are less frequently described. A recent study comparing repeat 2-stage revision to intramedullary arthrodesis reported 89% infection eradication in the arthrodesis group compared to 80% in the 2-stage revision TKA group.[60] Carr and colleagues compared outcomes of arthrodesis and AKA, reporting higher risk of postoperative infection with arthrodesis, likely a result of hardware presence in the knee.[61] Additionally, the risk of nonunion with arthrodesis may contribute to persistent pain with impaired quality of life and greater reoperation rates.[62] Hanssen and team reported nearly 25% pseudoarthrosis rate in 13 attempted arthrodeses after failed knee PJI.[53] However, the risk of death has been reported

28% higher than those who receive arthrodesis or repeat 2-stage revision, although this may be secondary to more significant patient comorbidities in patients undergoing amputation relative to other options.[54] Despite poor functional outcomes of AKA, the relative increase of AKA compared with arthrodesis may be the result of unsatisfactory outcomes of arthrodesis and better patient satisfaction with AKA.[63]

Salvage operations such as arthrodesis or AKA present obvious disadvantages with their association to poor function and activity limitation. Multiple studies report that no more than half of the patients who receive an AKA can walk.[64–66] Sierra and team reported on 25 AKA patients, finding that 9 were fitted with above-the-knee prosthesis, but only 5 were walking to a limited degree.[64] Fedorka reported on 35 patients who underwent AKA, with 14 of these fitted for prostheses and 8 functionally independent outside the home.[66] In contrast, Robinson and team reported on 20 patients with a successful arthrodesis, 16 of which were able to ambulate and perform their daily activities with minimal pain and only 6 which required walker or cane for ambulation.[67] Other studies have demonstrated improved functional outcome measures for arthrodesis when compared to amputation.[60,67,68] Attempted knee arthrodesis is not without complication, with reports of persistent infection, severe limb length discrepancy, and pseudoarthrosis.[53,60,67,68]

Clinical factors have been noted for pushing clinicians toward alternative management options, rather than repeat 2-stage revision. Son and colleagues in the same Medicare database study looking at patients over the age of 65 with TKA PJI reported patients who underwent arthrodesis were more likely to have associated obesity, advanced renal disease, and multiple prior failed revision attempts. Those who underwent amputation had higher Charlson Comorbidity Index score, obesity, existing deep vein thrombosis, and multiple prior failed revision attempts.[54] Patients with significantly high surgical risk are more often considered for salvage options in an effort to limit repeat surgical interventions.

The failure rate of index 2-stage revision with early failures due to the same organism reinfections emphasizes the importance of appropriate timing of the second stage procedure, whether that is reimplantation or implant-utilizing arthrodesis. Threshold values of ESR and CRP have been explored in an effort to establish proper timing of reimplantation; however, multiple studies have questioned the reliability and predictive value of these markers.[17,69,70] Stambough and team found in a large patient cohort that delta change in serum ESR and CRP before and after the 2-stage revision was not associated with reinfection risk, providing no reliable diagnostic accuracy for timing of reimplantation.[69] Antibiotic holiday of different durations is also commonly done in the United States; however, utility of this prior to reimplantation has not been reliably supported with improved preimplantation decision-making or postimplantation success.[17] Other crucial aspects of PJI treatment have been explored but yet to have established consensus, including IV versus oral antibiotics, use of adjuvant medications such as rifampin, duration of antibiotics, utility of drug holiday, intra-articular and intraosseous antibiotic infusions, intra-articular antibiotic beads, and many more.[70] These are outside the scope of this particular article.

MANAGEMENT RECOMMENDATIONS FOR RECURRENT PERIPROSTHETIC JOINT INFECTION

Optimizing Index 2-Stage Revision

With the reported increased failure rates of each subsequent attempt at 2-stage management, every effort should be made at a successful index 2-stage intervention. If available, a multidisciplinary team including the expert consultation with an infectious disease specialist is recommended to assist with appropriate microbial detection methods, antimicrobial management, and patient monitoring. Appropriate microbiological methods used to detect and grow pathogens are crucial, including standard specimen cultures as well as next-generation molecular methods such as rapid PCR diagnostics, 16s sequencing, and/or shotgun/targeted whole genome sequencing. Cultures must be held for at least 14 days, with culture media sensitive to all possible pathogens including gram-negative bacteria, gram-positive bacteria, AFB, and fungus. Surgically, limiting time off antibiotics prior to reimplantation, keeping operative times limited and efficient, and performing thorough debridement are supported.

Management of PJI is most successful at institutions that provide a higher volume of arthroplasty or infection-related revisions, with multidisciplinary teams of subspecialists and evidence-based protocols to guide management.

Surgical Management After Index 2-Stage Revision

While further investigation is necessary to better understand the relationship between infection eradication and functional outcome of the different management options after failed index 2-stage revision, a robust conversation with the patient and informed decision-making are paramount. The authors find that each patient situation is unique to such a degree that a reliable algorithm cannot be constructed.

It is the practice of the authors' institution to aggressively seek joint salvage when reasonable and possible. Patients with failure of index 2-stage revision undergo discussion with surgical team and infectious disease specialists as to their candidacy for prolonged antibiotic therapy and/or lifelong suppression after a second 2-stage attempt. In the event of multiple failed 2-stage revisions, serious discussion of salvage options is performed, with a preference for AKA or girdlestone in older, less healthy, and less functional patients.

The authors routinely work alongside their orthopedic infectious disease colleagues preoperatively to formulate the most effective methods of preoperative- and intraoperative bacterial identification in an effort to guide surgical management and postoperative antimicrobial selection and duration. Preoperative identification of pathogens assists in guiding the choices for surgical management and intraoperative decisions such as the selection of antibiotic or antifungal additives to cement, the aggressiveness of debridement and tissue resection, and implant choices.

In select patients who have been stratified as high risk for recurrent infection, attempts at joint salvage with the use of functional, durable antibiotic spacers and lifelong suppressive antibiotics are performed. In this instance, high-dose antibiotic cement is used to place an all-polyethylene tibia with cobalt chrome femur for knees or all-polyethylene–cemented cup with cemented stem for hips. Investigations are underway as to the outcomes of such technique in high-risk patient population with various antibiotic protocols in place.

Limited utilization of DAIR and double DAIR techniques are employed dependent on unique patient situations in which a favorable microorganism has been identified in acute hematogenous or the early postoperative period, when the morbidity of full implant removal is deemed too high.

NEW DEVELOPMENTS

Over the past decade, focus on advancements pertaining to infection prevention and treatment has become the forefront of research in the authors' field. Despite increased knowledge, diagnostic accuracy, and treatment algorithms, the needle has not signi cantly moved with patient outcomes and eradication rates in chronic PJI.[71] Currently, there are many promising novel developments that may improve the identification of infectious pathogens as well as prevention and treatment. Molecular diagnostics, including PCR diagnostics, 16s sequencing, and shotgun or targeted whole genome sequencing, have been shown to improve organism identification and resistant genes.[72–77] The current gold standard for organism and antimicrobial resistance relies on standard culture data which are inconclusive in over 30% of PJI.[78] Molecular diagnostics such as next-generation sequencing have shown promising early results with detection of an organism in 44% to 82% of CN PJIs.[74,79] Implant coatings, such as polymeric nanofibers or defensive antibacterial coatings, may have the potential to reduce the incidence of PJI.[80,81] Techniques such as rapid 2-stage exchange, intraosseous antibiotic delivery, and novel immunotherapy and bacteriophage therapy could help improve eradication rates and circumvent resistant pathways.[73,82] Although systemic antimicrobial therapy remains the gold standard in the treatment of PJI, bacteriophages have gained interest due to their ability to attack bacterial cells. Currently, there are a few case series showing success in infection eradication with the use of bacteriophages. There are ongoing investigations evaluating their potency as well as safety profile both locally and systemically.[82,83] Another approach currently being explored involves the activity of host immune cells at the site of infection and biofilm. This process involves the recruitment of MDSCs to create an antibacterial milieu at the site of bacterial infections that tend to release toxins locally.[84] These treatment adjuvants remain investigational; however, they show promising early results in difficult-to-treat cases.

SUMMARY

PJI remain one of the most common complications after TJA. It is challenging to manage, associated with signi cant morbidity and mortality, and is a nancial burden on the health care system. Failure of 2-stage management for chronic PJI, the current gold standard, is not uncommon. Repeat infections are oftentimes polymicrobial, multiple drug-resistant microorganisms, or new organisms. Optimizing the success of index 2-stage revision is the greatest prevention against failure of any subsequent management options, and requires a robust team-based approach. Efforts at joint salvage

with repeat 2-stage revision are most common; however, success rates plummet with each subsequent attempt. There are a plethora of other joint salvage or limb salvage procedures that providers may consider for each unique patient presentation. Future success at managing this challenging problem will rely on high-quality research providing guidance for multidisciplinary teams in optimized management and exploring novel pathogen identi cation methods, therapeutic modalities, and surgical protocols.

CLINICS CARE POINTS

- With poorer outcomes of each subsequent attempt at joint salvage after PJI, optimizing the success of index 2-stage revision is crucial.
- A multi-specialty team including hospitalists, infectious disease specialists, and orthopedic surgeons with experience in managing PJI results in the best outcomes for these patients.
- Use of next-generation molecular methods of antimicrobial detection, if available, helps guide appropriate intraoperative and postoperative surgical and medical decisions.
- Further work on the development and implementation of staging systems and predictive models for PJI will assist in the decision-making and counseling of patients.
- Novel medical treatment adjuvants remain investigational, but show early promise in improving outcomes of these difficult cases.

DISCLOSURE

The authors have nothing to disclose.

REFERENCES

1. Berend KR, Lombardi AVJ, Morris MJ, et al. Two-stage treatment of hip periprosthetic joint infection is associated with a high rate of infection control but high mortality. Clin Orthop Relat Res 2013; 471(2):510.
2. Boddapati V, Fu MC, Mayman DJ, et al. Revision total knee arthroplasty for periprosthetic joint infection is associated with increased postoperative morbidity and mortality relative to noninfectious revisions. J Arthroplasty 2018;33(2):521–6.
3. Kurtz SM, Lau E, Schmier J, et al. Infection burden for hip and knee arthroplasty in the United States. J Arthroplasty 2008;23(7):984–91.
4. Bozic KJ, Ries MD. The impact of infection after total hip arthroplasty on hospital and surgeon

resource utilization. J Bone Joint Surg Am 2005; 87(8):1746–51.

5. Hartman CW, Daubach EC, Richard BT, et al. Predictors of reinfection in prosthetic joint infections following two-stage reimplantation. J Arthroplasty 2022;37(7S):S674–7.

6. Kubista B, Hartzler RU, Wood CM, et al. Reinfection after two-stage revision for periprosthetic infection of total knee arthroplasty. Int Orthop 2012;36(1): 65–71.

7. Petis SM, Perry KI, Mabry TM, et al. Two-stage exchange protocol for periprosthetic joint infection following total knee arthroplasty in 245 knees without prior treatment for infection. JBJS 2019;101(3):239.

8. Sabry FY, Buller L, Ahmed S, et al. Preoperative prediction of failure following two-stage revision for knee prosthetic joint infections. J Arthroplasty 2014;29(1):115–21.

9. Garvin KL, Miller RE, Gilbert TM, et al. Late reinfection may recur more than 5 years after reimplantation of tha and tka: analysis of pathogen factors. Clin Orthop Relat Res 2018;476(2):345.

10. Kurd MF, Ghanem E, Steinbrecher J, et al. Two-stage exchange knee arthroplasty: does resistance of the infecting organism influence the outcome? Clin Orthop Relat Res 2010;468(8):2060.

11. Haleem AA, Berry DJ, Hanssen AD. Mid-term to long-term followup of two-stage reimplantation for infected total knee arthroplasty. Clin Orthop Relat Res 2004;428:35–9.

12. Ma CY, Lu YD, Bell KL, et al. Predictors of treatment failure after 2-stage reimplantation for infected total knee arthroplasty: a 2- to 10-year Follow-Up. J Arthroplasty 2018;33(7):2234–9.

13. McPherson EJ, Woodson C, Holtom P, et al. Periprosthetic total hip infection: outcomes using a staging system. Clin Orthop Relat Res 2002;403:8.

14. Mortazavi SMJ, Vegari D, Ho A, et al. Two-stage exchange arthroplasty for infected total knee arthroplasty: predictors of failure. Clin Orthop Relat Res 2011;469(11):3049–54.

15. Stambough JB, Curtin BM, Odum SM, et al. Does change in ESR and CRP guide the timing of two-stage arthroplasty reimplantation? Clin Orthop Relat Res 2019;477(2):364–71.

16. Steinicke AC, Schwarze J, Gosheger G, et al. Repeat two-stage exchange arthroplasty for recurrent periprosthetic hip or knee infection: what are the chances for success? Arch Orthop Trauma Surg 2023;143(4):1731–40.

17. Bejon P, Berendt A, Atkins BL, et al. Two-stage revision for prosthetic joint infection: predictors of outcome and the role of reimplantation microbiology. J Antimicrob Chemother 2010;65(3):569–75.

18. Zmistowski B, Fedorka CJ, Sheehan E, et al. Prosthetic joint infection caused by gram-negative organisms. J Arthroplasty 2011;26(6 Suppl):104–8.

19. Egbulefu FJ, Yang J, Segreti JC, et al. Recurrent failures after 2-stage exchanges are secondary to new organisms not previously covered by antibiotics. Arthroplasty Today 2022;17:186–91.e1.

20. Heim CE, Vidlak D, Odvody J, et al. Human prosthetic joint infections are associated with myeloid-derived suppressor cells (MDSCs): implications for infection persistence. J Orthop Res 2018;36(6): 1605–13.

21. Parvizi J, Tan TL, Goswami K, et al. The 2018 definition of periprosthetic hip and knee infection: an evidence-based and validated criteria. J Arthroplasty 2018; 33(5):1309–14.e2.

22. Zhang H, Xie S, Li Y, et al. The potential performance of serum albumin to globulin ratio, albumin and globulin in the diagnosis of periprosthetic joint infection and prediction of reinfection following reimplantation. BMC Muscoskel Disord 2022;23(1): 730.

23. Watts CD, Wagner ER, Houdek MT, et al. Morbid obesity: a significant risk factor for failure of two-stage revision total knee arthroplasty for infection. J Bone Joint Surg Am 2014;96(18):e154.

24. Pulido L, Ghanem E, Joshi A, et al. Periprosthetic joint infection: the incidence, timing, and predisposing factors. Clin Orthop Relat Res 2008;466(7):1710.

25. Houdek MT, Wagner ER, Watts CD, et al. Morbid obesity: a significant risk factor for failure of two-stage revision total hip arthroplasty for infection. J Bone Joint Surg Am 2015;97(4):326–32.

26. Cancienne JM, Granadillo VA, Patel KJ, et al. Risk factors for repeat debridement, spacer retention, amputation, arthrodesis, and mortality after removal of an infected total knee arthroplasty with spacer placement. J Arthroplasty 2018;33(2):515–20.

27. Patel R. Biofilms and antimicrobial resistance. Clin Orthop Relat Res 2005;437:41–7.

28. Schilcher K, Horswill AR. Staphylococcal biofilm development: structure, regulation, and treatment strategies. Microbiol Mol Biol Rev 2020;84(3). 000266-e119.

29. Stewart PS, Costerton JW. Antibiotic resistance of bacteria in biofilms. Lancet 2001;358(9276):135–8.

30. Kilgus DJ, Howe DJ, Strang A. Results of periprosthetic hip and knee infections caused by resistant bacteria. Clin Orthop Relat Res 2002;404:116–24.

31. Klemt C, Smith EJ, Tirumala V, et al. Outcomes and risk factors associated with 2-stage reimplantation requiring an interim spacer exchange for periprosthetic joint infection. J Arthroplasty 2021;36(3): 1094–100.

32. Maheshwari AV, Gioe TJ, Kalore NV, et al. Reinfection after prior staged reimplantation for septic total knee arthroplasty: is salvage still possible? J Arthroplasty 2010;25(6 Suppl):92–7.

33. Rosteius T, Jansen O, Fehmer T, et al. Evaluating the microbial pattern of periprosthetic joint infections of

the hip and knee. J Med Microbiol 2018;67(11): 1608–13.

34. Aggarwal VK, Bakhshi H, Ecker NU, et al. Organism profile in periprosthetic joint infection: pathogens differ at two arthroplasty infection referral centers in Europe and in the United States. J Knee Surg 2014;27(5):399–406.

35. Tan TL, Kheir MM, Rondon AJ, et al. Determining the role and duration of the "antibiotic holiday" period in periprosthetic joint infection. J Arthroplasty 2018;33(9):2976–80.

36. Puetzler J, Schulze M, Gosheger G, et al. Is long time to reimplantation a risk factor for reinfection in two-stage revision for periprosthetic infection? A systematic review of the literature. Front Surg 2023;10:1113006.

37. George J, Miller EM, Curtis GL, et al. Success of two-stage reimplantation in patients requiring an interim spacer exchange. J Arthroplasty 2018; 33(7S):S228–32.

38. Rajgopal A, Panjwani TR, Rao A, et al. Are the outcomes of revision knee arthroplasty for flexion instability the same as for other major failure mechanisms? J Arthroplasty 2017;32(10):3093–7.

39. Brimmo O, Ramanathan D, Schiltz NK, et al. Irrigation and debridement before a 2-stage revision total knee arthroplasty does not increase risk of failure. J Arthroplasty 2016;31(2):461–4.

40. Nodzo SR, Boyle KK, Nocon AA, et al. The influence of a failed irrigation and debridement on the outcomes of a subsequent 2-stage revision knee arthroplasty. J Arthroplasty 2017;32(8):2508–12.

41. Orland MD, Lee RY, Naami EE, et al. Surgical duration implicated in major postoperative complications in total hip and total knee arthroplasty: a retrospective cohort study. J Am Acad Orthop Surg Glob Res Rev 2020;4(11). e20.00043.

42. Wang Q, Goswami K, Shohat N, et al. Longer Operative Time Results in a Higher Rate of Subsequent Periprosthetic Joint Infection in Patients Undergoing Primary Joint Arthroplasty. J Arthroplasty 2019;34(5):947–53.

43. Ravi B, Croxford R, Reichmann WM, et al. The changing demographics of total joint arthroplasty recipients in the United States and Ontario from 2001 to 2007. Best Pract Res Clin Rheumatol 2012; 26(5):637–47.

44. Scigliano NM, Carender CN, Glass NA, et al. Operative time and risk of surgical site infection and periprosthetic joint infection: a systematic review and meta-analysis. Iowa Orthop J 2022;42(1):155–61.

45. Cierny G, Mader JT, Penninck JJ. A clinical staging system for adult osteomyelitis. Clin Orthop Relat Res 2003;414:7–24.

46. Hotchen AJ, McNally MA, Sendi P. The classification of long bone osteomyelitis: a systemic review of the literature. J Bone Jt Infect 2017;2(4):167–74.

47. Marais LC, Ferreira N, Aldous C, et al. A modified staging system for chronic osteomyelitis. J Orthop 2015;12(4):184–92.

48. Waldvogel FA, Medoff G, Swartz MN. Osteomyelitis: a review of clinical features, therapeutic considerations and unusual aspects. N Engl J Med 1970;282(4):198–206.

49. McPherson EJ, Tontz W, Patzakis M, et al. Outcome of infected total knee utilizing a staging system for prosthetic joint infection. Am J Orthop (Belle Mead NJ) 1999;28(3):161–5.

50. Coughlan A, Taylor F. Classifications in brief: The McPherson classification of periprosthetic infection. Clin Orthop Relat Res 2020;478(4):903–8.

51. Romanò CL, Romanò D, Logoluso N, et al. Bone and joint infections in adults: a comprehensive classification proposal. Eur Orthop Traumatol 2011; 1(6):207–17.

52. Amanatullah D, Dennis D, Oltra EG, et al. Hip and knee section, diagnosis, definitions: proceedings of international consensus on orthopedic infections. J Arthroplasty 2019;34(2):S329–37.

53. Hanssen AD, Trousdale RT, Osmon DR. Patient outcome with reinfection following reimplantation for the infected total knee arthroplasty. Clin Orthop Relat Res 1995;321:55–67.

54. Son MS, Lau E, Parvizi J, et al. What are the frequency, associated factors, and mortality of amputation and arthrodesis after a failed infected TKA? Clin Orthop Relat Res 2017;475(12):2905–13.

55. Bradbury T, Fehring TK, Taunton M, et al. The fate of acute methicillin-resistant Staphylococcus aureus periprosthetic knee infections treated by open debridement and retention of components. J Arthroplasty 2009;24(6 Suppl):101–4.

56. Marculescu CE, Berbari EF, Hanssen AD, et al. Outcome of prosthetic joint infections treated with debridement and retention of components. Clin Infect Dis 2006;42(4):471–8.

57. Deirmengian C, Greenbaum J, Lotke PA, et al. Limited success with open debridement and retention of components in the treatment of acute Staphylococcus aureus infections after total knee arthroplasty. J Arthroplasty 2003;18(7 Suppl 1):22–6.

58. Vahedi H, Aali-Rezaie A, Shahi A, et al. Irrigation, débridement, and implant retention for recurrence of periprosthetic joint infection following two-stage revision total knee arthroplasty: a matched cohort study. J Arthroplasty 2019;34(8):1772–5.

59. Azzam K, Parvizi J, Kaufman D, et al. Revision of the unstable total knee arthroplasty: outcome predictors. J Arthroplasty 2011;26(8):1139–44.

60. Gathen M, Wimmer MD, Ploeger MM, et al. Comparison of two-stage revision arthroplasty and intramedullary arthrodesis in patients with failed infected knee arthroplasty. Arch Orthop Trauma Surg 2018;138(10):1443–52.

61. Carr JB, Werner BC, Browne JA. Trends and outcomes in the treatment of failed septic total knee arthroplasty: comparing arthrodesis and above-knee amputation. J Arthroplasty 2016;31(7):1574–7.

62. Morrey BF, Westholm F, Schoifet S, et al. Long-term results of various treatment options for infected total knee arthroplasty. Clin Orthop Relat Res 1989;248:120–8.

63. Khanna V, Tushinski DM, Soever LJ, et al. Above knee amputation following total knee arthroplasty: when enough is enough. J Arthroplasty 2015;30(4):658–62.

64. Sierra RJ, Trousdale RT, Pagnano MW. Above-the-knee amputation after a total knee replacement: prevalence, etiology, and functional outcome. J Bone Joint Surg Am 2003;85(6):1000–4.

65. Isiklar ZU, Landon GC, Tullos HS. Amputation after failed total knee arthroplasty. Clin Orthop Relat Res 1994;299:173–8.

66. Fedorka CJ, Chen AF, McGarry WM, et al. Functional ability after above-the-knee amputation for infected total knee arthroplasty. Clin Orthop Relat Res 2011;469(4):1024–32.

67. Robinson M, Piponov HI, Ormseth A, et al. Knee arthrodesis outcomes after infected total knee arthroplasty and failure of two-stage revision with an antibiotic cement spacer. J Am Acad Orthop Surg Glob Res Rev 2018;2(1):e077.

68. Bargiotas K, Wohlrab D, Sewecke JJ, et al. Arthrodesis of the knee with a long intramedullary nail following the failure of a total knee arthroplasty as the result of infection. J Bone Joint Surg Am 2006;88(3):553–8.

69. Stambough JB, Majors IB, Oholendt CK, et al. Improvements in isokinetic quadriceps and hamstring strength testing after focused therapy in patients with flexion instability. J Arthroplasty 2020;35(8):2237–43.

70. Restrepo C, Schmitt S, Backstein D, et al. Antibiotic treatment and timing of reimplantation. J Orthop Res 2014;32(Suppl 1):S136–40.

71. Goswami K, Stevenson KL, Parvizi J. Intraoperative and postoperative infection prevention. J Arthroplasty 2020;35(3S):S2–8.

72. Indelli PF, Ghirardelli S, Violante B, et al. Next generation sequencing for pathogen detection in periprosthetic joint infections. EFORT Open Rev 2021;6(4):236–44.

73. Kildow BJ, Ryan SP, Danilkowicz R, et al. Next-generation sequencing not superior to culture in periprosthetic joint infection diagnosis. Bone Joint Lett J 2021;103-B(1):26–31.

74. Tarabichi M, Shohat N, Goswami K, et al. Can next generation sequencing play a role in detecting pathogens in synovial fluid? Bone Joint Lett J 2018;100-B(2):127–33.

75. Street TL, Sanderson ND, Atkins BL, et al. Molecular diagnosis of orthopedic-device-related infection directly from sonication fluid by metagenomic sequencing. J Clin Microbiol 2017;55(8):2334–47.

76. Echeverria AP, Cohn IS, Danko DC, et al. Sequencing of circulating microbial cell-free DNA can identify pathogens in periprosthetic joint infections. J Bone Joint Surg Am 2021;103(18):1705–12.

77. Garvin KL, Kildow BJ, Hewlett A, et al. The challenge of emerging resistant gram-positive pathogens in hip and knee periprosthetic joint infections. JBJS 2023. https://doi.org/10.2106/JBJS.22.00792.

78. Parvizi J, Erkocak OF, Della Valle CJ. Culture-negative periprosthetic joint infection. J Bone Joint Surg Am 2014;96(5):430–6.

79. Thoendel MJ, Jeraldo PR, Greenwood-Quaintance KE, et al. Identification of prosthetic joint infection pathogens using a shotgun metagenomics approach. Clin Infect Dis 2018;67(9):1333–8.

80. Esteves GM, Esteves J, Resende M, et al. Antimicrobial and antibiofilm coating of dental implants—past and new perspectives. Antibiotics (Basel) 2022;11(2):235.

81. Davidson DJ, Spratt D, Liddle AD. Implant materials and prosthetic joint infection: the battle with the biofilm. EFORT Open Rev 2019;4(11):633–9.

82. Ferry T, Kolenda C, Batailler C, et al. Phage Therapy as adjuvant to conservative surgery and antibiotics to salvage patients with relapsing s. aureus prosthetic knee infection. Front Med 2020;7:570572.

83. Tkhilaishvili T, Winkler T, Müller M, et al. Bacteriophages as adjuvant to antibiotics for the treatment of periprosthetic joint infection caused by multidrug-resistant pseudomonas aeruginosa. Antimicrob Agents Chemother 2019;64(1). e00924-19.

84. Gries CM, Kielian T. Staphylococcal biofilms and immune polarization during prosthetic joint infection. JAAOS 2017;25:S20.

85. Cancienne JM, Werner BC, Bolarinwa SA, Browne JA. Removal of an Infected Total Hip Arthroplasty: Risk Factors for Repeat Debridement, Long-term Spacer Retention, and Mortality. J Arthroplasty 2017;32(8):2519–22.

Trauma

The State of Local Antibiotic Use in Orthopedic Trauma

Carlo Eikani, BS[a,b,*], Aaron Hoyt, MD[b], Elizabeth Cho, MD[b],
Ashley E. Levack, MD, MAS[a,b]

KEYWORDS

- Local antibiotics • Fracture-related infection • Osteomyelitis • Orthopedic trauma
- Antibiotic-coated implants

KEY POINTS

- Antibiotic powder is time efficient and can be applied directly at the time of wound closure but lacks the ability of sustained release.
- Polymethylmethacrylate has the versatility to be used in different forms (bead, spacer, or implant) but is limited by early burst kinetics and need for removal.
- Biodegradable products such as calcium phosphate and calcium sulfate can deliver antibiotics over a longer period of time without the need for removal but have been associated with wound complications.
- Antibiotic-coated implants can act as a prophylactic option but are not approved in the United States.
- Novel carriers, such as hydrogels and nanoparticles, have shown promising preclinical results but have not been investigated enough to be used in a clinical setting.

INTRODUCTION

Fracture-related infection (FRI) is a challenging complication in orthopedic trauma that often necessitates multiple surgeries and can result in delayed bone healing, reduced function, and significant declines in patient quality of life.[1,2] Although the overall rate of FRI is reported to be around 1.8%, rates of infection are notably increased open fractures.[3,4] Despite modern prophylactic strategies, FRI rates after Gustilo Anderson type III fractures remain as high as 20% to 30%.[5–8] FRI also places significant burden on the health care system, generating financial costs to the patient that are 6.5 times higher than for noninfected cases.[9]

Early administration of systemic antibiotics and surgical intervention remain the gold standard for FRI care.[10] However, despite this, treatment failures can occur in 29% to 35% of cases,

with recurrence of infection described to be around 9%.[11–13] For these reasons, advances in prophylactic and treatment options are critical to improve outcomes. The introduction of antibiotics locally at the site of at-risk fractures has increased over the past decade and is the subject of numerous studies aimed at reducing the burden of infection. A 2018 meta-analysis revealed that the use of local antibiotics among all open fractures, in addition to standard systemic prophylaxis, reduced infection risk from 16.5% to 4.6%.[14] Nonetheless, indications, optimal carriers, and antibiotic dosing for local delivery of antibiotics remain a topic of investigation. To further complicate the decision-making, numerous carriers with widely varying properties can be used to deliver antibiotics locally, compounding the variation in clinical practice and research. The purpose of this review article is to outline the existing local

---

[a] Loyola University Stritch School of Medicine; [b] Department of Orthopaedic Surgery & Rehabilitation, Loyola University Medical Center, 2160 South 1st Avenue, Maguire Suite 1700, Maywood, IL, USA
* Corresponding author.
E-mail address: ceikani@luc.edu

antibiotic options used in the prevention and treatment of FRI and discuss the key considerations for each.

DISCUSSION

Antibiotic Powder

Lyophilized antibiotic powder can be applied directly into the wound bed, typically at the time of wound closure. Vancomycin powder first became popularized in orthopedics approximately 10 years ago when literature emerged demonstrating efficacy in reducing postoperative infections after spinal fusion.[15–17] However, in the orthopedic trauma setting, topical administration of antibiotic powder has more recently become a topic of interest and ongoing area of research.

Some clinical studies on the use of local antibiotics have demonstrated conflicting results in differing anatomic locations. Owen and colleagues evaluated 140 patients undergoing surgery of the pelvis and acetabulum, approximately half of whom received vancomycin and tobramycin topically at closure, finding no significant improvement in the rate of FRI with the use of antibiotic powder treatment after adjusting for estimated blood loss. They conclude that the protective effect of topical antibiotics may be limited to patients with minimal to low intraoperative blood loss of less than 1 L[18] In contrast, in a more recent retrospective study of 789 acetabular fractures, Cichos and colleagues found no improvement in infection rates with the use of topical vancomycin or a combination of vancomycin and tobramycin to a control group without topical antibiotic administration.[19]

The VANCO study, a multicenter randomized controlled trial across 36 institutions sponsored by the Major Extremity Trauma Research Consortium, was the first large-scale study to demonstrate the clinical benefit of using vancomycin antibiotic powder as a prophylactic agent against FRI.[20] This study specifically evaluated the efficacy of vancomycin powder in tibial plateau and pilon fractures that were deemed high risk for infection. They found that the administration of vancomycin powder in these wounds decreased the risk of deep infection by 3.7%, for a relative risk reduction of 35% driven by a decrease in gram-positive infections.[20] This study prompted the ongoing TOBRA study, which will compare the use of vancomycin powder versus a combination of vancomycin and tobramycin in high-risk tibial plateau and pilon fractures (ClinicalTrials. gov NCT 04597008).

The main advantages of using local antibiotics in the loose powder form (ie, without a carrier) are the ease of use and ability to apply the antimicrobial at high concentrations directly at wound closure. The resulting local concentrations are higher than would be attainable via systemic delivery due to drug toxicities that would be seen at these systemic levels. Although there were early concerns about the possible nephrotoxicity of topical application of aminoglycosides such as gentamycin and tobramycin and glycopeptides such as vancomycin, studies have demonstrated that antibiotic powder is safe to use and avoids the adverse effects associated with systemic administration.[18,21] Other advantages specific to topical vancomycin include widespread availability, low cost, efficacy against the most common pathogens involved in surgical site infection, and relatively low concern for osteogenic cytotoxicity that could hinder bone healing.[22,23] The main disadvantage of antibiotic powder is the lack of controlled delivery into target tissues as it can only applied as a single-burst dose.[24]

Overall, local antibiotic powder remains a low-risk and low-cost intervention for use in the prophylactic setting. However, there is limited evidence supporting its routine use beyond high-risk wounds in tibial plateau and pilon fractures as demonstrated by the VANCO study. The widespread use of antibiotic powders carries theoretic concern about promoting antimicrobial resistance, although there are no current data available to support this. The short-lived and high local concentrations of antibiotic may provide insufficient exposure to promote mutation and resistance. Last, although commonly used clinically, the efficacy of using antibiotic powder in treating infection remains unknown with little clinical evidence.

Polymethylmethacrylate

Polymethylmethacrylate (PMMA) has been used for decades as an antibiotic carrier in several forms including antibiotic laden beads, spacers, and coatings around implanted devices.[25] In some formulations, low doses of antibiotics are premixed into the PMMA, typically for prophylactic use in arthroplasty settings. However, higher doses of antibiotics can be added to the PMMA by mixing the antibiotic with the powdered polymer before adding the monomer. Although it is known that higher doses of antibiotics in PMMA degrade the mechanical properties, of the cement, antibiotic laden PMMA in the setting of orthopedic trauma is not intended to be a structural material.[26–29] Therefore, high doses, typically 5% to 10% of antibiotic by dry weight (ie, 2–4 g of antibiotic per 40 g of PMMA) are often used.

For nearly 30 years, antibiotic-loaded PMMA beads have been used in conjunction with surgical debridement to prevent soft tissue and bone infections and manage prosthetic joint infections and osteomyelitis.[30–34] The most commonly used antibiotics in PMMA are gentamicin, tobramycin, and vancomycin.[35] These antibiotics are available in powdered forms, are water soluble, and importantly are chemically stable and thus able to withstand the high temperatures during the exothermic reaction of PMMA polymerization.

Antibiotic beads can be implanted and wound closed over top if possible. However, if the wound is not amenable to primary closure, a "bead pouch" technique is an alternative option for short durations of time between repeated surgical debridements and before definitive coverage. In this technique, antibiotic-loaded beads are placed in the bony or soft tissue defect and the extremity is covered by an occlusive dressing such as Ioban (3M St Louis, MO).[35,36] This technique has been found to be effective in reducing infection in a few small retrospective studies. Warner and colleagues found that a bead pouch resulted in fewer late methicillin-resistant *Staphylococcus aureus* infections for extremity blast injuries but more unanticipated returns to the operating room for wound complications.[37] Recently, Patterson and colleagues found that the antibiotic bead pouch for initial coverage of type IIIB open tibial shaft fractures requiring flap coverage was associated with a lower risk of FRI.[38] A large-scale multicenter prospective clinical trial investigating the use of bead pouch versus wound vacuum therapy for type III open fractures is underway (ClinicalTrials.gov NCT05615844).

PMMA with or without antibiotics can be used to fill bone voids to manage dead space in the setting of bony defects. Often, this is a necessary step to achieve healing via the two-stage Masquelet technique.[39] In the setting of long bone infections, antibiotic-laden PMMA can also been used to coat intramedullary implants.[40] There are several techniques to accomplish this and a variety of implants can be used, including a long ball-tipped guidewire, threaded Ilizarov rod, or locked intramedullary nail. Thonse and colleagues treated 11 infected nonunion patients definitively with intramedullary nails coated with tobramycin and gentamycin PMMA cement.[31] They achieved infection control in 95% of patients with a union rate of 100%.[31] Similar studies have also found high infection control in patients treated definitively with intramedullary nails.[41,42] The drawbacks of

this technique are the technical challenges of adequately coating the nail and the concern for cement debonding from the implant during subsequent planned or unplanned nail removal. Cement debonding causes retained PMMA within the intramedullary canal which can be challenging to remove and can even become colonized with bacteria leading to persistence of infection.

Antibiotics are eluted from antibiotic-loaded cement with a predictable burst phenomenon that peaks in 24 to 48 hours post-implantation, followed by rapid decline in concentration.[43,44] Increased porosity can increase the rate of release and different cement manufacturers can also produce different elution profiles.[45] Shinsako and colleagues demonstrated that increased surface area-to-volume ratios in vancomycin-mixed PMMA beads yielded larger initial bursts of antibiotic release and increased percent of total antibiotic released.[44,46] Therefore, for the same volume of cement, a large number of small beads would have increased total concentration of antibiotic delivery compared with a single large spacer. The combinations of antibiotics can also affect release kinetics. Hsieh and colleagues investigated the release of both gentamicin and vancomycin, finding a synergistic relationship that increased vancomycin release by 145% and gentamicin by 45%.[47–49] Despite such synergistic effects, the total release of antibiotic from a PMMA carrier is at best limited to a small percentage of the total antibiotic included in the PMMA.[44] However, due to rapid declines in eluted concentrations, the use of antibiotic-laden PMMA for durations longer than 72 hours leads to the release of antibiotic at subtherapeutic levels. Exposure to subtherapeutic levels of antibiotics can theoretically promote bacterial resistance and provide an environment in which bacteria can colonize the PMMA.[45,50] Nuet and colleagues studied colonization of gentamicin-laden beads retrieved from 20 patients with periprosthetic joint infections. Ninety percent of patients with gentamicin beads had colonization with bacteria and 67% of bacterial strains that were isolated from these beads were gentamicin resistant.[51]

Despite its long-standing history of use and varying clinical applications, PMMA as a carrier for antibiotic release has significant limitations. The main pitfall of antibiotic-loaded PMMA is the fact that it is permanent until surgically removed. With the exception of PMMA-coated statically locked intramedullary nails or coated plate constructs and rare instances of fracture healing around PMMA spacers, most of the implanted antibiotic-laden PMMA is intended for a second stage removal procedure. This results in associated cost and risk of additional surgery. In addition to the above discussed inherent limitations of elution kinetics and concern of promoting antibiotic resistance as a result of subtherapeutic elution, there are also situations in which the infectious organism is already resistant to the antibiotics typically used in PMMA. Some patients may also have allergies to the antibiotics typically used. As a result, alternative antibiotic selections are necessary, but the choices are limited to those that can withstand the high polymerization temperatures. Overall, PMMA has played an important role in the management of orthopedic infection for decades; however, it is by no means an optimal antibiotic carrier.

Calcium Sulfate

Given the limitations of PMMA, commercially available biodegradable bone graft substitutes, such as calcium sulfate, have gained attention as an alternate method of local antibiotic delivery.[52] Calcium sulfate has become a desirable alternative because it is osteoconductive, lacks immunologic side effects, and promotes bone regeneration even during its degradation over a period of 4 to 12 weeks.[53]

Calcium sulfate is made in the operating room by mixing the calcium sulfate powder with an antibiotic power followed by sterile water. Alternatively, aqueous formulations of antibiotics can be mixed in, foregoing the addition of sterile water. Commercially available molds exist for preparing calcium sulfate beads of various sizes including STIMULAN (Biocomposites, Wilmington, NC) and OSTEOSET (Wright Medical Technology, Arlington, TN). Calcium sulfate has demonstrated improved elution kinetics compared with PMMA beads of similar size.[44,54,55] Importantly, the polymerization process of calcium sulfate occurs at room temperature, broadening the potential options for antibiotic usage in certain infections in which the typical antibiotics are not ideal.[54]

Several laboratory studies have demonstrated the efficacy of antibiotic-loaded calcium sulfate beads in preventing and treating implant associated infection. McConoughey and colleagues analyzed bacterial inhibition when PMMA and calcium sulfate beads were placed in agar and found equivalent results with both.[55–57] Despite success in preclinical studies, clinical studies to date are few. One randomized clinical trial of 30 patients with long bone osteomyelitis or infected nonunion comparing tobramycin-impregnated calcium sulfate versus PMMA beads found similar rates of infection eradication and union but higher rates of reoperation in the PMMA group.[58] The investigators concluded that the use of calcium sulfate may help eliminate the morbidity associated with additional surgery required with PMMA use.[58]

Calcium sulfate can also be inserted within the intramedullary canal. Rivera and colleagues presented a combined technique to prevent infection in long bone fractures by using an absorbable calcium sulfate depot and a concomitant intramedullary nail finding no exacerbation or recurrence of intramedullary infection in their 11 patient series.[59] Another retrospective study compared limb salvage procedures for infection cure or infection prophylaxis with a PMMA-intramedullary nail or calcium sulfate-intramedullary nail. When used for infection prophylaxis there was 100% prevention of infection rate and when used for infection cure there was 77.8% eradication.[41] Finally, a systematic review and meta-analysis found significant rates of infection eradication when comparing calcium sulfate to alternative methods of treatment for chronic osteomyelitis.[60]

Calcium sulfate has several disadvantages including inconsistent resorption rate and potential cytotoxicity.[53] In addition, curing times vary significantly with differing calcium sulfate antibiotic combinations, with some combinations taking up to 20 minutes to fully set. Calcium sulfate is not capable of load bearing.[52] However, similar to antibiotic-laden PMMA, its use in orthopedic trauma is not intended for structural support. Finally, the use of calcium sulfate can lead to wound drainage and excess fluid accumulation in the wound bed, leading to wound complications.[61] This fluid can often resemble purulence which may make it challenging to distinguish it from a recurrent infection and makes some clinicians hesitant to use it. Despite these limitations and lack of clinical evidence demonstrating efficacy, calcium sulfate remains an option that has some advantages over PMMA for treatment of FRI.

Calcium Phosphate

Calcium phosphate cement (CPC) is an absorbable biomaterial whose structural similarity to bone allows its use in the management of bone defects.[62] CPC shares advantages of calcium sulfate in that it polymerizes at room temperature, is resorbable, and is osteoconductive. Calcium phosphate has a slow resorption rate on the scale of months to years (6 months to several years depending on composition).[63] Similar to PMMA and calcium sulfate, the elution of antibiotics from CPCs also demonstrates burst kinetics.[64–67] However, the elution characteristics from CPCs have not been as extensively studied as in PMMA.

One such commercially available bio-composite product is CERAMENT (Bonesupport, Lund, Sweden), a liquid injectable product containing calcium sulfate crystals and hydroxyapatite (calcium phosphate) particles. In this mixture, calcium sulfate acts as a resorbable carrier for hydroxyapatite. The hydroxyapatite acts as a scaffold for bony ingrowth that also provides long-term structural support to newly formed bone. Further formulations for use in infection are loaded either with gentamycin (CERAMENT G) which is FDA-approved in the United States or vancomycin (CERAMENT V) which is not approved for use in the United States. In their series of 100 patients with chronic osteomyelitis treated with single-stage debridement, dead space management with Cerament G, and culture-specific systemic antibiotics, McNally and colleagues reported a 96% infection eradication rate in chronic osteomyelitis patients at a mean of 6 years' follow-up.[68] Similarly, Drampalos and colleagues achieved a 92.3% eradication rate in their series of 52 patients with implant-related chronic osteomyelitis.[69] Other studies using other off-label formulations of antibiotic-loaded CPC have also shown success in single-stage treatment of osteomyelitis.[64,70]

The disadvantages of calcium phosphate are similar to calcium sulfate, with wound complications and prolonged wound leakage being the most commonly cited. Wound problems including persistent leakage have been reported in 6% of McNally's study and 8% of patients in Dramapalos's study, all resolving without intervention.[69,71] In contrast, a smaller case series of 20 patients treated with Cerament G or V had a 40% revision surgery rate for wound problems related to prolonged secretion or leakage.[72] Overall, CPCs remain an option for treatment of septic nonunion and osteomyelitis associated with bone defects given its slow biodegradation profile, osteoinductive abilities, and structural integrity.

Antibiotic-Coated Implants

Manufactured antibiotic-coated implants are an emerging strategy to prevent and treat FRIs. Although implants may be coated with compounds that have antibacterial properties, such as silver coatings, for the purposes of this review on antibiotic carriers, focus will be placed on implants coated with antibiotics. As opposed to the off-label coating of definitive implants with antibiotic-loaded PMMA or other resorbable materials discussed previously, implants pre-coated with antibiotics save time associated with intraoperative coating of implants and further avoids variability in the dosing and mixing of antibiotics.

The only commercially available antibiotic-coated implant is the EXPERT Tibial Nail PROtect (DePuy Synthes, Raynham, MA), which is not currently approved for use in the United States. This device has been used in Europe since 2005 with multiple studies supporting its use. The coating that is applied to this device is a thin layer of poly(D,L-lactic acid) (PDLLA) containing gentamicin that releases antibiotic in a burst fashion followed by a slower release over a period of 2 weeks, intended to prevent biofilm formation on the implant. This gentamicin-coated tibial nail has been shown to be safe with minimal systemic exposure to the antibiotic.[73] However, there are theoretic concerns that the PDLLA layer used to carry the gentamicin may produce an acidic environment as it degrades which may lead to tissue inflammation and damage as well as have deleterious effects on fracture healing. A systematic review conducted by De Meo and colleagues demonstrated that a gentamicin-coated tibia nail was an effective method at reducing the rate of FRI in 114 open fractures and 89 nonunion revision cases. However, there was insufficient evidence to determine the effectiveness of preventing FRI in closed injuries.[74] Although promising results have been published, it is important to consider the small number of patients, the retrospective nature of all eight studies included and low levels of evidence in the studies included in this analysis.

Alternative antibiotic-coated implants are being developed and tested in animal models. One study investigating the effect of a tobramycin-periapatite coating on titanium implants in a rabbit model demonstrated not only effective prophylaxis against infection but also had the benefit of improved osseointegration.[75] In addition, another study found the use of a vancomycin-loaded phosphatidylcholine coating on titanium and stainless coupons in vitro resulted in significantly lower biofilm formation for both *S aureus* and *Pseudomonas aeruginosa*.[76] Another study used a polymer coating with either vancomycin or tigecycline in an animal model of open fractures where *S aureus* was directly inoculated into the fracture site finding significantly decreased bacterial burden with local drug concentrations above the minimal inhibitory concentration for over 7 days.[77]

Finally, Ghimire and colleagues conducted a study using a vancomycin coating on an intramedullary implant that is triggered for release when exposed to a micrococcal-nuclease present in *S aureus*, eradicating the bacteria from the implant surface in vitro and preventing invasion into the surrounding bone in vivo after inoculation into femoral canals of mice.[78] Although there are several promising technologies being developed for coating implants with antibiotics, including novel technologies allowing for a triggered release, further studies are necessary to evaluate their safety for use in humans and eventual clinical efficacy.

Novel Carriers

Several novel carriers are currently under investigation as potential alternatives to current methods of local antibiotic delivery, including hydrogels, collagens, and nanoparticles. Although many of these carriers have shown promise in early studies as effective antibiotic carriers, they are only in their preliminary stage of development. Further research is needed to optimize the design and delivery of antibiotics via these novel carriers and evaluate their safety and efficacy in clinical trials.

Hydrogels

Hydrogels are highly absorbent, biocompatible, and can be designed to release antibiotics in a controlled manner. By incorporating antibiotics into the hydrogel matrix, a sustained release of the drug can be achieved, allowing for high local concentrations while minimizing systemic exposure and reducing the risk of antibiotic resistance as a result of prolonged exposure to subtherapeutic antibiotics levels.[79] In addition, hydrogels can be formulated to adhere to tissue surfaces, providing prolonged contact time and enhancing the efficacy of the antibiotic. Several preclinical studies have investigated the use of hydrogels for local antibiotic delivery in orthopedics, with promising results. For example, a study by Jung and colleagues demonstrated that a hydrogel loaded with vancomycin and bone morphogenetic protein-2 was effective at suppressing bacterial proliferation in a rat model of osteomyelitis.[80] Overall, hydrogels represent a promising future strategy for localized antibiotic delivery in orthopedics, with the potential to improve patient outcomes, prevent FRI, and theoretically reduce the burden of antibiotic resistance.

Although hydrogels have several advantages for local antibiotic delivery, one limitation is the difficulty of achieving consistent and sustained drug release from the hydrogel matrix, which can vary depending on factors such as the composition of the gel, the method of drug incorporation, and the location of the implant. Another concern is the potential for immune reactions or inflammation caused by the hydrogel material itself. One study found that a hydrogel loaded with gentamicin increased the inflammatory response in vitro compared with the antibiotic alone, highlighting the need for careful evaluation of the biocompatibility of hydrogel formulations.[81] Further research is needed to optimize the delivery parameters and determine clinical effectiveness.

Collagens

Collagens are a family of fibrous proteins that are integral components of connective tissues in the body, including bone, cartilage, and tendons. They have been extensively studied as biomaterials for various applications in orthopedics, including as drug delivery vehicles. Collagen scaffolds have been shown to have high porosity and surface area, which makes them suitable for loading with antibiotics. Several studies have investigated the use of collagens as a carrier for antibiotics in the treatment of orthopedic infections. Preclinical studies have demonstrated that collagen sponges loaded with vancomycin and gentamicin can effectively inhibit the growth of *S aureus* in vitro and in vivo and reduce the incidence or severity of bone infections.[82,83]

Although collagens have been shown to have great potential as drug delivery vehicles for antibiotics, there are also some limitations to their use. One potential drawback of using collagen as an antibiotic delivery vehicle is the risk of immune reactions. Collagen is a naturally occurring protein in the body, but when used as a biomaterial, an immune response may be triggered in some patients. In addition, different types of collagens have varying degrees of purity and degradation rates, which can affect the release of antibiotics and their efficacy in treating infections. Furthermore, the processing methods used to extract and purify collagen can also affect its properties and performance as an antibiotic carrier. Additional clinical data are needed before the widespread adoption of this method of antibiotic delivery.

Nanoparticles

Nanoparticles are emerging as promising carriers for antibiotics in orthopedics due to their small size, high surface area-to-volume ratio, and potential for targeted delivery to a specific location over an extended time period. Several studies have investigated the use of nanoparticles as antibiotic carriers, including for the treatment of osteomyelitis and implant-related infections. In vitro and in vivo studies have demonstrated the efficacy of nanoparticle-based antibiotic delivery systems against a range of bacterial strains, including multidrug-resistant bacteria. One study by Rukavina and colleagues evaluated the efficacy of silver nanoparticles loaded with gentamicin in a mouse model of osteomyelitis caused by methicillin-resistant S aureus, demonstrating reduced bacterial load and inflammation in the infected bone compared with traditional gentamicin treatment.[84] Another study by Hou and colleagues developed a hydroxyapatite nanoparticle-based antibiotic delivery system for the treatment of prosthetic joint infections caused by Staphylococcus epidermidis.[85] The investigators found that the nanoparticle-based therapy provided sustained release of antibiotics over a period of 14 days and was effective at reducing bacterial load in vitro and in a rat model of prosthetic joint infection.

Although nanoparticles have shown promise as antibiotic delivery vehicles in orthopedics, there are also some downsides to their use. Some types of nanoparticles can be toxic to cells and tissues, which can limit their clinical use. In addition, nanoparticles can be excreted from the body quickly, reducing the duration of their therapeutic effect. The immune system may recognize nanoparticles as foreign bodies and clear them from the body before they have a chance to deliver the antibiotic in sufficient amounts and may lead to an immunogenic response. Finally, the production of nanoparticles can be expensive, and the scaling up of nanoparticle manufacturing for clinical use may be challenging. Further translational research is necessary to optimize the technology before venturing into clinical use.

SUMMARY

There is evolving evidence that supports the use of local antibiotics as a prophylactic measure, but evidence for efficacy in FRI treatment is significantly lacking. Each local antibiotic discussed in this review is associated with its own advantages and disadvantages. Antibiotic powder is easy to use, time efficient, and can be applied directly and diffusely to a wound before closure but lacks the option for sustained release. PMMA has the versatility to be used as a spacer, bead or as an implant coating, but is limited by early burst kinetics and need for removal. The biodegradable products such as calcium sulfate and calcium phosphate are able to deliver antibiotics over a longer period of time without the need for removal. These have the added theoretic function of promoting bone growth; however, they have been associated with wound drainage and other complications. Antibiotic-coated implants provide prophylaxis that has the potential to reduce infection rates, but manufactured devices are not approved for use in the United States. Finally, novel carriers such as hydrogels, collagens, and nanoparticles are future tools with early preclinical results that have not yet been investigated enough for routine use in a clinical setting. The decision for which local antibiotic method to use is determined by patient, injury, and surgeon factors. Higher level evidence-based research is limited, and further studies are needed before clinical recommendations can be made.

CLINICS CARE POINTS

- There is evolving clinical evidence that supports the use of local antibiotics as a prophylactic measure, but high level evidence for efficacy in fracture-related infection treatment is lacking.

- The highest level evidence regarding local antibiotic use in orthopedic trauma stems from the VANCO trial, in which local vancomycin powder administered at wound closure during definitive fixation-reduced gram positive infection rates in high-risk tibial plateau and pilon fractures.

- Polymethylmethacrylate has historically been the most widely used local antibiotic delivery device, however drawbacks include early burst kinetics, subtherapeutic levels of antibiotic delivery with prolonged use, and permanence of the material often necessitating surgical removal.

- Emerging biomaterials such as antibiotic-coated implants, hydrogels, collagens, and nanoparticles require further investigation before clinical use.

DISCLOSURE

A.E. Levack is a board or committee member on the Orthopedic Trauma Association. All other authors have nothing to disclose.

REFERENCES

1. Walter N, Rupp M, Hierl K, et al. Long-term patient-related quality of life after fracture-related infections of the long bones. Bone Jt Res 2021;10(5):321–7.

2. Iliaens J, Onsea J, Hoekstra H, et al. Fracture-related infection in long bone fractures: A comprehensive analysis of the economic impact and influence on quality of life. Injury 2021;52(11):3344–9.

3. Redfern J, Wasilko SM, Groth ME, et al. Surgical site infections in patients with type 3 open fractures: comparing antibiotic prophylaxis with cefazolin plus gentamicin versus piperacillin/tazobactam. J Orthop Trauma 2016;30(8):415–9.

4. Metsemakers W, Kuehl R, Moriarty T, et al. Infection after fracture fixation: current surgical and microbiological concepts. Injury 2018;49(3):511–22.

5. Birt MC, Anderson DW, Toby EB, et al. Osteomyelitis: recent advances in pathophysiology and therapeutic strategies. J Orthop 2017;14(1):45–52.

6. Hadizie D, Kor Y, Ghani S, et al. The Incidence of Fracture-Related Infection in Open Tibia Fracture with Different Time Interval of Initial Debridement. Malays Orthop J 2022;16(3):24–9.

7. Dunkel N, Pittet D, Tovmirzaeva L, et al. Short duration of antibiotic prophylaxis in open fractures does not enhance risk of subsequent infection. Bone Jt J 2013;95(6):831–7.

8. Li J, Wang Q, Lu Y, et al. Relationship between time to surgical debridement and the incidence of infection in patients with open tibial fractures. Orthop Surg 2020;12(2):524–32.

9. O'Connor O, Thahir A, Krkovic M. How Much Does an Infected Fracture Cost? Arch Bone Jt Surg 2022;10(2):135.

10. Chang Y, Kennedy SA, Bhandari M, et al. Effects of antibiotic prophylaxis in patients with open fracture of the extremities: a systematic review of randomized controlled trials. JBJS Rev 2015;3(6):e2.

11. Horton SA, Hoyt BW, Zaidi SM, et al. Risk factors for treatment failure of fracture-related infections. Injury 2021;52(6):1351–5.

12. Berkes M, Obremskey WT, Scannell B, et al. Maintenance of hardware after early postoperative infection following fracture internal fixation. JBJS 2010;92(4):823–8.

13. Bezstarosti H, Van Lieshout E, Voskamp L, et al. Insights into treatment and outcome of fracture-related infection: a systematic literature review. Arch Orthop Trauma Surg 2019;139:61–72.

14. Morgenstern M, Vallejo A, McNally M, et al. The effect of local antibiotic prophylaxis when treating open limb fractures: a systematic review and meta-analysis. Bone Jt Res 2018;7(7):447–56.

15. Sweet FA, Roh M, Sliva C. Intrawound application of vancomycin for prophylaxis in instrumented thoracolumbar fusions: efficacy, drug levels, and patient outcomes. Spine 2011;36(24):2084–8.

16. O'Neill KR, Smith JG, Abtahi AM, et al. Reduced surgical site infections in patients undergoing posterior spinal stabilization of traumatic injuries using vancomycin powder. Spine J 2011;11(7):641–6.

17. Molinari RW, Khera OA, Molinari WJ III. Prophylactic intraoperative powdered vancomycin and postoperative deep spinal wound infection: 1,512 consecutive surgical cases over a 6-year period. Eur Spine J 2012;21:476–82.

18. Owen MT, Keener EM, Hyde ZB, et al. Intraoperative topical antibiotics for infection prophylaxis in pelvic and acetabular surgery. J Orthop Trauma 2017;31(11):589–94.

19. Cichos KH, Spitler CA, Quade JH, et al. Intrawound antibiotic powder in acetabular fracture open reduction internal fixation does not reduce surgical site infections. J Orthop Trauma 2021;35(4):198–204.

20. The Major Extremity Trauma Research Consortium (METRC). Effect of Intrawound Vancomycin Powder in Operatively Treated High-risk Tibia Fractures: A Randomized Clinical Trial. JAMA Surg 2021;156(5):e207259. https://doi.org/10.1001/jamasurg.2020.7259.

21. O'Toole RV, Degani Y, Carlini AR, et al. Systemic absorption and nephrotoxicity associated with topical vancomycin powder for fracture surgery. J Orthop Trauma 2021;35(1):29–34.

22. O'Toole RV, Joshi M, Carlini AR, et al. Local antibiotic therapy to reduce infection after operative treatment of fractures at high risk of infection: a multicenter, randomized, controlled trial (VANCO study). J Orthop Trauma 2017;31:S18–24.

23. Lawing CR, Lin FC, Dahners LE. Local injection of aminoglycosides for prophylaxis against infection in open fractures. J Bone Joint Surg Am 2015;97(22):1844.

24. ter Boo GJA, Grijpma DW, Moriarty TF, et al. Antimicrobial delivery systems for local infection prophylaxis in orthopedic-and trauma surgery. Biomaterials 2015;52:113–25.

25. Jaeblon T. Polymethylmethacrylate: properties and contemporary uses in orthopaedics. J Am Acad Orthop Surg 2010;18(5):297–305.

26. Duncan C, Masri BA. The role of antibiotic-loaded cement in the treatment of an infection after a hip replacement. Instr Course Lect 1995;44:305–13.

27. Tai CL, Lai PL, Lin WD, et al. Modification of mechanical properties, polymerization temperature, and handling time of polymethylmethacrylate cement for enhancing applicability in vertebroplasty. BioMed Res Int 2016;2016.

28. Meyer P Jr, Lautenschlager E, Moore B. On the setting properties of acrylic bone cement. JBJS 1973;55(1):149–56.

29. Preininger B, Matziolis G, Pfitzner T, et al. In situ tele-thermographic measurements during PMMA spacer augmentation in temporary arthrodesis after periprosthetic knee joint infection. Technol Health Care 2012;20(4):337–41.

30. Van Vugt TA, Arts JJ, Geurts JA. Antibiotic-loaded polymethylmethacrylate beads and spacers in

treatment of orthopedic infections and the role of biofilm formation. Front Microbiol 2019;10:1626.

31. Thonse R, Conway J. Antibiotic cement-coated interlocking nail for the treatment of infected non-unions and segmental bone defects. J Orthop Trauma 2007;21(4):258–68.

32. Ristiniemi J, Lakovaara M, Flinkkilä T, et al. Staged method using antibiotic beads and subsequent autografting for large traumatic tibial bone loss: 22 of 23 fractures healed after 5–20 months. Acta Orthop 2007;78(4):520–7.

33. DeCoster TA, Bozorgnia S. Antibiotic beads. J Am Acad Orthop Surg 2008;16(11):674–8.

34. Diefenbeck M, Mückley T, Hofmann GO. Prophylaxis and treatment of implant-related infections by local application of antibiotics. Injury 2006; 37(2):S95–104.

35. Popham G, Mangino P, Seligson D, et al. Antibiotic-impregnated beads. Part II: Factors in antibiotic selection. Orthop Rev 1991;20(4):331–7.

36. Henry SL, Ostermann PA, Seligson D. The Antibiotic Bead Pouch Technique: The Management of Severe Compound Fractures. Clin Orthop Relat Res 1976-2007 1993;295:54–62.

37. Warner M, Henderson C, Kadrmas W, et al. Comparison of vacuum-assisted closure to the antibiotic bead pouch for the treatment of blast injury of the extremity. Orthopedics 2010;33(2):77–82.

38. Patterson JT, Becerra JA, Brown M, et al. Antibiotic bead pouch versus negative pressure wound therapy at initial management of AO/OTA 42 type IIIB open tibia fracture may reduce fracture related infection: A retrospective analysis of 113 patients. Injury 2023;54(2):744–50.

39. Masquelet A, Fitoussi F, Begue T, et al. Reconstruction of the long bones by the induced membrane and spongy autograft. Ann Chir Plast Esthet 2000; 45:346–53.

40. Riel RU, Gladden PB. A simple method for fashioning an antibiotic cement-coated interlocking intramedullary nail. Am J Orthop 2010;39(1):18–21.

41. Downey EA, Jaime KM, Reif TJ, et al. Prophylaxis and treatment of infection in long bones using an antibiotic-loaded ceramic coating with interlocking intramedullary nails. J Bone Jt Infect 2022;7(2):101–7.

42. Ismat A, Walter N, Baertl S, et al. Antibiotic cement coating in orthopedic surgery: a systematic review of reported clinical techniques. J Orthop Traumatol 2021;22:1–20.

43. Lee SH, Tai CL, Chen SY, et al. Elution and mechanical strength of vancomycin-loaded bone cement: in vitro study of the influence of brand combination. PLoS One 2016;11(11):e0166545.

44. Levack AE, Turajane K, Yang X, et al. Thermal stability and in vitro elution kinetics of alternative antibiotics in polymethylmethacrylate (PMMA) bone cement. JBJS 2021;103(18):1694–704.

45. Van de Belt H, Neut D, Uges D, et al. Surface roughness, porosity and wettability of gentamicin-loaded bone cements and their antibiotic release. Biomaterials 2000;21(19):1981–7.

46. Shinsako K, Okui Y, Matsuda Y, et al. Effects of bead size and polymerization in PMMA bone cement on vancomycin release. Bio Med Mater Eng 2008;18(6):377–85.

47. Hsieh PH, Tai CL, Lee PC, et al. Liquid gentamicin and vancomycin in bone cement: a potentially more cost-effective regimen. J Arthroplasty 2009;24(1):125–30.

48. Penner MJ, Masri BA, Duncan CP. Elution characteristics of vancomycin and tobramycin combined in acrylic bone—cement. J Arthroplasty 1996; 11(8):939–44.

49. Klekamp J, Dawson JM, Haas DW, et al. The use of vancomycin and tobramycin in acrylic bone cement: biomechanical effects and elution kinetics for use in joint arthroplasty. J Arthroplasty 1999; 14(3):339–46.

50. Kendall RW, Duncan CP, Smith JA, et al. Persistence of bacteria on antibiotic loaded acrylic depots: a reason for caution. Clin Orthop Relat Res 1996;329:273–80.

51. Neut D, van de Belt H, Stokroos I, et al. Biomaterial-associated infection of gentamicin-loaded PMMA beads in orthopaedic revision surgery. J Antimicrob Chemother 2001;47(6):885–91.

52. Lewis KN, Thomas M, Puleo D. Mechanical and degradation behavior of polymer-calcium sulfate composites. J Mater Sci Mater Med 2006;17:531–7.

53. El-Husseiny M, Patel S, MacFarlane R, et al. Biodegradable antibiotic delivery systems. J Bone Joint Surg Br 2011;93(2):151–7.

54. Levack AE, Turajane K, Driscoll DA, et al. Identifying alternative antibiotics that elute from calcium sulfate beads for treatment of orthopedic infections. J Orthop Res 2022;40(5):1143–53.

55. McConoughey SJ, Howlin RP, Wiseman J, et al. Comparing PMMA and calcium sulfate as carriers for the local delivery of antibiotics to infected surgical sites. J Biomed Mater Res B Appl Biomater 2015;103(4):870–7.

56. Knecht CS, Moley JP, McGrath MS, et al. Antibiotic loaded calcium sulfate bead and pulse lavage eradicates biofilms on metal implant materials in vitro. J Orthop Res 2018;36(9):2349–54.

57. Thomas DB, Brooks DE, Bice TG, et al. Tobramycin-impregnated calcium sulfate prevents infection in contaminated wounds. Clin Orthop Relat Res 2005;441:366–71.

58. McKee MD, Li-Bland EA, Wild LM, et al. A prospective, randomized clinical trial comparing an antibiotic-impregnated bioabsorbable bone substitute with standard antibiotic-impregnated cement beads in the treatment of chronic osteomyelitis and infected nonunion. J Orthop Trauma 2010;24(8):483–90.

59. Rivera JC, McClure PK, Fragomen AT, et al. Intra-medullary antibiotic depot does not preclude successful intramedullary lengthening or compression. J Orthop Trauma 2021;35(8):e309.

60. Sheridan GA, Falk DP, Fragomen AT, et al. Calcium sulfate in the management of osteomyelitis: A systematic review and meta-analysis of comparative studies. Medicine (Baltim) 2022;101(45):e31364.

61. McPherson E, Dipane M, Sherif S. Dissolvable antibiotic beads in treatment of periprosthetic joint infection and revision arthroplasty-the use of synthetic pure calcium sulfate (Stimulan®) impregnated with vancomycin & tobramycin. Reconstr Rev 2013;3(1).

62. FRAKENBURG EP, Goldstein SA, Bauer TW, et al. Biomechanical and histological evaluation of a calcium phosphate cement. JBJS 1998;80(8):1112–24.

63. Fernandez de Grado G, Keller L, Idoux-Gillet Y, et al. Bone substitutes: a review of their characteristics, clinical use, and perspectives for large bone defects management. J Tissue Eng 2018;9. 2041731418776819.

64. Mukai M, Uchida K, Sugo K, et al. Long-term antibacterial activity of vancomycin from calcium phosphate cement in vivo. Bio Med Mater Eng 2022;33(1):41–50.

65. Niikura T, Lee SY, Iwakura T, et al. Antibiotic-impregnated calcium phosphate cement as part of a comprehensive treatment for patients with established orthopaedic infection. J Orthop Sci 2016;21(4):539–45.

66. Urabe K, Naruse K, Hattori H, et al. In vitro comparison of elution characteristics of vancomycin from calcium phosphate cement and polymethylmethacrylate. J Orthop Sci 2009;14:784–93.

67. Waterman P, Barber M, Weintrob AC, et al. The elution of colistimethate sodium from polymethylmethacrylate and calcium phosphate cement beads. Am J Orthop 2012;41(6):256–9.

68. McNally M, Ferguson J, Lau A, et al. Single-stage treatment of chronic osteomyelitis with a new absorbable, gentamicin-loaded, calcium sulphate/hydroxyapatite biocomposite: a prospective series of 100 cases. Bone Jt J 2016;98(9):1289–96.

69. Drampalos E, Mohammad HR, Pillai A. Augmented debridement for implant related chronic osteomyelitis with an absorbable, gentamycin loaded calcium sulfate/hydroxyapatite biocomposite. J Orthop 2020;17:173–9.

70. Freischmidt H, Armbruster J, Reiter G, et al. Individualized techniques of implant coating with an antibiotic-loaded, hydroxyapatite/calcium sulphate bone graft substitute. Ther Clin Risk Manag 2020;689–94.

71. McNally MA, Ferguson JY, Scarborough M, et al. Mid-to long-term results of single-stage surgery for patients with chronic osteomyelitis using a bio-absorbable gentamicin-loaded ceramic carrier. Bone Jt J 2022;104(9):1095–100.

72. Niemann M, Graef F, Ahmad SS, et al. Outcome Analysis of the Use of Cerament® in Patients with Chronic Osteomyelitis and Corticomedullary Defects. Diagnostics 2022;12(5):1207.

73. Moghaddam A, Graeser V, Westhauser F, et al. Patients' safety: is there a systemic release of gentamicin by gentamicin-coated tibia nails in clinical use? Ther Clin Risk Manag 2016;1387–93.

74. De Meo D, Cannari FM, Petriello L, et al. Gentamicin-coated tibia nail in fractures and nonunion to reduce fracture-related infections: A systematic review. Molecules 2020;25(22):5471.

75. Moojen DJF, Vogely HC, Fleer A, et al. Prophylaxis of infection and effects on osseointegration using a tobramycin-periapatite coating on titanium implants—An experimental study in the rabbit. J Orthop Res 2009;27(6):710–6.

76. Jennings JA, Carpenter DP, Troxel KS, et al. Novel antibiotic-loaded point-of-care implant coating inhibits biofilm. Clin Orthop Relat Res 2015;473:2270–82.

77. Stavrakis A, Zhu S, Loftin A, et al. Controlled release of vancomycin and tigecycline from an orthopaedic implant coating prevents Staphylococcus aureus infection in an open fracture animal model. BioMed Res Int 2019;2019.

78. Ghimire A, Skelly JD, Song J. Micrococcal-nuclease-triggered on-demand release of vancomycin from intramedullary implant coating eradicates Staphylococcus aureus infection in mouse femoral canals. ACS Cent Sci 2019;5(12):1929–36.

79. Schwarz EM, McLaren AC, Sculco TP, et al. Adjuvant antibiotic-loaded bone cement: concerns with current use and research to make it work. J Orthop Res 2021;39(2):227–39.

80. Jung SW, Oh SH, Lee IS, et al. In situ gelling hydrogel with anti-bacterial activity and bone healing property for treatment of osteomyelitis. Tissue Eng Regen Med 2019;16:479–90.

81. Hernandez-Gordillo V, Kassis T, Lampejo A, et al. Fully synthetic matrices for in vitro culture of primary human intestinal enteroids and endometrial organoids. Biomaterials 2020;254:120125.

82. Friess W, Uludag H, Foskett S, et al. Characterization of absorbable collagen sponges as rhBMP-2 carriers. Int J Pharm 1999;187(1):91–9.

83. Shahi A, Ritter M, Elmallah R, et al. Collagen sponges for antibiotic delivery in orthopaedic surgery. J Am Acad Orthop Surg 2021;29(1):e28–36.

84. Rukavina Z, Vranic S, Brcic I, et al. Silver nanoparticles loaded with gentamicin for the treatment of osteomyelitis caused by methicillin-resistant Staphylococcus aureus in a mouse model. Int J Nanomed 2020;15:4847–59.

85. Hou Y, Lin Q, Shan Y, et al. Hydroxyapatite nanoparticles loaded with vancomycin and rifampicin for the treatment of Staphylococcus epidermidis-induced prosthetic joint infection. J Orthopaedic Translation 2021;29:84–91.

Pediatrics

Navigating the Enigma of Pediatric Musculoskeletal Infections: A Race Against Time

Stephanie N. Moore-Lotridge, PhD[a,b],
Brian Q. Hou, BA[c], Katherine S. Hajdu, BS[c],
Malini Anand, BS[c], William Hefley, BS[c],
Jonathan G. Schoenecker, MD, PhD[a,b,d,e,f],*

KEYWORDS

- Musculoskeletal infections • Acute phase response • Septic arthritis • Osteomyelitis
- Pyomyositis • Sepsis • Multiorgan dysfunction syndrome

KEY POINTS

- The primary objective of caring for a child with a musculoskeletal infection (MSKI) is to prevent multiorgan dysfunction that can result in fatality.
- The four questions in infection that must be addressed are: where is it, what is it, how severe is it, and how to treat it
- The acute phase response is crucial for fighting a bacterial infection, but dysregulation of this response can lead to complications including multiorgan dysfunction
- Multifocal infections must be considered by using fast sequence MRI and interpreting measures of the acute phase response, such as C-reactive protein levels
- Primary treatment for MSKI is antibiotics. Discretion about withholding antibiotics for success of cultures must be used in children at risk of disease dissemination.

INTRODUCTION

Few conditions in pediatric orthopedics are as enigmatic or carry higher stakes for a child than potential musculoskeletal infections (MSKIs). Pediatric orthopedic surgeons are frequently consulted to evaluate children with suspected MSKI. For example, the Children's Orthopedic Trauma and Infection Consortium for Evidence-based Studies (CORTICES) group determined that pediatric MSKI accounts for nearly 1 in 10 pediatric orthopedic consultations at academic pediatric tertiary care centers.[1] Fortunately, modern medicine and the advent of antibiotics have dramatically reduced the mortality of MSKI in children, which was estimated as high as 40% in the pre-antibiotic era.[2,3] Although few pediatric patients now succumb to MSKI in the United States, it continues to cause significant morbidity in children, including the potential for long-term negative impacts on the growing skeleton.[4–7] Thus, it is essential that pediatric orthopedic surgeons are armed with the best tools to provide an efficient and accurate workup with up-to-date knowledge of the optimal treatment for each organism and presentation of infection they encounter.

To ensure proper care for children with suspected MSKI, all members of the medical and surgical team should prioritize completing four

---

[a] Department of Orthopedics, Vanderbilt University Medical Center, Nashville, TN, USA; [b] Vanderbilt Center for Bone Biology, Vanderbilt University Medical Center, Nashville, TN, USA; [c] School of Medicine, Vanderbilt University Medical Center, Nashville, TN, USA; [d] Department of Pathology, Microbiology and Immunology, Vanderbilt University Medical Center, Nashville, TN, USA; [e] Department of Pharmacology, Vanderbilt University Medical Center, Nashville, TN, USA; [f] Department of Pediatrics, Monroe Carell Jr. Children's Hospital at Vanderbilt, Nashville, TN, USA
* Corresponding author. 1155 MRB4, 2215-B Garland Avenue, Nashville, TN 37232.
E-mail address: Jon.schoenecker@vumc.org

Orthop Clin N Am 55 (2024) 217–232
https://doi.org/10.1016/j.ocl.2023.09.004
0030-5898/24/© 2023 Elsevier Inc. All rights reserved.

tasks. The team should determine: (1) where is the infection, (2) is it an infection and if so, what is the pathogen, (3) how severe is the infection, and (4) how to treat the infection. Importantly, during the workup for a suspected MSKI, these tasks are being assessed in a temporally concordant manner, where ndings from one can in uence another, and therefore should not be conducted in isolation. This review discusses the tools and philosophy behind these four tasks, emphasizing current best practices and advancements. It is worth noting that although this review primarily focuses on the most common MSKIs and causative organisms, the principles discussed can be applied to all MSKI cases, even those involving less common organisms.

TASK 1: WHERE IS THE INFECTION?

The developing musculoskeletal system is particularly vulnerable to "spontaneous" bacterial infections, as bacteria can bind and thrive in the microenvironments of damaged and regenerating tissues (8, 9), which is mimicked in growing bones. The unique characteristics of the physis, such as robust "tortuous" vascularity,[8] its relative immune privileged nature,[9] and concentration of growth factors and binding sites further predispose these tissue sites to initiation of infection. For reasons not completely understood, lower extremities are far more susceptible to spontaneous MSKI than upper extremities, with the femur (hip and knee) being the most susceptible.

Armed with the understanding that bacteria can thrive in the developing musculoskeletal tissue, the most important goal of the medical and surgical team is to quickly determine which tissues and/or joint(s) are involved. In the past, an irritable joint with other diagnostic criteria suggesting MSKI was thought to be an intra-articular process, primarily septic arthritis. As MRI has become a more accessible and commonly used tool in arsenal of MSKI workup (Table 1), it is now understood that the perceived prevalence of intra-articular pathology was likely driven by "anatomic ascertainment bias," associated with the use of x-ray and ultrasound. These imaging modalities are excellent at revealing intra-articular effusions, but poor at detecting early osteomyelitis or pyomyositis or distinguishing concurrent infections (Fig. 1). For example, just 1 decade ago, pericapsular hip pyomyositis was considered a tropical infection; however, due to MRI use, it is now a common diagnosis in temperate

climates.[10–14] Furthermore, the routine use of MRI has similarly revealed heterogeneity of infectious pathologies around the knee with synovitis, isolated osteomyelitis, and bursitis occurring at a greater frequency than isolated septic arthritis.[4] Taken together, these studies illustrate the clear inferiority of prior imaging approaches and support for MRI being suggested as the gold standard for accurately determining the anatomic location(s) and burden of MSKI.

Although MRI provides superior spatial resolution and sensitivity to capture the extent of the infection, routine implementation may not be possible at all centers due to the availability of scanners, access to train technicians, or limited capacity to integrate this technology with the current hospital system and billing practices. Thus, until these barriers can routinely be overcome, the most impactful tool in an orthopedic surgeon's toolbox remains is his or her ability to perform a thorough physical examination and delineate musculoskeletal pain generators to help direct the clinical workup. In conjunction with a thorough physical examination and knowledge that tissues other than the intra-articular space may be involved, physicians can apply appropriate aspiration of all suspected tissue (see Task 2) in the emergency room (ER) or operating room (OR) with the intent of assaying muscle, bone, or intra-articular uid from the maximum point of tenderness in the child. Therefore, even if advanced imaging is not available, the medical team can work to ensure sources of infection are not missed.

TASK 2: IS IT AN INFECTION, AND IF SO, WHAT IS THE PATHOGEN?

Rapid diagnosis of infection and identi cation of the causative organism is essential to properly treat pediatric patients with suspected MSKI. First, identi cation of noninfectious mimicries of MSKI in pediatric patients, such as in ammatory conditions or cancer, is essential to both prevent unneeded treatment and direct critical therapy. Second, in cases of presumed MSKI, rapid identi cation of the causative organisms allows for earlier narrowing of antibiotic therapy, thus decreasing the overuse of broad-spectrum antibiotics. However, methodology and the tools available for rapid identi cation of infectious organisms still require improvement. Prior studies have reported culture positivity rates for patients with con rmed MSKI ranging between ~40% and 80%.[15–17] In the recent multicenter

Table 1
Snapshot of fast-sequence MRI for pediatric musculoskeletal infection

	Suspected Focus of Pathology	MSKI Screening Protocol	Initial Field of View	First Sequence	Second Sequence	Third Sequence	Fourth Sequence	Estimated Time (min)
Lower Body	Pelvis	Pelvis	Iliac crest to mid-femur	Coronal STIR	Coronal T1	Axial T2 fat sat		10–15
	Hip	Pelvis	Iliac crest to mid-femur	Coronal STIR	Coronal T1	Axial T2 fat sat		10–15
	Femur	Femur	Hip joint to knee joint	Coronal STIR	Coronal T1	Axial T2 fat sat		10–15
	Knee	Knee	Mid-femur to mid-tibia	Coronal STIR	Coronal T1	Axial T2 fat sat		10–15
	Tibia	Tibia	Knee joint to ankle joint	Coronal STIR	Coronal T1	Axial T2 fat sat		10–15
	Ankle	Ankle and Foot	Mid-tibia to toes/plantar foot	Coronal STIR	Coronal T1	Axial T2 fat sat	Sagittal STIR	12–18
	Foot	Ankle and Foot	Mid-tibia to toes/plantar foot	Coronal STIR	Coronal T1	Axial T2 fat sat	Sagittal STIR	12–18
	Unknown LE	Screening LE with CTLS spine	Iliac crest to plantar foot	Coronal STIR	Coronal T1	Axial T2 fat sat		10–15
			Occiput to coccyx	Sagittal STIR	Sagittal T1	Axial T2		10–15
Axial	Spine	CTLS spine	Occiput to coccyx	Sagittal STIR	Sagittal T1	Axial T2		10–15
Upper Body	Shoulder	Shoulder	Shoulder joint to mid-humerus	Coronal STIR	Coronal T1	Axial T2 fat sat		10–15
	Humerus	Humerus	Shoulder joint to elbow joint	Coronal STIR	Coronal T1	Axial T2 fat sat		10–15
	Elbow	Elbow	Mid-humerus to mid-forearm	Coronal STIR	Coronal T1	Axial T2 fat sat	Sagittal STIR	12–18
	Forearm	Forearm	Elbow joint to wrist joint	Coronal STIR	Coronal T1	Axial T2 fat sat		10–15
	Wrist	Wrist & Hand	Mid-forearm to finger tips	Coronal STIR	Coronal T1	Axial T2 fat sat		10–15
	Hand	Wrist and Hand	Mid-forearm to finger tips	Coronal STIR	Coronal T1	Axial T2 fat sat		10–15
	Unknown UE	Screening UE	Shoulder joint to finger tips	Coronal STIR	Coronal T1	Axial T2 fat sat		10–15

Abbreviations: CTLS, cervical, thoracic, lumbar, sacral; LE, lower extremity; STIR, short tau inversion recovery; UE, upper extremity.

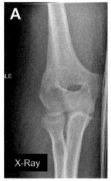
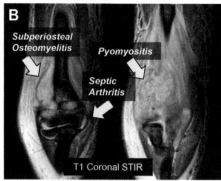
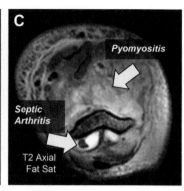

Fig. 1. Advantages of fast-sequence MRI over x-ray and ultrasound. A 16-year-old patient presented with a painful elbow joint. X-ray (A) did not reveal diagnostic information and ultrasound (not shown) was suggestive of a septic joint. The elbow fast-sequence MRI was performed non-sedated in less than 15-minutes which revealed invaluable diagnostic information for culture and debridement. (B) MRI (T1 coronal STIR sequence) and (C) (axial T2 fat sat), illustrates evidence of simultaneous subperiosteal osteomyelitis, septic arthritis, and pyomyositis. Without this information, culture and surgical debridement would have been primarily focused on the intra-articular space and potentially intraosseous, whereas the primary focus of the infection was extra-articular in the muscle and subperiosteal space. (Figure permission: Schoenecker Laboratory.)

CORTICES study, it was found that only one in three pediatric MSKI-related consultations, on average, produced a culture-positive identification at the time of orthopedic consultation.[1] Negative culture results may occur because the child does not have an infection, the causative organism is difficult to culture, the incorrect tissue was sampled, or the infection is disseminated without abscess. In addition, the methodology of identifying organisms still primarily relies on bacterial culture, which can take days, or weeks in cases such as *Kingella kingae*, to produce results. Clearly, this is an area of pediatric MSKI care that requires improvement. Working within these shortcomings, an important role of the pediatric orthopedic surgeon is to provide a sufficient sample of the most likely infected tissue.

The Usual Suspects

Pyogenic organisms are the most common causative pathogens of pediatric MSKI with *Staphylococcus aureus* being responsible for 40% to 90% of cases.[3,18] However, epidemiologic patterns of pediatric MSKI are regularly changing, attributable to dynamic mutations in the bacterial genome, use of antibiotics, and vaccinations. For example, with the advent of routine infant vaccination against *Haemophilus influenza* and the pneumococcal conjugate vaccines, the incidence of MSKI caused by *H influenza* and *Staphylococcus pneumo* has decreased substantially.[19] *K kingae* has replaced *H influenza* as the predominant cause of septic arthritis in younger children and has become more common than *S aureus* in children aged 1 to 2 years.[20,21] In another

example, a 2008 study found that zero children were treated for a Methicillin-resistant *S* (MRSA) infection in 1982; yet from 2002 to 2004, MRSA was isolated as the causative organism in 30% of children.[22] In a recent multicenter study of pediatric tertiary care centers conducted by the CORTICES group, it was found that *S aureus* accounted for ~65% of all culture-positive infections at the time of consultation by orthopedic providers, of which 37.4% of confirmed staphylococcal infections were methicillin resistant (ie, MRSA)[1] (Fig. 2).

It is important to note that the most common causative pathogens of MSKI can vary regionally as well. Thus, it is important that the medical team be aware of these trends, especially in individuals who may have trained in a different location. A retrospective study by the CORTICES group found that the proportion of causative pathogens identi ed at the time of consultation varied not only across regions but also between sites within the same region (Table 2).[1] Although *Staphylococcus* remained the primary cause of culture-positive MSKI across all regions, a significantly higher total *S aureus* rate (methicillin sensitive staphylococcus aureus [MSSA] + MRSA) was observed in the southern region at the time of consultation compared with all other regions (P = .039) (see Fig. 2). Although interinstitutional variability was detected within the same region, the average proportion of MRSA between regions was fairly consistent, ranging from 20% to 29%. *Staphylococcus pyogenes* was observed at comparable rates across regions (4%–11%), with the greatest proportion being

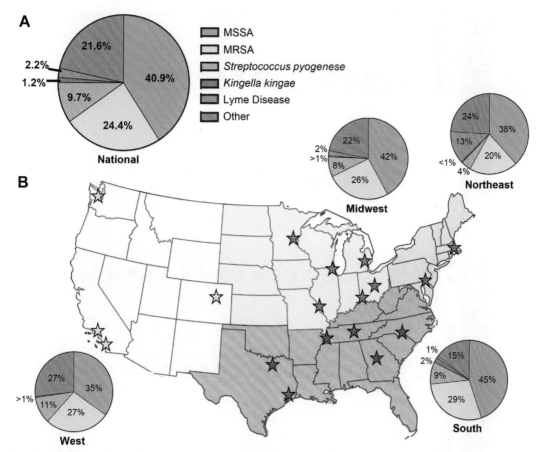

Fig. 2. Causative pathogen proportions in the United States as published by Schoenecker and colleagues. (*A*) Culture-positive results from orthopedic consultations for MSKI across all 18 CORTICES sites. (*B*) Proportion of positive cultures by region: West (*n* = 4, yellow), Midwest (*n* = 6, green), South (*n* = 6, red), and Northeast (*n* = 2, blue). (Figure permission: Schoenecker Laboratory as presented in https://doi.org/10.1371/journal.pone. 0234055.g001)

found in the West, where a single institution reported that 25% of annual consults were positive for *S pyogenes*. Likewise, the proportion of *K kingae* observed was fairly equal across all regions (<1%–2% of culture positive cases), with the greatest proportion being found in the South, where a single institution reported a rate of 7%. Finally, as previously reported,[23] Lyme disease was primarily seen in the Northeast and at select sites in the Midwest (Northeast vs all other regions: *P* = .007) (see Table 2). Together, these studies illustrate that the epidemiology of MSKIs is ever-changing and up-to-date data on the common pathogens and their genetic variations must be considered when diagnosing and directing treatments.

Sample Early and Sample Often
Tissue and blood cultures are routinely used to identify pathogens responsible for an MSKI. Blood cultures should be taken as soon as an

intravenous (IV) is placed in the child. Tissue cultures can be obtained either in the ER or OR with signi cantly improved success after a thorough physical examination in combination with a fast-sequence MRI to localize the source of infection (Task 1). In addition to increasing the culture positivity rates of the sampled tissue, the MRI may prevent inoculating sterile tissue by inadvertently passing through infected tissue (such as muscle) on the way to the bone or intra-articular space. Reiterating the point above, the most important role for the pediatric orthopedic surgeon in tissue sampling is to assure that (1) the proper tissue is sampled and (2) suf cient sample is collected in a timely manner to optimize care of the child.

Do Not Hold the Antibiotics…If You Are Headed to the OR "Soon"
With the anticipated bene t of improving culture yields, it has long been suggested that antibiotics

Table 2
Pathogen variance per region of the United States

Site	Region	% MSSA	% MRSA	% Streptococcus Pyogenes	% Kingella Kingae	% Borrelia burgdorferi	% Other	Ratio of MSSA/MRSA
1	Northeast	38%	20%	0%	1%	9%	32%	1.91
2	Northeast	39%	20%	8%	0%	17%	16%	1.89
3	Midwest	31%	39%	8%	0%	0%	22%	0.79
4	Midwest	35%	25%	4%	0%	0%	36%	1.37
5	Midwest	39%	31%	0%	1%	0%	30%	1.23
6	Midwest	47%	18%	13%	2%	7%	13%	2.67
7	Midwest	46%	21%	13%	0%	3%	18%	2.14
8	Midwest	52%	21%	10%	0%	0%	17%	2.44
9	South	36%	29%	4%	7%	0%	24%	1.26
10	South	32%	42%	5%	0%	0%	21%	0.78
11	South	36%	36%	7%	5%	2%	14%	1.00
12	South	56%	13%	20%	0%	0%	11%	4.18
13	South	57%	30%	3%	0%	0%	10%	1.89
14	South	51%	26%	12%	0%	1%	10%	1.96
15	West	40%	28%	25%	2%	0%	5%	1.43
16	West	35%	9%	4%	0%	0%	51%	3.77
17	West	27%	50%	7%	0%	0%	17%	0.53
18	West	38%	19%	9%	0%	0%	34%	2.00
Comparison between Regions		$P = .654$, ns	$P = .590$, ns	$P = .767$, ns	$P = .970$, ns	$P = .022$, *	$P = .451$, ns	$P = .969$, ns

Figure permission: Schoenecker Laboratory as presented in https://doi.org/10.1371/journal.pone.0234055.g001

are held until a culture was obtained. Recent reports have challenged this long-held tenant, demonstrating that prior antibiotic administration had no effect on culture sensitivity in patients with either local or disseminated MSKI. Furthermore, in patients with local infections, earlier antibiotic administration was found to be correlated with shorter length of stay.[16] Likewise, in pediatric patients diagnosed with osteomyelitis, prior antibiotic administration did not impact positive identification of the pathogen in bone biopsy cultures, though the overall culture yields were found to be lower and inversely correlated with the duration of antibiotic therapy.[24] For these reasons, the current recommendation is to refrain from delaying antibiotics, particularly in patients experiencing an exuberant acute phase response (APR) (see Task 3) given (1) the limited impact on tissue culture success and (2) the clear benefit of antibiotic administration in reducing the risk for complications.[25] The caveat to this recommendation is that it is unknown how long before culturing antibiotics can be administered before having a negative effect on cultures. In most of the previously mentioned studies, the time from antibiotic administration to culture was less than 24 hours.

Technical Improvements in Pathogen Identification

Although traditional blood and tissue culture support the identi cation of many common pathogens, standard techniques (which are almost a century old) can take days or weeks to propagate a result. Furthermore, it is now well understood that a myriad of causative pathogens for MSKI remain difficult to culture under standard conditions. For these reasons, innovative tools for identifying pathogens with greater efficacy have been examined, many of which are based on genetic amplification of bacterial DNA. For example, one such pathogen, K kingae, has been rising in incidence as a causative pathogen for septic arthritis in children younger than 2 years old in part due to improved detection methods.[20,26,27] Unlike the more virulent Staphylococcus species, K kingae is a less virulent gram-negative bacillus that is difficult to culture under standard conditions and if successful can often for 2 weeks to produce growth. In cases where K kingae is suspected, PCR-based testing is now commonly used to detect the pathogen DNA within tissue samples. Although currently outsourced by many hospitals, PCR-based testing for identification of pathogens is increasing in prevalence to meet the diagnostics needs for children with MSKI.

Given the clear utility of standard polymerase chain reaction (PCR) for rapid identi cation of fastidious pathogens, Wood and colleagues recently examined the utility of target-enriched multiplex PCR (TEM-PCR) for identi cation of pathogens in pediatric patients with suspected MSKI. TEM-PCR, which was rst described in 2006,[28] is a highly flexible, dynamic, platform capable of identifying a large spectrum of pathogens in a single sample with high sensitivity and specificity.[29] When compared with standard culturing techniques, TEM-PCR was found to be concordant in 100% of cases and able to detect pathogens in three cases deemed negative by standard culture (two of which were K kingae). Likewise, TEM-PCR reliably detected methicillin and clindamycin resistance in S aureus isolates. Therefore, in addition to outperforming traditional culture techniques, these results suggest that TEM-PCR may serve as a rapid diagnostic tool for identifying the causative pathogens in children with MSKI.

Although not yet commonly used in the evaluation of pediatric MSKIs, next-generation sequencing (NGS) and other high-throughput, "omics"-based techniques have been examined as ultra-sensitive means of diagnosing infections. Like the genetic assessment tools described above, these tools have the potential to identify a bacterium and its susceptibilities within hours as opposed to days required for traditional culturing. While powerful, NGS and omics-based analyses generate a large quantity of data that require specialized analysis to be applied clinically. Furthermore, the data generated are broad and "hypothesis-free" and therefore likely include more information than what is necessary to make a diagnosis. Finally, these methods can still be costly for many institutions to perform if infrastructure and trained personnel are not provided. Therefore, although these data can be very helpful in terms of research aimed at improving care for patients with MSKI, its use in clinical care must be weighed relative to the clinical burden and cost associated with such measures compared with standard assessments. Given these factors, the broad application of these techniques for diagnosing pediatric MSKIs remains inapplicable at this time but holds promise for the future.

TASK 3: HOW SEVERE IS THE MUSCULOSKELETAL INFECTION

Perhaps the most important consideration the medical team must make when working up a child with suspected MSKI is determining how severe the infection is. This information is critical, as it can help predict the risk of a local infection becoming disseminated, as well as the risk of adverse medical and musculoskeletal outcomes including multiorgan dysfunction and death.

Morbidity and Mortality Is Relative to a Prolonged or Exuberant Acute Phase Response

Unlike an acute injury (Fig. 3), in the context of an MSKI, tissue damage is continual as the infection worsens or spreads. As a result, the regulated and coordinated nature of the APR can be lost.[30,32] After invading the body, bacterial proliferation and the expression of virulence factors allow pathogens to evade the host containment mechanisms (fibrin/DNA webs) and migrate through tissue planes causing damage to neighboring tissue. Thus, as opposed to single isolated infections, the APR in combinatory infections is more exuberant, correlating with the amount of tissue infected and the duration of the infection. Furthermore, in addition to the "volume" of an infection, the bacteria's capacity to hijack many of the acute phase reactants can further drive an exuberant "survival" APR (Fig. 4A).

When dysregulated, an exuberant survival APR can drive inflammation and coagulation to pathologic levels. Clinically, this can present as tachypnea and/or a swollen extremity indicating possible thrombotic complications, such as septic pulmonary emboli or deep vein thrombosis,

as well as systemic inflammatory response syndrome (SIRS), which together increase the risk of multiorgan dysfunction and death.[30] Furthermore, given the essential role for vascularity in developing bone, coagulopathy following an exuberant APR can also impact the vascular supply to bone, leading to avascular necrosis, potential loss of joint function, and abnormal limb development. For these reasons, rapid diagnosis and treatment of an infection is essential to mitigate an exuberant or prolonged APR, thus reducing the risk of complications, patient morbidity, and mortality (see Fig. 4B).

Measuring the Acute Phase Response to Assess Musculoskeletal Infection Severity

Accurately determining the severity of an MSKI is essential to managing patient morbidity and mortality. Clinically, this can be accomplished through the combined assessment of a patient's presenting symptoms, vitals, laboratory values, culture results, and imaging. Previously, laboratory values, such as C-reactive protein (CRP), were primarily used at admission to assist with diagnosis of MSKI with little use after the initial diagnosis. Over the past ~10 years, studies have demonstrated the clinical utility of measuring the CRP serially throughout a case to assess disease severity, monitor the patient's response to treatment, and prognosticate the risk for complications (Fig. 5). In addition to CRP, thrombocytopenia has

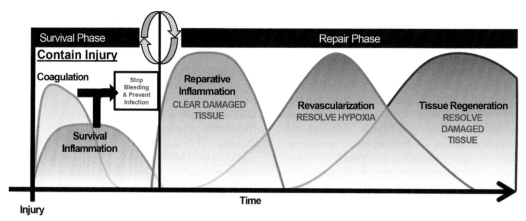

Fig. 3. The acute phase response: The Body's Response to Injury. In proportion to the amount of injury, the acute phase response (APR) is activated to achieve two goals: (1) ensure survival and (2) promote tissue repair. (A) These objectives are tackled in a temporal order: during the "survival" phase, damage control is initiated by a coordinated effort between coagulation and the survival inflammatory response to temporarily seal off compartments with a fibrin/platelet seal. In addition to stopping bleeding, this sealant promotes ingress of survival inflammatory cells which help reduce the susceptibility to infection. For example, neutrophils, in cooperation with the host's coagulation response, work to trap bacteria in DNA neutrophil extracellular traps (NETs) and fibrin webs and release chemotaxis to kill pathogens. Meanwhile, macrophages clear the trapped bacteria. Once survival is ensured, the APR transitions to a reparative inflammatory response that paves the way for revascularization and regeneration of the damaged tissues. In an acute injury, this series of events occurs over several weeks, allowing for a timely recovery.[30,31] (Figure permission: Schoenecker Laboratory.)

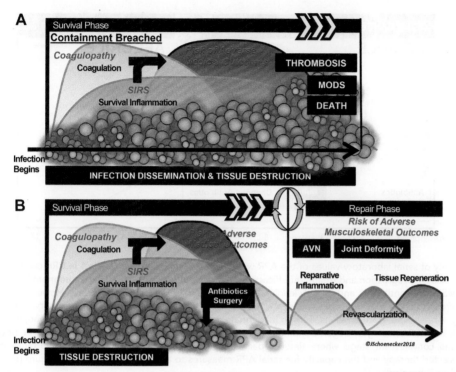

Fig. 4. The acute phase response during infection. (*A*) As infection progresses, the survival phase of the APR will progressively increase in magnitude as it attempts to respond to the growing infection and tissue destruction. The duration and severity of activation of coagulation and survival inflammation proportionally increases the patient's risk for complications such as thrombosis (AVN), acute respiratory distress syndrome (ARDS), multiorgan dysfunction (MODS), and even death. (*B*) Through intervention with surgical debridement and antibiotic administration, the pathogen onslaught can be reduced, allowing the survival phase of the APR to be sufficient to stop bleeding and trap the remaining bacteria. However, as a result of the exuberant survival APR activated in response to infection, patients may still experience impaired tissue healing following the resolution of the infection (B-repair phase). (Figure permission: Schoenecker Laboratory.)

been suggested as a prognostic measure of critical illness, morbidity, and mortality in pediatric patients with MSKI.[33] This is reported to be in part due to the sequestration of platelets in microvessels, which can be reflected as thrombocytopenia in circulation, contributing to the pathogenesis of organ dysfunction. Although a patient's presenting symptoms, such as fever, indicate the activation of the APR, more sensitive measures of plasma reactants (ie, CRP and others) and cellular effectors (such as platelets and inflammatory cells) can aid in discerning the severity of the APR and accurately prognosticate the risk for complication. This is discussed in length in the following articles.[34–39]

Virulence factors drive disease severity through attacking the cellular acute phase response

As highlighted above, pyogenic organisms are the most common causative pathogens of pediatric MSKI with *S aureus* being responsible for 40% to

90% of cases.[3,18] In addition to antibacterial resistance genes, *S aureus* has acquired virulence factors to help the pathogen evade the host's cellular APR[40,41] and as a result have been associated with elevated inflammatory responses in pediatric MSKI.[42] Although the incidence varies between patient populations,[43–52] two examples of virulence factors observed in community-associated MSSA and MRSA are Pantone-Valentine Leukocidin (PVL) and leukocidin AB (LukAB). The expression of either PVL or LukAB promotes host leukocyte destruction through toxin-mediated pore formation and cellular lysis.[53–56] By evading the host's cellular APR, PVL and LukAB can drive *S aureus* infection severity by promoting dissemination, tissue necrosis, and elevating the inflammatory response.[53,55,57–59] Thus, treating physicians should consider the presence of acquired virulence factors, particularly in cases of community-associated *S aureus* infections (both MSSA and MRSA), to better prognosticate MSKI disease severity and patient outcomes.

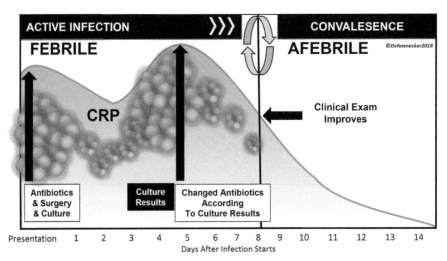

Fig. 5. Utility of serial laboratory values of the APR within a case. Trends, or the "Delta," in CRP can be useful in assessing disease progression and treatment efficacy in pediatric patients with MSKI. Early treatment is essential in treating MSKI, with antibiotics and surgery leading to a decrease in CRP over the first 2 days. However, when CRP begins increasing again over day 3 and 4, this can indicate to the treating physician that further intervention may be necessary. At this time, culture results showed inadequate antibiotic therapy and antibiotics were adjusted. After this point, the CRP once again began trending downward and the clinical examination improved. The body then entered the convalescent stage where tissue repair can begin. This case highlights the importance of both culture-directed therapy and the capacity for serial APR measures to assist with patient care. (Figure permission: Schoenecker Laboratory.)

TASK 4: HOW TO TREAT THE MUSCULOSKELETAL INFECTION

Antibiotics and surgical debridement are paramount for cessation of the continuous injury caused by an MSKI[30,32] (see Fig. 4B). In cases of local infections, treatment includes administration of antibiotics and the use of surgical debridement to reduce the source of the infection. In cases of disseminated infections, antibiotics continue to be paramount, but the medical care team must also consider medical management of organ dysfunction that can result from an exuberant APR.[30] In this final section, the authors highlight common treatment modalities, focusing on those aimed at combatting the MSKI and therapeutic options to combat an exuberant host APR.

Common Antibiotics Used in Pediatric Orthopedics

Before the advent of antibiotics, the mortality rate of acute hematogenous osteomyelitis in children was as high as 40%.[2,3] Fortunately, in current day medicine, the mortality rate from pediatric infections has dropped tremendously in recent years.[5,22,60] Antibiotics continue to be the first line of therapy for MSKI. In addition to culture results, patient factors can also inform antibiotic selection. As discussed above, a rapid

identification of the causative organisms is important given that it allows for earlier narrowing of antibiotic therapy, thereby decreasing the overuse of broad-spectrum antibiotics. Thus, in addition to collaborating with colleagues who specialize in infectious disease, it is important for pediatric orthopedic surgeons to have a broad understanding of the advantages and disadvantages of common antibiotics used to treat MSKI including beta-lactams, glycopeptides, lincosamides, lipopeptides, rifampin, and to a lesser degree, aminoglycosides.

Intravenous Versus Oral Administration: Is a Peripherally Inserted Central Catheter Line a Thing of the Past?

Traditionally, the duration and route of antibiotics administered depends on the institutional experience, the patient's response, and the type of tissue affected. For example, 2 to 4 weeks of IV antibiotics is often recommended for osteomyelitis followed by oral antibiotics for a total of 6 to 8 weeks. Some institutions have promoted shorter durations of IV antibiotics until CRP has decreased by 50% followed by 2 to 4 weeks of oral antibiotics.[61] In either case, IV antibiotics are commonly administered through a peripherally inserted central catheter (PICC). Beyond providing a secure route for vascular delivery of antibiotics, the use of a PICC line in pediatric patients is riddled with complications ranging from occlusion of the line to more serious complications such as infection or thrombosis.[62–64] For these reasons, physicians have begun to compare the effectiveness (ie, treatment failure) of oral versus IV antibiotic administration in pediatric patients with MSKI. A retrospective cohort study by Karen *and colleagues* in *JAMA Pediatric* illustrated that across 36 participating Children's Hospitals, PICC and oral antibiotic administration after discharge were equally as effective in patients with acute hematogenous osteomyelitis, yet patients with a PICC had a higher risk of returning to the emergency room or hospitalization for an adverse outcome.[65] This study highlights the need for physicians to challenge the long-standing belief that a PICC is essential for antibiotic care. As oral antibiotics continue to improve in efficacy and tissue penetration, IV administration beyond the time of hospitalization may not offer increased efficacy. Future prospective studies in cases of more severe, disseminated, infections will be essential for understanding the true potential for negating use of a PICC and their associated complications in pediatric patients with MSKI.

Antibacterial Resistance Impact on Musculoskeletal Infection Severity

As previously highlighted, physicians are now observing an increased rate of patients with MRSA-associated MSKI because of antibiotic administration and pathogen evolution. Although this trend brought great concern to the medical community, the relative severity of infections caused by MRSA versus MSSA remains controversial. Clinically, reports have suggested that compared with non-MRSA MSKI, patients with MRSA endure a more robust APR, have a longer hospital stay, and experience a higher rate of complications such as deep vein thrombosis, septic pulmonary emboli, and pathologic fractures.[66–70] Furthermore, in adult patients hospitalized for MRSA or MSSA infections, those with MRSA were reported to have poorer outcomes, including longer hospital stays, greater rates of complications, and increased mortality.[71] Alternatively, a recent retrospective study by An and colleagues demonstrated that in pediatric MSKI patients with *S aureus* infections, no significant difference in length of stay, days with a fever, or duration of antibiotics was observed between patients with MSSA versus MRSA.[72] In this retrospective study, although patients with MRSA underwent more operative interventions than MSSA; CRP (as a measure of the APR), temperature, white blood cell count (WBC) count, pulse,

and respiratory rate were all unable to differentiate patients with MRSA from those with MSSA.[72] This finding aligns with other studies reporting a variable success of prediction algorithms for distinguishing between MRSA versus MSSA by assessing four predictive parameters: a temperature higher than 100.4°F, a WBC count greater than 12,000 cells/μL, a hematocrit level less than 34%, and a CRP level greater than 13 mg/L.[73] Although initial reports found that 92% of all patients with all four predictors suffered from MRSA, subsequent studies have found diminished success (50%) using this algorithm.[74] As MSSA continues to gain the virulence factors that were once only prevalent in MRSA, the relative virulence of MRSA and MSSA and the associated severity of disease are likely becoming more comparable in certain regions then previously anticipate. Thus, although at one time it was beneficial to determine the difference between MRSA and MSSA to prognosticate disease severity, the dynamic genetic evolutions of these infectious organisms are quickly rendering this to be an arguable point.

Indications for Surgical Management: Culture, Excise, and Source Control

In collaboration with antibiotic administration to obtain cultures, reduce the infectious burden, and mitigate the associated APR, surgical debridement of the infected tissue can be required. Numerous factors should be considered when directing surgical intervention in these patients. For example, relative to assessing the severity of disease, any patient who is physiologically unstable secondary to an MSKI should be considered for urgent surgical debridement. This is particularly important in cases of rapidly progressing and destructive infections, such as necrotizing fasciitis.[75] Beyond these cases, the indications for surgery become less defined. In general, abscesses will not resolve on their own; thus, drainage and debridement are required. Depending on the location and severity of the MSKI, drainage, irrigation, and debridement can be done at the bedside, as a small radiographically guided procedure or may require an open approach to reach the source of the infection. This is particularly true when the infection lies deeper within tissues behind vital structures, involves multiple tissues, or has formed more complex fluid collections.[76] As highlighted above, a clear understanding of the location of the infection and the involvement of surrounding tissues from MRI can help guide surgical management and the prevention of inoculating noninfected tissues or joint spaces via the surgical or aspiration approach.

Pharmacologic Management of the Acute Phase Response

As highlighted above, overactivation of the APR in response to a severe and/or disseminated MSKI can result in marked changes in inflammation and coagulation. Thus, the most effective means to prevent and treat an exuberant APR is to mitigate the infection with antibiotics and surgical debridement, as highlighted above. To compliment these efforts, numerous studies in the adult population have begun to examine the therapeutic benefit of correcting hyperinflammation and the coagulopathies with the aim of reducing the morbidity and mortality of infection.[34,77–80] For example, prior studies have examined either the use of intravenous immunoglobulin (IVIG) or corticosteroids as a means to combat hyperinflammation associated with severe MSKI. In adult cases of Group A Streptococcus infections, including cases of severe necrotizing fasciitis, IVIG was theorized to help clear bacteria from the body and neutralize the superantigens, thereby reducing the rate of SIRS[81–85] Corticosteroid use is cases of severe infection or sepsis remains controversial in terms of efficacy.[86,87] In cases of severe infections like necrotizing fasciitis, corticosteroid administration has been suggested as a therapeutic means to reduce SIRS and improve patient outcomes.[75] Although the number of studies is limited,[88] in pediatric patients with septic arthritis use of corticosteroids as an adjunct to antibiotic administration, has been suggested to reduce patient pain, improve function of the infected joint at 12 months, reduce the number of days antibiotics are required, reduce the number of hospitalized days, and expedite the time to a normalized CRP. Together, these studies suggest that future controlled studies are required to identify the patient populations and clinical scenarios of MSKI where therapies will be most efficacious.

To combat coagulopathy driven by an MSKI, one of the most logical means is to replace the consumed coagulation factors. This has been attempted clinically by multiple pharmacologic means, including administration of fresh frozen plasma, administration of antithrombin and recombinant thrombomodulin, or supplementation with vitamin K.[89–91] Given that vitamin K is an essential cofactor for factors II, VII, IX, and X, protein C, and protein S, vitamin K supplementation has been examined in the setting of infection for the treatment of both hyper- and hypocoagulability with no reported adverse events.[75,77,92,93] In the authors' opinion, when considering potential morbidity associated with severe disseminated MSKI and the potential benefits (with minimal side effects) of vitamin K, administration may be worthwhile in cases of severe disease.

SUMMARY

Pediatric orthopedic surgeons are commonly consulted for cases of suspected MSKIs. Unlike other emergent consultations, such as fracture care, MSKIs can present with marked heterogeneity in disease location, causative organism, disease severity, and required treatment. Given that time is often the essence to promote optimal patient outcomes and reduce complication rates, there are four paramount tasks that all members of the medical and surgical team should set out to complete in cases of suspected pediatric MSKI. The team should determine: (1) where is the infection, (2) is it an infection and if so, what is the pathogen, (3) how severe is the infection including the risk of multiorgan dysfunction syndrome and death, and (4) how to treat the infection.

This review discussed the tools available to accomplish these four tasks in cases of pediatric MSKIs, highlighting current best practices and recent medical advancements. Importantly, physicians should be vigilant and never underestimate the pathogen, given that an exuberant APR can increase the risk of patient morbidity and mortality. Going forward, these tools should give treating physicians more confidence when evaluating patients with suspected MSKI.

CLINICS CARE POINTS

- The primary objective of caring for a child with a musculoskeletal infection (MSKI) is to prevent multiorgan dysfunction that can result in fatality.

- When evaluating a child for suspect MSKI focus should be on answering the following four questions, where is it, what is it, how severe is it, and how to treat it.

- Especially in children more than the age of 4 years, MSKI can be multifocal including bone, muscle, and intra-articular space. A fast-sequence MRI can be an invaluable tool in making this distinction.

- The acute phase response is a crucial aspect of fighting a bacterial infection in MSKI cases. However, excessive activation of this response can lead to the development of micro- and macro-thrombosis, which in turn can contribute to the development of adverse outcomes associated with MSKI.

- Laboratory values, such as C-reactive protein (CRP), are powerful indicators of MSKI severity. If repeated serially, measures of CRP can also help determine if an infection is worsening or improving.

- The primary mode of treatment for MSKI is antibiotics. Therefore, it is important to exercise caution and avoid withholding antibiotics to enhance the success of cultures in severely infected children or those susceptible to disease dissemination.

FUNDING

Funding for this work was supported by the Caitlin Lovejoy Fund, the Vanderbilt University Medical Center Department of Orthopaedics, the Vanderbilt School of Medicine Research Immersion program, and the Burroughs Wellcome Fund Physician-Scientist Institutional Award to Vanderbilt University (ID: 1018894). The Schoenecker laboratory is likewise supported in part by the NIH (5R01GM126062-05, 1R21AR080914-01, 1R21AR07908-01, 1R01AI173795-01), Department of Defense (W81XWH-18-1-0536), and Veterans Administration BLRD (1 IO1 BX005062).

ACKNOWLEDGMENTS

The authors would like to thank their Pediatric Orthopedic partners, as well as members of the Schoenecker laboratory, for their assistance in critically reviewing this work. As always, the authors would like to thank their families for their continued support. Finally, the authors would like to thank the physicians and medical staff who care for pediatric patients with MSKI at our institution—this work would not have bene possible without their dedication.

DISCLOSURE

The authors have nothing to disclose.

REFERENCES

1. Schoenecker JG, Shore BJ, Hedequest D, et al. The Children's Orthopaedic T, Infection Consortium for Evidence Based Study G. Defining the volume of consultations for musculoskeletal infection encountered by pediatric orthopaedic services in the United States. PLoS One 2020;15(6):e0234055.

2. Ciampolini J, Harding KG. Pathophysiology of chronic bacterial osteomyelitis. Why do antibiotics fail so often? Postgrad Med J 2000;76(898):479–83.

3. Song KM, Sloboda JF. Acute hematogenous osteomyelitis in children. J Am Acad Orthop Surg 2001; 9(3):166–75.

4. Gibian JT, Daryoush JR, Wollenman CC, et al. The Heterogeneity of Pediatric Knee Infections: A Retrospective Analysis. Journal of pediatric orthopedics 2019. https://doi.org/10.1097/bpo.0000000000001425.

5. Mignemi ME, Benvenuti MA, An TJ, et al. A Novel Classification System Based on Dissemination of Musculoskeletal Infection is Predictive of Hospital Outcomes. Journal of pediatric orthopedics 2018; 38(5):279–86.

6. Benvenuti MA, An TJ, Mignemi ME, et al. A Clinical Prediction Algorithm to Stratify Pediatric Musculoskeletal Infection by Severity. Journal of pediatric orthopedics 2019;39(3):153–7.

7. Alshryda S, Huntley JS, Banaszkiewicz PA. Paediatric orthopaedics: an evidence-based approach to clinical questions. Switzerland: Springer International Publishing; 2016.

8. Hobo T. Zur Pathogenese der akuten haematogenen Osteomyelitis. Acta Sch Med Univ Kioto 1921;4:1–29.

9. Cunningham R, Cockayne A, Humphreys H. Clinical and molecular aspects of the pathogenesis of *Staphylococcus aureus* bone and joint infections. J Med Microbiol 1996;44(3):157–64.

10. Mignemi ME, Menge TJ, Cole HA, et al. Epidemiology, diagnosis, and treatment of pericapsular pyomyositis of the hip in children. Journal of pediatric orthopedics 2014;34(3):316–25.

11. Comegna L, Guidone PI, Prezioso G, et al. Pyomyositis is not only a tropical pathology: a case series. J Med Case Rep 2016;10(1):1–6.

12. Shuler FD, Buchanan GS, Stover C, et al. Pyomyositis mistaken for septic hip arthritis in children: the role of MRI in diagnosis and management. Marshall Journal of Medicine 2018;4(2):22.

13. Chotai PN, Hsiao MS, Pathak I, et al. Pediatric pelvic pyomyositis: initial MRI can be misleading. J Pediatr Orthop B 2016;25(6):520–4.

14. Levitt DL, Byer R, Miller AF. Point-of-Care Ultrasound to Diagnose Pyomyositis in a Child. Pediatr Emerg Care 2019;35(1):69–71.

15. Section J, Gibbons SD, Barton T, et al. Microbiological Culture Methods for Pediatric Musculoskeletal Infection: A Guideline for Optimal Use. JBJS 2015;97(6):441–9.

16. Benvenuti MA, An TJ, Mignemi ME, et al. Effects of Antibiotic Timing on Culture Results and Clinical Outcomes in Pediatric Musculoskeletal Infection. J Pediatr Orthop 2019;39(3):158–62.

17. Arkader A, Brusalis C, Warner WC, et al. Update in Pediatric Musculoskeletal Infections: When It Is, When It Isn't, and What to Do. J Am Acad Orthop Surg 2016;24(9):e112–21.

18. Blyth MJ, Kincaid R, Craigen MA, et al. The changing epidemiology of acute and subacute

haematogenous osteomyelitis in children. J Bone Joint Surg Br 2001;83(1):99–102.

19. Peltola H, Kallio MJ, Unkila-Kallio L. Reduced incidence of septic arthritis in children by Haemophilus influenzae type-b vaccination. Implications for treatment. J Bone Joint Surg Br 1998;80(3):471–3.

20. Wong M, Williams N, Cooper C. Systematic Review of Kingella kingae Musculoskeletal Infection in Children: Epidemiology, Impact and Management Strategies. Pediatric Health Med Ther 2020;11: 73–84.

21. Masters EA, Ricciardi BF, Bentley KLdM, et al. Skeletal infections: microbial pathogenesis, immunity and clinical management. Nat Rev Microbiol 2022; 20(7):385–400.

22. Gafur OA, Copley LA, Hollmig ST, et al. The impact of the current epidemiology of pediatric musculoskeletal infection on evaluation and treatment guidelines. Journal of pediatric orthopedics 2008; 28(7):777–85.

23. Schwartz AM, Hinckley AF, Mead PS, et al. Surveillance for Lyme Disease - United States, 2008-2015. MMWR Surveill Summ 2017;66(22):1–12.

24. Zhorne DJ, Altobelli ME, Cruz AT. Impact of antibiotic pretreatment on bone biopsy yield for children with acute hematogenous osteomyelitis. Hosp Pediatr 2015;5(6):337–41.

25. Schoenecker J, Daryoush J, Gibian JT, et al, editors. Can CRP predict the need to esclate care after initial debridement for musculoskeltal infection? Virtual: POSNA; 2020.

26. Adebiyi EO, Ayoade F. Kingella kingae. Treasure Island (FL): StatPearls Publishing; 2019.

27. Yagupsky P, Erlich Y, Ariela S, et al. Outbreak of Kingella kingae skeletal system infections in children in daycare. Pediatr Infect Dis J 2006;25(6): 526–32.

28. Han J, Swan DC, Smith SJ, et al. Simultaneous amplification and identification of 25 human papillomavirus types with Templex technology. J Clin Microbiol 2006;44(11):4157–62.

29. Wood JB, Sesler C, Stalons D, et al. Performance of TEM-PCR vs Culture for Bacterial Identification in Pediatric Musculoskeletal Infections. Open Forum Infect Dis 2018;5(6). https://doi.org/10.1093/ofid/ofy119.

30. Benvenuti M, An T, Amaro E, et al. Double-Edged Sword: Musculoskeletal Infection Provoked Acute Phase Response in Children. Orthop Clin N Am 2017;48(2):181–97.

31. Mignemi NA, Yuasa M, Baker CE, et al. Plasmin prevents dystrophic calcification after muscle injury. J Bone Miner Res 2017;32(2):294–308.

32. An TJ, Benvenuti MA, Mignemi ME, et al. Pediatric Musculoskeletal Infection: Hijacking the Acute-Phase Response. JBJS Rev 2016;4(9). https://doi.org/10.2106/JBJS.RVW.15.00099.

33. Moore-Lotridge SN, Gibson BH, Duvernay MT, et al. Pediatric Musculoskeletal Infection. JPOSNA 2020;2(2).

34. Moore-Lotridge SN, Gibson BHY, Duvernay MT, et al. Pediatric Musculoskeletal Infection : An Update Through the Four Pillars of Clinical Care and Immunothrombotic Similarities With COVID-19. Journal of the Pediatric Orthopaedic Society of North America 2020;2(2). https://doi.org/10.55275/JPOSNA-2020-124.

35. Hysong AA, Posey SL, Blum DM, et al. Current concepts review necrotizing fasciitis: pillaging the acute phase response. J Bone Jt Surg Am Vol 2020;102(6):526.

36. Benvenuti M, An T, Amaro E, et al. Double-edged sword: musculoskeletal infection provoked acute phase response in children. Orthopedic Clinics 2017;48(2):181–97.

37. Amaro E, Marvi TK, Posey SL, et al. C-reactive protein predicts risk of venous thromboembolism in pediatric musculoskeletal infection. J Pediatr Orthop 2019;39(1):e62–7.

38. Benvenuti MA, An TJ, Mignemi ME, et al. A clinical prediction algorithm to stratify pediatric musculoskeletal infection by severity. Journal of pediatric orthopedics 2019;39(3):153.

39. Johnson SR, Benvenuti T, Nian H, et al. Measures of Admission Immunocoagulopathy as an Indicator for In-Hospital Mortality in Patients with Necrotizing Fasciitis: A Retrospective Study. JBJS Open Access 2023;8(1).

40. David MZ, Daum RS. Community-associated methicillin-resistant Staphylococcus aureus: epidemiology and clinical consequences of an emerging epidemic. Clin Microbiol Rev 2010;23(3):616–87.

41. Bennett MR, Thomsen IP. Epidemiological and Clinical Evidence for the Role of Toxins in S. aureus Human Disease. Toxins 2020;12(6):408.

42. Bocchini CE, Hulten KG, Mason EO, et al. Panton-Valentine leukocidin genes are associated with enhanced inflammatory response and local disease in acute hematogenous Staphylococcus aureus osteomyelitis in children. Pediatrics 2006;117(2): 433–40.

43. Huber H, Koller S, Giezendanner N, et al. Prevalence and characteristics of meticillin-resistant Staphylococcus aureus in humans in contact with farm animals, in livestock, and in food of animal origin, Switzerland, 2009. Euro Surveill 2010;15(16): 19542.

44. Zhang K, McClure J-A, Elsayed S, et al. Coexistence of Panton-Valentine Leukocidin—Positive and—Negative Community-Associated Methicillin-Resistant Staphylococcus aureus USA400 Sibling Strains in a Large Canadian Health-Care Region. The Journal of infectious diseases 2008; 197(2):195–204.

45. Wardyn SE, Forshey BM, Smith TC. High prevalence of Panton-Valentine leukocidin among methicillin-sensitive *Staphylococcus aureus* colonization isolates in rural Iowa. Microb Drug Resist 2012;18(4):427–33.

46. Cabrera EC, Ramirez-Argamosa DT, Rodriguez RD. Prevalence of community-acquired methicillin-resistant *Staphylococcus aureus* from inmates of the Manila City Jail, characterization for SCCmec type and occurrence of Panton-Valentine leukocidin gene. Philipp Sci Letters 2010;3(1):4–12.

47. Shore AC, Tecklenborg SC, Brennan GI, et al. Panton-Valentine leukocidin-positive *Staphylococcus aureus* in Ireland from 2002 to 2011: 21 clones, frequent importation of clones, temporal shifts of predominant methicillin-resistant S. aureus clones, and increasing multiresistance. J Clin Microbiol 2014;52(3):859–70.

48. Neela V, Ehsanollah GR, Zamberi S, et al. Prevalence of Panton–Valentine leukocidin genes among carriage and invasive *Staphylococcus aureus* isolates in Malaysia. Int J Infect Dis 2009;13(3):e131–2.

49. Krziwanek K, Luger C, Sammer B, et al. PVL-positive MRSA in Austria. Eur J Clin Microbiol Infect Dis 2007;26(12):931–5.

50. Wannet W, Heck M, Pluister G, et al. Panton-Valentine leukocidin positive MRSA in 2003: the Dutch situation. Euro Surveill 2004;9(11):3–4.

51. Brown ML, O'Hara FP, Close NM, et al. Prevalence and sequence variation of Panton-Valentine leukocidin in methicillin-resistant and methicillin-susceptible *Staphylococcus aureus* strains in the United States. J Clin Microbiol 2012;50(1):86–90.

52. Mediavilla JR, Chen L, Mathema B, et al. Global epidemiology of community-associated methicillin resistant *Staphylococcus aureus* (CA-MRSA). Curr Opin Microbiol 2012;15(5):588–95.

53. Daskalaki M, Rojo P, Marin-Ferrer M, et al. Panton–Valentine leukocidin-positive *Staphylococcus aureus* skin and soft tissue infections among children in an emergency department in Madrid, Spain. Clin Microbiol Infection 2010;16(1):74–7.

54. Melles DC, van Leeuwen WB, Boelens HAM, et al. Panton-Valentine leukocidin genes in *Staphylococcus aureus*. Emerg Infect Dis 2006;12(7):1174–5.

55. C S EG. Two cases of panton-valentine leukocidin (PVL) toxin positive *staphylococcus aureus* (MSSA) osteomyelitis in children. Orthopaedic Proceedings 2009;91-B(SUPP_II):213.

56. DuMont AL, Yoong P, Day CJ, et al. *Staphylococcus aureus* LukAB cytotoxin kills human neutrophils by targeting the CD11b subunit of the integrin Mac-1. Proc Natl Acad Sci USA 2013;110(26):10794–9.

57. Powers ME, Wardenburg JB. Igniting the fire: *Staphylococcus aureus* virulence factors in the pathogenesis of sepsis. PLoS Pathog 2014;10(2):e1003871.

58. Yoong P, Torres VJ. The effects of *Staphylococcus aureus* leukotoxins on the host: cell lysis and beyond. Curr Opin Microbiol 2013;16(1):63–9.

59. DuMont AL, Yoong P, Surewaard BG, et al. *Staphylococcus aureus* elaborates leukocidin AB to mediate escape from within human neutrophils. Infect Immun 2013;81(5):1830–41.

60. Dodwell ER. Osteomyelitis and septic arthritis in children: current concepts. Curr Opin Pediatr 2013;25(1):58–63.

61. Castellazzi L, Mantero M, Esposito S. Update on the Management of Pediatric Acute Osteomyelitis and Septic Arthritis. Int J Mol Sci 2016;17(6). https://doi.org/10.1097/MOP.0b013e32835c2b42.

62. Jumani K, Advani S, Reich NG, et al. Risk factors for peripherally inserted central venous catheter complications in children. JAMA Pediatr 2013;167(5):429–35.

63. Barrier A, Williams DJ, Connelly M, et al. Frequency of peripherally inserted central catheter complications in children. Pediatr Infect Dis J 2012;31(5):519–21.

64. Venkataraman ST. To PICC or Not to PICC, That Is the Question. Pediatr Crit Care Med 2018;19(12).

65. Keren R, Shah SS, Srivastava R, et al. Comparative Effectiveness of Intravenous vs Oral Antibiotics for Postdischarge Treatment of Acute Osteomyelitis in Children. JAMA Pediatr 2015;169(2):120–8.

66. Saavedra-Lozano J, Mejias A, Ahmad N, et al. Changing trends in acute osteomyelitis in children: impact of methicillin-resistant *Staphylococcus aureus* infections. Journal of pediatric orthopedics 2008;28(5):569–75.

67. Chiappini E, Mastrangelo G, Lazzeri S. A Case of Acute Osteomyelitis: An Update on Diagnosis and Treatment. Int J Environ Res Public Health 2016;13(6):539.

68. Saavedra-Lozano J, Mejías A, Ahmad N, et al. Changing Trends in Acute Osteomyelitis in Children: Impact of Methicillin-Resistant *Staphylococcus aureus* Infections. J Pediatr Orthop 2008;28(5).

69. Belthur MV, Phillips WA, Kaplan SL, et al. Letters to the editor. J Pediatr Orthop 2010;30(8):942.

70. Ryu DJ, Kang JS, Moon KH, et al. Clinical Characteristics of Methicillin-resistant *Staphylococcus aureus* Infection for Chronic Periprosthetic Hip and Knee Infection. Hip Pelvis 2014;26(4):235–42.

71. Chatterjee A, Rai S, Guddattu V, et al. Is methicillin-resistant *Staphylococcus aureus* infection associated with higher mortality and morbidity in hospitalized patients? A cohort study of 551 patients from South Western India. Risk Manag Healthc Pol 2018;11:243–50.

72. An TJ, Benvenuti MA, Mignemi ME, et al. Similar Clinical Severity and Outcomes for Methicillin-Resistant and Methicillin-Susceptible *Staphylococcus aureus*

Pediatric Musculoskeletal Infections. Open Forum Infect Dis 2017;4(1):ofx013–.

73. Ju KL, Zurakowski D, Kocher MS. Differentiating between methicillin-resistant and methicillin-sensitive *Staphylococcus aureus* osteomyelitis in children: an evidence-based clinical prediction algorithm. J Bone Jt Surg Am Vol 2011;93(18):1693–701.

74. Shrader MW, Nowlin M, Segal LS. Independent analysis of a clinical predictive algorithm to identify methicillin-resistant *Staphylococcus aureus* osteomyelitis in children. J Pediatr Orthop 2013;33(7): 759–62.

75. Hysong AA, Posey SL, Blum DM, et al. Necrotizing Fasciitis: Pillaging the Acute Phase Response. JBJS 2020;102(6):526–37.

76. Mignemi M, Copley L, Schoenecker J. Evidence-Based Treatment for Musculoskeletal Infection. Paediatric orthopaedics 2017;403–18. Springer.

77. Saracco P, Vitale P, Scolfaro C, et al. The coagulopathy in sepsis: significance and implications for treatment. Pediatr Rep 2011;3(4).

78. Fisher VR, Scott MK, Tremblay CA, et al. Disseminated intravascular coagulation: laboratory support for management and treatment. Lab Med 2013; 44(suppl_1):e10–4.

79. Levi M, Opal SM. Coagulation abnormalities in critically ill patients. Crit Care 2006;10(4):222.

80. Stutz CM, Lynda D, O'Neill KR, et al. Coagulopathies in orthopaedics: links to inflammation and the potential of individualizing treatment strategies. J Orthop Trauma 2013;27(4):236–41.

81. Morgan MS. Diagnosis and management of necrotising fasciitis: a multiparametric approach. J Hosp Infect 2010;75(4):249–57.

82. Rietveld JA, Pilmore HL, Jones PG, et al. Necrotising fasciitis: a single centre's experience. N Z Med J 1995;108(995):72–4.

83. Cawley MJ, Briggs M, Haith LR Jr, et al. Intravenous immunoglobulin as adjunctive treatment for streptococcal toxic shock syndrome associated with necrotizing fasciitis: case report and review. Pharmacotherapy 1999;19(9):1094–8.

84. Chiu C, Ou J, CHANG KS, et al. Successful treatment of severe streptococcal toxic shock syndrome with a combination of intravenous immunoglobulin, dexamethasone and antibiotics. Infection 1997; 25(1):47–8.

85. Lamothe F, D'Amico P, Ghosn P, et al. Clinical usefulness of intravenous human immunoglobulins in invasive group A streptococcal infections: case report and review. Clin Infect Dis 1995;21(6):1469–70.

86. Mason PE, Al-Khafaji A, Milbrandt EB, et al. CORTICUS: the end of unconditional love for steroid use? Crit Care 2009;13(4):309.

87. Marik PE, Pastores SM, Annane D, et al, American College of Critical Care Medicine. Recommendations for the diagnosis and management of corticosteroid insufficiency in critically ill adult patients: consensus statements from an international task force by the American College of Critical Care Medicine. Crit Care Med 2008;36(6):1937–49.

88. Delgado-Noguera MF, Forero Delgadillo JM, Franco AA, et al. Corticosteroids for septic arthritis in children. Cochrane Database Syst Rev 2018; 11(11):Cd012125.

89. Iba T, Levy JH, Raj A, et al. Advance in the management of sepsis-induced coagulopathy and disseminated intravascular coagulation. J Clin Med 2019; 8(5):728.

90. Nishida O, Ogura H, Egi M, et al. The Japanese clinical practice guidelines for management of sepsis and septic shock 2016 (J-SSCG 2016). Journal of intensive care 2018;6(1):1–77.

91. Arishima T, Ito T, Yasuda T, et al. Circulating activated protein C levels are not increased in septic patients treated with recombinant human soluble thrombomodulin. Thromb J 2018;16(1):24.

92. Levi M, de Jonge E, van der Poll T. Plasma and plasma components in the management of disseminated intravascular coagulation. Best Pract Res Clin Haematol 2006;19(1):127–42.

93. Azar FM, Calandruccio JH, Grear BJ, et al. Perioperative pain management, an issue of orthopedic clinics. Elsevier Health Sciences; 2017.

Sequestration and Involucrum

Understanding Bone Necrosis and Revascularization in Pediatric Orthopedics

Katherine S. Hajdu, BS[a], Courtney E. Baker, MD[b],
Stephanie N. Moore-Lotridge, PhD[b,c],
Jonathan G. Schoenecker, MD, PhD[b,c,d,e,f,*]

KEYWORDS

• Sequestration • Osteomyelitis • Involucrum • Induced membrane technique
• Immunocoagulopathy

KEY POINTS

• Sequestration is an infection-induced avascular necrosis of the diaphysis and/or metaphysis of bone.
• The body's acute phase response calls on cells, toxins, and matrices to trap and destroy microorganisms. This response is proportional to the extent of the infection and, if severe enough, the acute phase response may be upregulated to a point termed immunocoagulopathy where platelets and neutrophils use fibrin and DNA neutrophil extracellular traps (DNAnets) to contain the infection. While beneficial, by trapping the microorganism, it is speculated that this leads to immunothrombosis which impedes vascular flow in bone leading to sequestration.
• In the first stage of healing the avascular bone, when the periosteum remains viable, stem cells "shunt" vascularity and bone around the sequestration through a combination of intramembranous or endochondral ossification, similar as to how a fracture heals. This process is called involucrum.
• In the second stage of healing, the sequestration is removed from the intraosseous space and replaced with new vasculature and bone through predominately creeping substitution.
• If either of these processes fails, the induced membrane technique is a two-stage surgical procedure designed to heal sequestration. Like involucrum, the induced membrane technique creates a highly vascularized membrane, akin to periosteum, which promotes revascularization and bone formation.

INTRODUCTION

Sequestration and involucrum are terms frequently used in the context of osteomyelitis to describe the processes of avascular necrosis (AVN) and subsequent healing within the metaphysis or diaphysis. Sequestration refers to bone necrosis caused by a loss of blood supply

[a] School of Medicine, Vanderbilt University, Nashville, Tennessee, USA; [b] Department of Orthopedics, Vanderbilt University Medical Center, Nashville, Tennessee, USA; [c] Vanderbilt Center for Bone Biology, Vanderbilt University Medical Center, Nashville, Tennessee, USA; [d] Department of Pathology, Microbiology and Immunology, Vanderbilt University Medical Center, Nashville, Tennessee, USA; [e] Department of Pharmacology, Vanderbilt University, Nashville, Tennessee, USA; [f] Department of Pediatrics, Monroe Carell Jr. Children's Hospital at Vanderbilt, Nashville, Tennessee, USA
* Corresponding author. 1155 MRB4, 2215-B Garland Avenue, Nashville, TN 37232.
E-mail address: Jon.schoenecker@vumc.org

Orthop Clin N Am 55 (2024) 233–246
https://doi.org/10.1016/j.ocl.2023.09.005

secondary to thrombosis.[1] The blood supply can be disrupted from a pathologically exuberant immune and coagulation system response—termed immunocoagulopathy—or from surgical debridement to address the infection.[2–5] The necrotic bone, known as a sequestrum, is structurally compromised, prone to pathologic fractures, and causes pain.

As part of the healing process in response to sequestrum, the body forms new bone first shunting around the necrotic area. This new bone is termed involucrum. Periosteum or endosteum drives this healing process by establishing a vascular network that surrounds the avascular sequestrum. From this initial vascular network, new bone is formed in the intraosseous space, mostly through creeping substitution.

This review explores the pathophysiology of sequestration and involucrum with an emphasis on fundamental bone biology principles. A thorough understanding of bone biology and the pathology of sequestration provides a clear picture for how to treat this process when the body is unsuccessful and offers clues to potential therapies for the future.

Bone Is a Highly Vascular Organ

Understanding the pathologic process of sequestration and involucrum begins with an appreciation of bone's anatomy and blood supply as sequestration results from a loss of blood flow in the diaphysis and/or metaphysis (Figs. 1 and 2). Osteoblasts, the primary bone-forming cells, are dependent on a steady supply of oxygen and nutrients for energy and bone-building substrates. These cells cannot survive more than 1 to 2 days without vascularity.[6] Owing to the limited diffusion of oxygen and nutrients through calcified tissue, osteoblasts must be within 200 μm of a fenestrated capillary to survive.[7] Consequently, bone is a highly vascular organ that is perfused via a combination of metaphyseal/epiphyseal (Fig. 2), diaphyseal, endosteal, and periosteal arteries.[8] These arteries create a vast, open-sinusoidal vascular network within the medullary space that supplies both cortical and medullary bone.[9,10] Nutrient arteries (see Fig. 2A) are the primary blood supply to long bones.[11,12] They enter the medullary canal through the diaphysis in a centripetal fashion ("outside to in"), branching out into medullary vessels that supply the endosteum

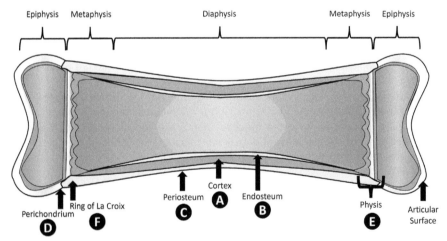

Fig. 1. Skeletally immature bone anatomy. (A) Cortical bone, referred to as the cortex, is a thick external shell of compact bone that contains Haversian canals allowing for blood vessel passage. Two fibrovascular layers surround the cortex. (B) The innermost layer is the endosteum which separates the cortical bone from the medullary space. The medullary space contains trabecular, spongy bone that is less dense and haematopoietically active. (C) The periosteum surrounds the external side of the cortex except at the articular surface of the epiphysis. The periosteum is a highly vascularized reservoir of stem cells known as pericytes. (D) The periosteum is contiguous with the perichondrium, another thick fibrovascular tissue. The perichondrium circumferentially surrounds the cartilage of the developing bone at the physis and articular surface in children. (E) The physis is a bone-forming machine of multiple layers spanning from the zone of ossification to the epiphyseal plate. Within the physis is a cartilaginous, avascular area that separates the metaphyseal and epiphyseal vascularity as no blood vessels cross this structure. Adjacent to the germinal cells of the physis is the epiphyseal plate, which mechanically supports the physis and prevents epiphyseal blood vessels from touching the physeal germinal cells. (F) The ring of La Croix is an area near the physis containing perivascular stem cells that proliferate and migrate into the physis to promote longitudinal bone growth. Copyright Schoenecker 2023

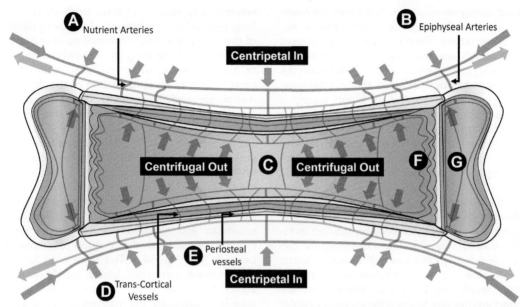

Fig. 2. Vascular anatomy of developing bone. Bone is a highly vascular organ. (*A*) Nutrient arteries are large caliber blood vessels, which penetrate the diaphysis and metaphysis of developing bone. (*B*) Alternatively, epiphyseal arteries must enter at the epiphysis, where they centripetally provide blood pumped from the heart to bone. (*C*) Once inside of the bone, this external blood supply combined with blood produced from the medullary cavity and is recycled to the rest of bone in a centrifugal fashion. (*D*) Transcortical vessels (TCVs) facilitate centrifugal perfusion. These vessels (both arterial and venous) traverse the endosteum and cortex to connect the bone marrow to the periosteum (*E*) and are an important facilitator of bone perfusion and venous drainage. At the ends of long bone, the physis separates the blood supply of the epiphysis from the metaphysis. Abutting the metaphyseal side of the physis are (*F*) metaphyseal vessels that end at the growth plate as large capillary loops with slow flow. The ingress of these blood vessels into the physis enables the production of primary spongiosum creating the zone of ossification. (*G*) Subchondral bone of the epiphysis is supplied solely by epiphyseal arteries which additionally provide nutrients and oxygen to the germinal cells of the physis via diffusion across the epiphyseal plate. Therefore, a disruption in the epiphyseal vasculature can also affect the germinal cells of the physis. Copyright Schoenecker 2023

and penetrate the cortex following the Haversian canal system. These transcortical vessels (see Fig. 2D) supply the cortex of bone in a centrifugal fashion ("inside to out") and connect the periosteum directly to the bone marrow.[13–18]

During skeletal development, the growth plate or physis (see Fig. 1E) separates the epiphysis from the metaphysis. The physis is composed of chondrocytes which, unlike osteoblasts, thrive in hypoxia.[19] The physis is therefore avascular. However, the subchondral bone of the epiphysis, adjacent to the physis, is very vascular as a result of the formation of a secondary ossification center. Chondrocytes at the physis receive nutrients from the epiphyseal vasculature via diffusion across the epiphyseal plate.[20,21] Within the physis, the chondrocytes are arranged in longitudinal columns in the direction of growth. The physis generates a steady state of new chondrocytes which hypertrophy until they are met by the metaphyseal vasculature. The metaphyseal vasculature is drawn into the physis via vascular endothelial growth factor

(VEGF) signaling produced by hypertrophic chondrocytes. This ingress of vessels disrupts the chondrocyte's hypoxic microenvironment and results in the transition from cartilage anlage to new bone.[22,23] Thus, the metaphysis of the growing skeleton, due to its high activity, is the most vascularized area of bone. Furthermore, as described by Hobo,[24] the vascularity at the metaphysis ends as a system of capillary loops where flow is slower. Therefore, the metaphysis is the most common site for osteomyelitis initiation due to its abundant vascularity and slow flow (see Fig. 2F).[9,24] The avascular chondrocytic physis is thus surrounded by invading metaphyseal vasculature and epiphyseal vessels that are physically separated from the physis via the epiphyseal plate. Once skeletal maturity is reached, the steady-state production of new chondrocytes by the physis slows and is then exceeded by the rate of invading vessels which overtakes and obliterates the physis.

Contiguous with the physis, periosteum is a multilayered tissue enveloping bone and most robust during development. It is a massive reservoir for bone-forming stem cells and a key vascular structure. The outer brous layer houses blood vessels, and the inner cambium layer contains pericyte progenitor cells.[25,26] Although the periosteum has both external and internal sources of perfusion, most of its blood supply is derived from centrifugal flow from blood within the intramedullary canal.[27] The periosteum is most robust in the metaphysis/diaphysis and thinner within the epiphysis, leading to distinct pathologic processes in these regions.[28]

Infection Causes a Vascular Insult

Following an infection, when vascularity to the diaphysis or metaphysis is disrupted, an avascular area of bone forms. Osteomyelitis can also affect the epiphysis as in the case of septic arthritis, leading to epiphyseal AVN. Importantly, epiphyseal AVN and sequestrum are distinct entities due to the differences in vascular anatomy, periosteum quantity, and the role of the physis in separating metaphyseal vascularity from the epiphysis. These differences in uence how necrotic bone heals in various locations and the unique complications they may cause (see below for more detail).

Osteomyelitis Induces Immunocoagulopathy and Immunothrombosis

The precise cause of vascular disruption in osteomyelitis that leads to sequestrum remains uncertain, though it is likely multifactorial and in large part related to the body's response to the infectious agent. The coagulation and innate immune systems are the body's primary defenses for containing an infection. Containment is achieved through the formation of a "damage matrix," primarily composed of fibrin (Fig. 3B).[29–31] In addition to containing the microorganisms, this matrix serves as a pathway for innate immune cells, such as neutrophils and macrophages, to enter the zone of infection and eliminate or engulf the pathogens.[2,3,32]

In severe osteomyelitis, standard containment mechanisms may prove insuf cient, particularly against virulent organisms like *Staphylococcus aureus* that can evade or manipulate the fibrin-laden damage matrix.[33] In response to this breach of containment, the body reinforces the fibrin matrix with neutrophil extracellular traps (NETs) composed of DNA and histones from in flammatory cells to better contain and trap the bacteria (see Fig. 3C).[32,34] This fortified damage matrix supports containment by being more resistant to degradation; however, this makes the damage matrix more thrombotic and

inflammatory which can drive both short- and long-term adverse outcomes. This upregulation of the damage matrix is referred to as *immunocoagulopathy*, indicating the intertwined activity of the innate immune and coagulation systems.[1,35] Although upregulation of the damage matrix successfully contains the infection, it also leads to vascular disruption or obstruction and subsequent avascularity (see Fig. 3D).

Furthermore, formation of a subperiosteal abscess can further contribute to vascular obstruction and AVN. As described by Trueta, either direct accumulation of purulence from the infection or vascular congestion causing indirect exudate accumulation can form an abscess that separates and elevates the periosteum from the cortex due to the buildup of material beneath (see Fig. 3A).[9] This separation further compromises periosteal blood supply to the adjacent cortical bone.[36] Interestingly, recent studies challenging this pathomechanism suggest that subperiosteal abscess formation may occur irrespective of osteomyelitis.[37] However, our current understanding suggests hematogenous seeding of the subperiosteal space most likely comes from bacteria in the blood stream following the centrifugal flow through bone into the periosteal space.

Once the infection has been eliminated, the body begins repairing itself. Before revascularization or ossi cation, the damage matrix needs to be removed. This process requires plasminogen activation to plasmin for brin degradation and macrophage clearance of NETs (see Fig. 3E).[38] Following removal, large areas of devascularized bone need to be resolved, and the repair mechanisms that the body uses are the same as those used to heal a fracture.

Sequestrum, Such as Fractures, Heal via Coordinated Teams of Cells

Sequestrum creates a zone of hypoxia and structural weakness—which is akin to a fracture. As such, the regenerative processes that resolve sequestrum are best characterized in the context of fracture healing. A thorough review on this topic and the speci c cells involved can be found in the recent publication by Baker and colleagues.[19]

Fractures typically heal through a process of secondary bone healing. Secondary bone healing is a mix of intramembranous angiogenesis/ossi cation and endochondral angiogenesis/ossi cation as determined by the local fracture microenvironment. Once bone fractures, blood ow increases to the periosteum in a centrifugal manner. Yuasa and colleagues demonstrated

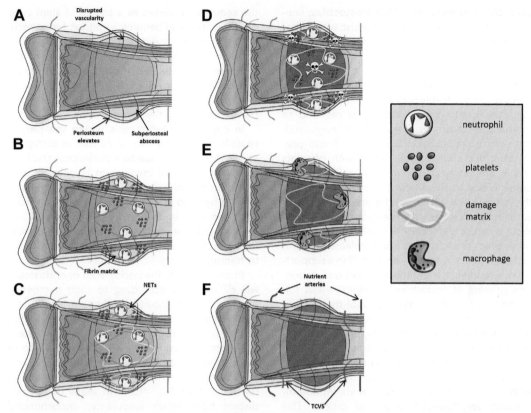

Fig. 3. Osteomyelitis can lead to sequestration. (*A*) Infection most commonly first initiates in the metaphysis, in the zone of ossification, due to large capillary loops and slow flow. The bacteria travels through the intraosseous circulation where they can seed anywhere within the metaphysis or diaphysis. As the infection progresses, exudate and purulence build up within the bone. When exuberant amounts of purulence are formed, it will continue through the cortex and build up under the fibrovascular periosteum which elevates off the cortex. Separation of the periosteum and cortex disrupts the continuity of the TCVs compounding avascularity to the underlying bone. (*B*) The innate immune (lymphocytes such as the neutrophils and macrophages) and coagulation systems (platelets) are activated in response to the infection. The coagulation system lays down a fibrin matrix to contain the infection and facilitate the infiltration of immune cells. (*C*) To further support containment of the infection, neutrophils expel neutrophil extracellular traps (NETs) during their death to fortify the fibrin creating an antiseptic damage matrix that is more resistant to degradation. (*D*) Owing to a combination of the infection itself and the body's response to the infection, vessels supplying bone become disrupted or obstructed leading to avascularity and ultimately, bone necrosis. (*E*) As the body shifts to repair these areas of necrotic bone, plasmin and other enzymes work to break down the damage matrix allowing macrophages to phagocytose and clear out the debris. (*F*) Left behind is sequestration, an area of necrotic bone in either the metaphysis or diaphysis. The nutrient artery and TCVs surrounding the area of sequestrum have remained intact. Copyright Schoenecker 2023

the elegantly linked temporal and spatial development of vascularity in a healing displaced fracture.[39] Following a displaced fracture, there is a vascular shunt through transcortical vessels to the periosteum. At the edge of a fracture blood is shunted where vascularity is intact, creating high oxygen tension and low strain, such that intramembranous ossification can occur to create new bone directly. Alternatively, in the center of a fracture where all vessels are disrupted and displacement is greater, hypoxia and strain are in abundance and osteoblasts cannot survive. Instead, an intermediate structure, a callus composed of chondrocytes, must be formed to resolve strain and hypoxia before osteoblasts can repopulate. This is the process of endochondral ossification, the formation of bone through a cartilage intermediate. The major cell types involved in secondary bone healing include prehypertrophic chondrocytes, hypertrophic chondrocytes, endothelial cells, and osteoblasts. These cells differentiate from pericytes that migrate into the area of injury from one of two dominant sources—periosteum and endosteum. In both fracture healing and sequestration depending on the microenvironment, these stem cells can progress into the osteoblast lineage or chondrocyte lineage to assist with either intramembranous or endochondral ossification, respectively.[4,40–42]

Chondrocytes thrive in hypoxic environment and thus predominate at the fracture gap. Two types of chondrocytes play a role in fracture healing. Pre-hypertrophic chondrocytes respond to mechanical strain by creating an organized, force-absorbing extracellular matrix. These pre-hypertrophic chondrocytes along with platelets and inflammatory cells form a soft callus proportional in size to the amount of strain present at the fracture site. Once interfragmentary strain is sufficiently reduced by the pre-hypertrophic chondrocyte, these chondrocytes grow, becoming hypertrophic chondrocytes that release growth factors to direct vascularity and creating a supportive environment for osteoblasts and ossification. This process of endochondral angiogenesis followed by ossification continues until the fracture is bridged and union occurs. This newly formed bone then begins the remodeling phase to return the cortical bone to a pre-injury state.

At the periphery of the fracture, where there is less strain and the bone's centrifugal vascularity is intact, the bone will heal via intramembranous angiogenesis and ossification. This occurs outside the cortex of bone in the subperiosteal space. Stem cells from the endosteum or periosteum can directly differentiate into osteoblasts due to microenvironmental conditions and availability. The intact transcortical vessels at the periphery increase in size as new bone is laid down. Furthermore, this initial healing process helps to initiate the endochondral angiogenesis and ossification to follow in the fracture gap.

Sequestration's avascular microenvironment imitates the hypoxic fracture gap. Therefore, sequestration following infection heals similarly to a fracture using a combination of intramembranous angiogenesis and ossification and endochondral angiogenesis and ossification.

Involucrum, Derived from Periosteum, Creates a Vascular Shunt Around Sequestration

In sequestration, the medullary and cortical bone of the metaphysis and diaphysis become devascularized, increasing blood flow to the periosteum, similar to the shunting of blood observed in fractures (Fig. 4A).[14,18,43] However, unlike fractures, where the periosteum is physically torn and displaced due to the injury, the continuity and vascular integrity of the surrounding periosteum may be maintained in sequestration.[44] In this way, the periosteum that is remaining around the sequestrum serves as a source of stem cells, pericytes, and can become a conduit for revascularization and ossification (see Fig. 4B–G).[45] Furthermore, the new bone forming from the engorged periosteum in response to sequestrum is referred to as involucrum (see Fig. 4H). Radiologically, the involucrum can be seen as thick new bone surrounding the sequestration (Fig. 5).[45]

In cases of osteomyelitis where the periosteum is significantly devascularized or disrupted either surgically or due to a pathologic fracture, the appearance of involucrum is delayed at a minimum and often never forms at all. The large area of hypoxia stimulates production of VEGF, which drives endochondral angiogenesis to create a vascular anastomosis between the proximal and distal sites of the sequestration similar to fracture healing.

Stem cells from the periosteum or endosteum will differentiate according to their microenvironment. Areas around involucrum have intact vascularity and relatively low strain at the edge of the necrotic region. In these locations, stem cells from the periosteum or endosteum can promote rapid resorption of the dead bone and subsequent intramembranous ossification to replace it (see Fig. 4C).[40] In areas of hypoxia distant from intact vascularity, endochondral ossification is the preferred mechanism of bone formation. Periosteal-derived stem cells in this area can differentiate into chondrocytes, which resolve the microenvironment, undergo hypertrophy, and release growth factors that promote endochondral angiogenesis and ossification (see Fig. 4D–F).

As opposed to the subperiosteal space where new bone can be made unimpeded, bone necrosis in the area of sequestration must be cleared before vascular invasion and bone formation can begin. Without surgical intervention to clear away the dead bone, the body must resorb the necrosis via creeping substitution, a slow process of simultaneous bone resorption and deposition along with gradual vascular ingress.[46,47] Hypoxia as well as other factors in bone upregulates osteoclastogenesis, which introduces osteoclasts to help breakdown and remove sequestration.[48–50] As osteoclasts clear the necrotic bone, vessels can begin to invade the hypoxic microenvironment bringing with them new stem cells to lay down bone via intramembranous ossification (Fig. 6). We speculate the bone marrow and endosteum are most likely providing the stem cells for new bone formation within the medullary canal as they are anatomically adjacent. Therefore, the mechanism by which bone is made in sequestration is probably

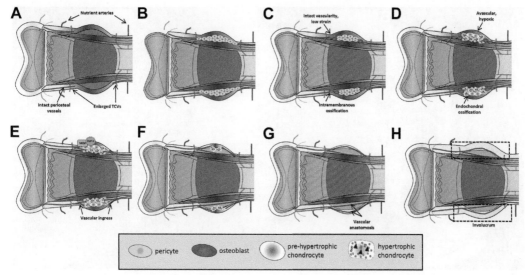

Fig. 4. Revascularization and ossification of the subperiosteal space via periosteum. (*A*) Osteomyelitis is accompanied by an increase in perfusion of the periosteum from the TCVs and nutrient artery. It is important to acknowledge that although this figure displays intact yet avascular periosteum, periosteum may retain its vascularity depending on the severity of infection. (*B*) Vascular disruption and injury from the infection stimulates the release of growth factors and chemoattractant that support the recruitment of stem cells. In the subperiosteal space, (*C*) these undifferentiated stem cells can directly become osteoblast in areas of low strain and intact vascularity at the necrotic edge. (*D–F*) In areas distant from vascularity, the hypoxic microenvironment promotes stem cell differentiation into a chondrocyte lineage, which supports endochondral ossification. Two populations of chondrocytes facilitate endochondral ossification. Pre-hypertrophic chondrocytes mechanically resolve the strain within the microenvironment to make it suitable for vascular ingress. Once the microenvironment is suitable for endothelial cell migration and vascular ingress, the pre-hypertrophic chondrocytes transition into hypertrophic chondrocytes. These hypertrophic chondrocytes release growth factors, vascular endothelial growth factor (VEGF) and bone morphogenetic protein 2 (BMP-2), to promote angiogenesis and subsequent ossification. (*G*) This process continues until there is vascular anastomosis between the proximal and distal sites of the sequestration. (*H*) Following, the periosteum lays down new bone via intramembranous ossification to form involucrum, vascularized bone circumventing sequestration. Copyright Schonecker 2023

distinctly different than in the subperiosteal space.

Strain is an important stimulus for endochondral ossi cation. In fracture healing, strain promotes the progression of endochondral ossi cation and the formation of a fracture callus.[51–53] Specifically, cyclic tensile strain has been demonstrated to promote both endochondral ossification and intramembranous ossification of mesenchymal stem cells (MSCs), derived from bone marrow.[54] However, too little or too much strain can lead to delayed healing, nonunion, or fracture. The importance of mechanical stimulation to promote and speedup revascularization is also true in healing sequestration. However, if the bone remains mechanically intact, there is little stimulus for endochondral angiogenesis and the healing process occurs more slowly. Sequestrum that leads to a non- or minimally-displaced pathologic fracture may ultimately accelerate the overall healing process because of this increased stimulus.

CLINICAL IMPLICATIONS
Identify Involucrum
Injured tissues cannot move on to the healing phase of the acute phase response until the risk of bleeding and infection is resolved.[19] Therefore, when managing and treating sequestration, clinicians must identify where the infection is located and how severe the infection is to determine how best to treat it.[55] Physical examination, laboratory assessment, and imaging are used to determine the location of the infection as well as the adequacy of infection control. Treatment will almost always involve antibiotic therapy with or without the aid of surgical debridement.

Once the infection is appropriately managed, further treatment decisions to support repair are in uenced by the status of the periosteum. Advanced imaging techniques such as MRI or PET scans can help determine indirectly whether the periosteum is viable and if involucrum is forming or has already formed. As highlighted

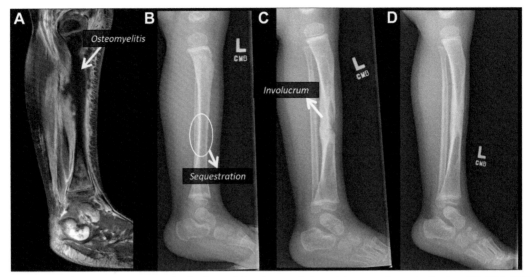

Fig. 5. Clinical case: sequestration heals through involucrum followed by creeping substitution. (A) STIR MRI sequence of a child with osteomyelitis of the mid-diaphysis tibia (*yellow arrow*). (B) Lateral radiograph of the leg demonstrating an area of lucency which is sequestration, devascularized bone of the diaphysis (*yellow arrow*). (C) Circumventing sequestration is involucrum which has formed through a combination of intramembranous angiogenesis and ossification and endochondral angiogenesis and ossification (yellow *arrow*). (D) The gradual process of creeping substitution fills in the area of sequestration until it is healed. STIR, short tau inversion recovery. Copyright Schoenecker 2023

above, on radiographs and CT scans, involucrum appears as thick, sclerotic bone,[45] whereas enhancement on MRI or PET scan within this area suggests intact vascularity (**Fig. 7**).[56]

If involucrum is present, it is reasonable to allow the bone to heal without surgical intervention, even in the presence of sequestration. Unlike fractures, which often require surgical intervention for quicker recovering and deformity prevention, sequestration alone many times does not necessitate operative management if involucrum is also present. In fact, encouraging weight-bearing and activity can expedite the healing process in certain cases as it stimulates strain and subsequent endochondral angiogenesis.[53,57–60] Clinical judgment and practice-based intuition is crucial to determine which patients should be allowed to weight bear, as significant pathologic fractures following osteomyelitis in children can occur if the bone and/or involucrum is mechanically insufficient.[61] Although non- or minimally-displaced pathologic fractures may speed up healing, they should be avoided as they can also lead to other complications and require further surgical treatment.

A study on the rate of pathologic fractures in children following S aureus osteomyelitis reported that 4.7% (364/17) experienced a fracture within 3 months after their injury.[62] The primary risk factor for fracture was the severity and complexity of the infection and its subsequent inflammatory response. Patients in the fracture group had a longer average hospital stay, longer duration of antibiotics, more inpatient complications, and a higher number of surgical procedures. A subperiosteal abscess extending more than 50% of the bone circumference was associated with an increased risk of fracture. These findings align with the intuition that a more severe infection leads to a large immunothrombosis, resulting in a larger area of devascularized bone and significant biomechanical compromise. Future research into methods of assessing the *in vivo* mechanical strength of bone and the developing involucrum would be invaluable for treating these patients. Methods such as finite elemental analysis from CT imaging have been used for research settings to assess bone quality,[63,64] but its clinical application in this setting is yet to be fully understood.

WHAT TO DO WHEN INVOLUCRUM DOES NOT FORM

Involucrum may not form when the periosteum has been disrupted due to an extremely virulent organism, following thrombosis secondary to immunocoagulopathy or after surgical debridement. In these cases, treatment modalities such as induced membrane technique can be considered to accelerate healing and promote bony union. Otherwise, the sequestrum may fracture

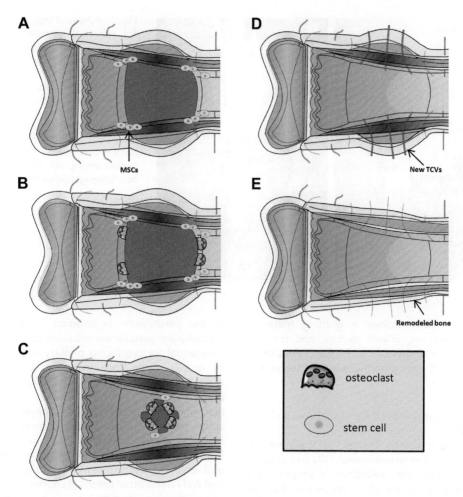

Fig. 6. Revascularization and ossification through creeping substitution. (*A*) Mesenchymal stem cells (MSCs), pericytes, are recruited to the area of injury caused by the prior infection to resolve bone necrosis. (*B*, *C*) Osteoclasts are upregulated to resolve the necrotic bone, whereas phagocytic cells work to clear the debris making way for vascular ingress and bone formation. (*D*) Eventually, new TCVs form reinstating the vascular connection between the medullary space and periosteum in the injured bone. (*E*) Following, as bone remodels, bone circulation resumes homeostatic conditions, and the medullary space resumes hematopoietic activity. Copyright Schoenecker 2023

from biomechanically compromised bone, premature load-bearing, or failure to revascularize and heal.

The induced membrane technique has shown considerable success for treatment of sequestration that fails to heal through involucrum.[65] This technique, first introduced by Professor Masquelet in 1986, is a two-stage surgical procedure.[66,67] The first stage of the procedure involves the thorough removal of the sequestrum until healthy, bleeding tissue is exposed. This is followed by the placement of a polymethylmethacrylate cement spacer into the defect, along with either temporary or permanent fixation. The cement spacer prevents fibrous tissue from invading the defect, instead triggering a local reaction that forms a highly vascularized

pseudosynovial membrane, rich in growth factors, essentially acting as a periosteum.[68] After a period of 6 to 8 weeks, the induced membrane is carefully incised, the spacer is removed, and the membrane is packed with morselized cancellous bone graft, typically sourced from the iliac crest, before definitive fixation is applied. The induced membrane serves to prevent the resorption of the graft and promotes revascularization and bone formation, much like the periosteum. Despite its overall success rate of 91% in children, the technique comes with a high rate of complications (54%), including fractures, joint stiffness, and deformities.[69] There is also a risk of significant graft resorption, even though the induced membrane is designed to protect against it. This technique has been widely

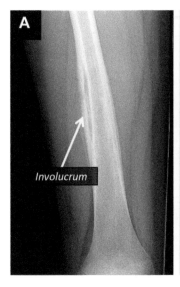 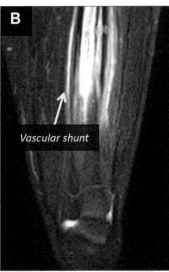

Fig. 7. Advanced imaging to assess for periosteal vascularity. (*A*) AP radiograph of the femur diaphysis demonstrating involucrum (*yellow arrow*) shunting around an area of sequestration. (*B*) Hyperintensity on this MRI sequence suggests vascularity is intact within the involucrum creating a vascular shunt and anastomosis between the proximal and distal portions of the affected bone (*yellow arrow*). AP, anterior-posterior. Copyright Schoenecker 2023

modified with variations in grafting material, bone substitutes, growth factors, and the use of vascularized grafts.[70,71] Further research is needed to fully compare these various technique modifications.

Sequestration Versus Epiphyseal Avascular Necrosis

It is important to acknowledge that there are key differences between epiphyseal AVN and sequestration within the metaphysis/diaphysis that significantly influence their respective healing processes. Although both are caused by a loss of vascular supply to bone, the unique vascular anatomy of these regions impacts their pathology and treatment. The epiphysis, as a result of its intra-articular location, has a limited number of nutrient arteries and less periosteum making it more susceptible to a loss of blood supply and less capable of forming involucrum. As previously discussed, the physis depends on epiphyseal vasculature for its nutrients and oxygen, which diffuse across the epiphyseal plate to nourish the adjacent germinal cells.[72] Disruption of the epiphyseal vasculature can lead to the death of these cells, resulting in a shortened physis, slower bone growth, and potentially a physeal arrest or physeal bar. This is especially true if the epiphysis revascularizes through a metaphyseal to epiphyseal mechanism, which obliterates the physis.

In contrast, the metaphysis and diaphysis benefit from a robust, often redundant, blood supply, and ample periosteum. These regions of bone are therefore more resilient to AVN and are much more capable of healing through the formation of involucrum, which is stimulated by the periosteum. In addition, although the metaphyseal vascular contribution to the physis is essential for producing primary spongiosum, its loss is more likely to cause a reversible widening of the physis due to a failure to form bone, as opposed to a devastating physeal arrest, which occurs with loss of epiphyseal vascularity. These differences likely account for the observation that sequestration typically heals faster and leads to no change in limb length, or if anything, overgrowth.[9] In contrast, epiphyseal AVN more often results in shorter angulated limbs following infection.

Future Directions

Improving diagnostic techniques is a crucial area for future research. Specifically, the development of imaging modalities that can accurately assess the integrity and viability of the periosteum would be invaluable. The improved use of current imaging data to assess structural integrity of the bone and risk of pathologic fractures is warranted. Such tools would enable clinicians to identify which patients are most likely to heal without intervention from those at risk for further complication, thereby sparing those unnecessary treatments or interventions. This would represent a significant step forward in personalized medicine, allowing for more targeted and effective treatment strategies.

Enhancing the induced membrane technique to create a new periosteum could significantly improve the management of sequestration. Currently, this procedure requires two stages and comes with a high rate of complication. Efforts should be directed toward refining this technique, with the ultimate goal of developing a single-stage procedure. This would not only reduce the burden on patients but also potentially improve outcomes by minimizing the risk of complications associated with multiple surgeries. Alternative bioengineered materials or growth factors to enhance the formation and function of the induced membrane are actively being explored.[73–76] Together, these modifications could markedly improve outcomes of the induced membrane technique for the treatment of sequestration and potentially new applications to other orthopedic conditions.

Prevention still remains the most effective approach in managing sequestration. If sequestration originates from an immunocoagulopathy leading to immunothrombosis, then prophylactic anticoagulation or targeted immune modulators could be bene cial. If found true, this therapeutic approach could represent a signi cant leap forward in managing sequestration, bringing us closer to a future where prevention becomes a feasible option.

In conclusion, the future of sequestration management lies in improving diagnostics, medical management, and surgical techniques. By focusing our efforts on these areas, we can markedly improve the prognosis for patients suffering from this challenging condition.

SUMMARY

Sequestration is an area of devascularized bone that heals through the same coordinated team of cells as a fracture to resolve hypoxia, promote vascular ingress, and nally, ensure mechanical stability through bone formation. Sequestration differs from fracture healing in its drastically reduced strain to stimulate endochondral angiogenesis/ossi cation for repair and typically, an intact periosteum. Intact periosteum, when present, acts as a vascular anastomosis around the avascular space and is a robust supply of vessels for arborization and stem cells, which helps to improve healing. Understanding the bone and vascular biology underlying the sequestration healing has direct implications for clinical management and treatment.

CLINICS CARE POINTS

- Sequestration is a condition where a section of metaphyseal or diaphyseal bone becomes necrotic due to a thrombotic state, known as immunocoagulopathy, leading to vascular obstruction and subsequent bone death.

- Involucrum, which is produced by a viable periosteum, forms around the sequestrum to serve as a vascular and bony shunt. Involucrum promotes healing of sequestration by facilitating vascular arborization and deploying stem cells to replace the necrotic bone.

- The induced membrane technique is a two-stage surgical procedure designed to heal sequestration that fails to correct through involucrum. It involves creating a highly vascularized membrane, akin to periosteum.

FUNDING

Caitlin Lovejoy Fund, the Vanderbilt University Medical Center Department of Orthopaedics, the Vanderbilt School of Medicine Research Immersion program, and the Vanderbilt Supporting Careers in Research for Interventional Physicians and Surgeons (SCRIPS) fellowship.

DISCLOSURE

The authors have nothing to disclose relevant to this work.

REFERENCES

1. Phemister DB. Necrotic bone and the subsequent changes which it undergoes. Journal of the American Medical Association 1915;LXIV(3):211–6.
2. Bauernfeind FG, Horvath G, Stutz A, et al. Cutting edge: NF-kappaB activating pattern recognition and cytokine receptors license NLRP3 inflammasome activation by regulating NLRP3 expression. J Immunol 2009;183(2):787–91.
3. Locke M, Longstaff C. Extracellular histones inhibit fibrinolysis through noncovalent and covalent interactions with fibrin. Thromb Haemost 2021;121(4):464–76.
4. Colnot C. Skeletal cell fate decisions within periosteum and bone marrow during bone regeneration. J Bone Miner Res 2009;24(2):274–82.
5. Zhang X, Xie C, Lin AS, et al. Periosteal progenitor cell fate in segmental cortical bone graft transplantations: implications for functional tissue engineering. J Bone Miner Res 2005;20(12):2124–37.
6. Manolagas SC. Birth and death of bone cells: basic regulatory mechanisms and implications for the pathogenesis and treatment of osteoporosis. Endocr Rev 2000;21(2):115–37.
7. Ham AW, Cormack DH. Ham's histology. 9th edition. Philadelphia: Lippincott; 1987.
8. Johnson EO, Soultanis K, Soucacos PN. Vascular anatomy and microcirculation of skeletal zones

vulnerable to osteonecrosis: vascularization of the femoral head. Orthop Clin North Am 2004;35(3): 285–91, viii.

9. Trueta J. The 3 types of acute hematogenous osteomyelitis. Schweiz Med Wochenschr 1963;93: 306–12.

10. Cowin SC, Cardoso L. Blood and interstitial flow in the hierarchical pore space architecture of bone tissue. J Biomech 2015;48(5):842–54.

11. Mysorekar VR. Diaphysial nutrient foramina in human long bones. J Anat 1967;101(Pt 4):813–22.

12. Brookes M. Cortical vascularization and growth in foetal tubular bones. J Anat 1963;97(Pt 4):597–609.

13. Grüneboom A, Hawwari I, Weidner D, et al. A network of trans-cortical capillaries as mainstay for blood circulation in long bones. Nat Metab 2019;1(2):236–50.

14. Trueta J, Cavadias AX. Vascular changes caused by the Küntscher type of nailing; an experimental study in the rabbit. J Bone Joint Surg Br 1955;37-b(3):492–505.

15. Trueta J, Morgan JD. The vascular contribution to osteogenesis. I. Studies by the injection method. J Bone Joint Surg Br 1960;42-b:97–109.

16. Trueta J. Appraisal of the vascular factor in the healing of fractures of the femoral neck. J Bone Joint Surg Br 1957;39-b(1):3–5.

17. Rhinelander FW. The normal microcirculation of diaphyseal cortex and its response to fracture. J Bone Joint Surg Am 1968;50(4):784–800.

18. Rhinelander FW, Baragry R. Microangiography in bone healing. I. Undisplaced closed fractures. J Bone Joint Surg Am 1962;44-a:1273–98.

19. Baker CE, Moore-Lotridge SN, Hysong AA, et al. Bone fracture acute phase response-a unifying theory of fracture repair: clinical and scientific implications. Clin Rev Bone Miner Metab 2018;16(4):142–58.

20. Williams RM, Zipfel WR, Tinsley ML, et al. Solute transport in growth plate cartilage: in vitro and in vivo. Biophys J 2007;93(3):1039–50.

21. Trueta J, Amato VP. The vascular contribution to osteogenesis. III. Changes in the growth cartilage caused by experimentally induced ischaemia. J Bone Joint Surg Br 1960;42-b:571–87.

22. Arsenault AL. Microvascular organization at the epiphyseal-metaphyseal junction of growing rats. J Bone Miner Res 1987;2(2):143–9.

23. Morini S, Pannarale L, Franchitto A, et al. Microvascular features and ossification process in the femoral head of growing rats. J Anat 1999;195(Pt 2):225–33.

24. Hobo T. Zur Pathogenese der akuten haematogenen Osteomyelitis. Acta Sch Med Univ Kioto 1921; 4:1–29.

25. Diaz-Flores L, Gutierrez R, Lopez-Alonso A, et al. Pericytes as a supplementary source of osteoblasts in periosteal osteogenesis. Clin Orthop Relat Res 1992;275:280–6.

26. Uddströmer L. The osteogenic capacity of tubular and membranous bone periosteum. A qualitative and quantitative experimental study in growing rabbits. Scand J Plast Reconstr Surg 1978;12(3): 195–205.

27. Johnson RW Jr. A physiological study of the blood supply of the diaphysis. Clin Orthop Relat Res 1968; 56:5–11.

28. Allen MR, Hock JM, Burr DB. Periosteum: biology, regulation, and response to osteoporosis therapies. Bone 2004;35(5):1003–12.

29. Benvenuti M, An T, Amaro E, et al. Double-edged sword: musculoskeletal infection provoked acute phase response in children. Orthop Clin North Am 2017;48(2):181–97.

30. An TJ, Benvenuti MA, Mignemi ME, et al. Similar clinical severity and outcomes for methicillin-resistant and methicillin-susceptible *Staphylococcus aureus* pediatric musculoskeletal infections. Open Forum Infect Dis 2017;4(1):ofx013.

31. Krautgartner WD, Klappacher M, Hannig M, et al. Fibrin mimics neutrophil extracellular traps in SEM. Ultrastruct Pathol 2010;34(4):226–31.

32. Longstaff C, Varjú I, Sótonyi P, et al. Mechanical stability and fibrinolytic resistance of clots containing fibrin, DNA, and histones. J Biol Chem 2013; 288(10):6946–56.

33. Nasser A, Azimi T, Ostadmohammadi S, et al. A comprehensive review of bacterial osteomyelitis with emphasis on *Staphylococcus aureus*. Microb Pathog 2020;148:104431.

34. Brinkmann V, Reichard U, Goosmann C, et al. Neutrophil extracellular traps kill bacteria. Science 2004;303(5663):1532–5.

35. Johnson SR, Benvenuti T, Nian H, et al. Measures of admission immunocoagulopathy as an indicator for in-hospital mortality in patients with necrotizing fasciitis: a retrospective study. JBJS Open Access 2023;8(1).

36. Chanavaz M. Anatomy and histophysiology of the periosteum: quantification of the periosteal blood supply to the adjacent bone with 85Sr and gamma spectrometry. J Oral Implantol 1995;21(3):214–9.

37. Labbé JL, Peres O, Leclair O, et al. Acute osteomyelitis in children: the pathogenesis revisited? Orthop Traumatol Surg Res 2010;96(3):268–75.

38. Farrera C, Fadeel B. Macrophage clearance of neutrophil extracellular traps is a silent process. J Immunol 2013;191(5):2647–56.

39. Yuasa M, Mignemi NA, Barnett JV, et al. The temporal and spatial development of vascularity in a healing displaced fracture. Bone 2014;67:208–21.

40. Debnath S, Yallowitz AR, McCormick J, et al. Discovery of a periosteal stem cell mediating intramembranous bone formation. Nature 2018; 562(7725):133–9.

41. Méndez-Ferrer S, Michurina TV, Ferraro F, et al. Mesenchymal and haematopoietic stem cells form

a unique bone marrow niche. Nature 2010; 466(7308):829–34.

42. Chan CK, Seo EY, Chen JY, et al. Identification and specification of the mouse skeletal stem cell. Cell 2015;160(1–2):285–98.

43. Tomlinson RE, Silva MJ. Skeletal blood flow in bone repair and maintenance. Bone Res 2013;1(4):311–22.

44. Daoud A, Saighi-Bouaouina A. Treatment of sequestra, pseudarthroses, and defects in the long bones of children who have chronic hematogenous osteomyelitis. J Bone Joint Surg Am 1989; 71(10):1448–68.

45. Pineda C, Espinosa R, Pena A. Radiographic imaging in osteomyelitis: the role of plain radiography, computed tomography, ultrasonography, magnetic resonance imaging, and scintigraphy. Semin Plast Surg 2009;23(2):80–9.

46. Khan SN, Cammisa FP Jr, Sandhu HS, et al. The biology of bone grafting. J Am Acad Orthop Surg 2005;13(1):77–86.

47. Roberts TT, Rosenbaum AJ. Bone grafts, bone substitutes and orthobiologics: the bridge between basic science and clinical advancements in fracture healing. Organogenesis 2012;8(4):114–24.

48. Boyle WJ, Simonet WS, Lacey DL. Osteoclast differentiation and activation. Nature 2003;423(6937):337–42.

49. Tang Y, Zhu J, Huang D, et al. Mandibular osteotomy-induced hypoxia enhances osteoclast activation and acid secretion by increasing glycolysis. J Cell Physiol 2019;234(7):11165–75.

50. Zhao Y, Chen G, Zhang W, et al. Autophagy regulates hypoxia-induced osteoclastogenesis through the HIF-1α/BNIP3 signaling pathway. J Cell Physiol 2012;227(2):639–48.

51. Neidlinger-Wilke C, Wilke HJ, Claes L. Cyclic stretching of human osteoblasts affects proliferation and metabolism: a new experimental method and its application. J Orthop Res 1994;12(1):70–8.

52. Ehrlich PJ, Lanyon LE. Mechanical strain and bone cell function: a review. Osteoporos Int 2002;13(9): 688–700.

53. Rubin J, Rubin C, Jacobs CR. Molecular pathways mediating mechanical signaling in bone. Gene 2006;367:1–16.

54. Carroll SF, Buckley CT, Kelly DJ. Cyclic Tensile Strain Can Play a Role in Directing both Intramembranous and Endochondral Ossification of Mesenchymal Stem Cells. Front Bioeng Biotechnol 2017;5:73.

55. Moore-Lotridge SN, Gibson BHY, Duvernay MT, et al. Pediatric musculoskeletal infection : an update through the four pillars of clinical care and immunothrombotic similarities With COVID-19. Journal of the Pediatric Orthopaedic Society of North America 2020;2(2).

56. Pineda C, Vargas A, Rodríguez AV. Imaging of osteomyelitis: current concepts. Infectious Disease Clinics 2006;20(4):789–825.

57. Rueff-Barroso CR, Milagres D, do Valle J, et al. Bone healing in rats submitted to weight-bearing and non-weight-bearing exercises. Med Sci Monit 2008;14(11): Br231–B236.

58. Boyde A. The real response of bone to exercise. J Anat 2003;203(2):173–89.

59. Huang TH, Lin SC, Chang FL, et al. Effects of different exercise modes on mineralization, structure, and biomechanical properties of growing bone. J Appl Physiol (1985) 2003;95(1):300–7.

60. Kubiak EN, Beebe MJ, North K, et al. Early weight bearing after lower extremity fractures in adults. J Am Acad Orthop Surg 2013;21(12): 727–38.

61. Belthur MV, Birchansky SB, Verdugo AA, et al. Pathologic fractures in children with acute Staphylococcus aureus osteomyelitis. J Bone Joint Surg Am 2012;94(1):34–42.

62. Fractures in Children With Staphylococcus aureus Osteomyelitis. AAP Grand Rounds 2012;27(4):40.

63. Collins CJ, Atkins PR, Ohs N, et al. Clinical observation of diminished bone quality and quantity through longitudinal HR-pQCT-derived remodeling and mechanoregulation. Sci Rep 2022;12(1): 17960.

64. Keaveny TM, Adams AL, Fischer H, et al. Increased risks of vertebral fracture and reoperation in primary spinal fusion patients who test positive for osteoporosis by Biomechanical Computed Tomography analysis. Spine J 2023;23(3):412–24.

65. Donegan DJ, Scolaro J, Matuszewski PE, et al. Staged bone grafting following placement of an antibiotic spacer block for the management of segmental long bone defects. Orthopedics 2011; 34(11):e730–5.

66. Masquelet AC, Fitoussi F, Begue T, et al. Reconstruction of the long bones by the induced membrane and spongy autograft. Ann Chir Plast Esthet 2000;45(3):346–53.

67. Apard T, Bigorre N, Cronier P, et al. Two-stage reconstruction of post-traumatic segmental tibia bone loss with nailing. Orthop Traumatol Surg Res 2010;96(5):549–53.

68. Pelissier P, Masquelet AC, Bareille R, et al. Induced membranes secrete growth factors including vascular and osteoinductive factors and could stimulate bone regeneration. J Orthop Res 2004;22(1): 73–9.

69. Morelli I, Drago L, George DA, et al. Managing large bone defects in children: a systematic review of the induced membrane technique. J Pediatr Orthop B 2018;27(5):443–55.

70. Morelli I, Drago L, George DA, et al. Masquelet technique: myth or reality? A systematic review and meta-analysis. Injury 2016;47(Suppl 6): S68–s76.

71. Giannoudis PV, Faour O, Goff T, et al. Masquelet technique for the treatment of bone defects:

tips-tricks and future directions. Injury 2011;42(6): 591–8.

72. Young MH. Epiphysial infarction in a growing long bone. The Journal of Bone & Joint Surgery British 1966;48-B(4):826–40.

73. Roberts SJ, van Gastel N, Carmeliet G, et al. Uncovering the periosteum for skeletal regeneration: the stem cell that lies beneath. Bone 2015;70:10–8.

74. Breitbart AS, Grande DA, Kessler R, et al. Tissue engineered bone repair of calvarial defects using cultured periosteal cells. Plast Reconstr Surg 1998; 101(3):567–74 [discussion: 75-6].

75. Perka C, Schultz O, Spitzer RS, et al. Segmental bone repair by tissue-engineered periosteal cell transplants with bioresorbable fleece and fibrin scaffolds in rabbits. Biomaterials 2000;21(11):1145–53.

76. Chang H, Knothe Tate ML. Concise review: the periosteum: tapping into a reservoir of clinically useful progenitor cells. Stem Cells Transl Med 2012;1(6):480–91.

Shoulder and Elbow

The Septic Elbow Joint
Treatment Approaches for Improved Patient Outcomes

Heather L. Mercer, PhD[a], Diego Rodriguez, BS[b],
Elizabeth Mikola, MD[b], Deana Mercer, MD[c],*

KEYWORDS

- Elbow joint • Septic • Infection • Arthrotomy • Arthroscopy • Antibiotic

---

KEY POINTS

- Arthrocentesis is the most effective way to diagnose septic arthritis of the elbow and should be done immediate and with a low threshold in cases of suspected joint infection.
- The joint fluid studies should include cultures for acid-fast bacillus, fungal, Gram stain, aerobic/anaerobic culture with sensitivities, and evaluation for crystalline arthropathies.
- Prompt broad-spectrum antibiotic administration followed by targeted antibiotic treatment after cultures are finalized is important.
- Two options for surgical intervention in cases of septic elbow joint are (1) arthroscopic irrigation and debridement and (2) open arthrotomy with joint irrigation and debridement.
- *Staphylococcus aureus* is the most common offending agent. Other possible organisms include nongonococcal and gonococcal bacterium, *Streptococci*, *Mycobacterium tuberculosis*, and fungal species.

INTRODUCTION

Septic elbow, or septic arthritis of the elbow, is a condition that affects about 12 per 100,000 people per year.[1,2] Risk factors are multiple and include age 80 or older, the presence of a joint prosthesis, open growth plates, inflammatory arthropathies, osteoarthritis, intravenous (IV) drug usage, alcoholism, diabetes, cutaneous ulcers, low socioeconomic status, and intra-articular corticosteroid injections.[3–6] Septic elbow is characterized by the invasion of pathogenic microorganisms into the elbow joint. When left untreated, septic elbow can cause severe joint destruction, cartilage degradation, bone erosion, periarticular soft tissue damage, systemic infection, and long-term disability owing to severe disruption of the elbow articular anatomy.[4,7]

Septic elbow is commonly caused by bacterial infection, including *Staphylococcus aureus*, *Streptococcus* species, or gram-negative organisms.[8] The most common offending organism is *S. aureus*.[9] The infection may arise from hematogenous spread, local trauma that violates the elbow joint, direct intra-articular injections, or contiguous spread from adjacent tissues.

Although relatively infrequent compared with other joint infections, the prevalence of septic elbow has shown regional variations, with certain populations, such as children, immunocompromised individuals, or those with preexisting joint diseases, being at a higher risk. Children with open physis have a higher risk of joint hematogenous spread, as anatomically, they contain small capillaries that run across the growth plate, increasing the risk of joint space seeding and subsequent infection.[10]

Timely diagnosis and intervention are crucial in mitigating the consequences of the septic elbow.

---

[a] Institute of Microbiology and Infection, School of Biosciences, University of Birmingham, Edgbaston, B15 2TT, Birmingham, England, United Kingdom; [b] Department of Orthopaedics and Rehabilitation, University of New Mexico Health Sciences Center, MSC10 5600, Albuquerque, New Mexico 87131, USA; [c] University of New Mexico Health Sciences Center, 1 University of New Mexico MSC 10-5600, Albuquerque, New Mexico 87131, USA
* Corresponding author. UNMHSC, 1 University of New Mexico MSC 10-5600, Albuquerque, New Mexico 87131.
E-mail address: dmercer@salud.unm.edu

0030-5898/24/© 2023 Elsevier Inc. All rights reserved.

The nonspeci c nature of initial symptoms often leads to delayed diagnosis. When elbow joint infection is clinically suspected, the history and physical examination should be comprehensive. A radiograph is important to rule out trauma and may have radiographic ndings consistent with infection, including periarticular erosion and juxta-articular osteopenia. Pain with active range of motion of the elbow and/or pain with axial load should heighten suspicion for infection. There should be a low threshold for joint aspiration; joint aspiration should be performed when the clinical examination and history are worrisome for joint infection. Blood work, including complete blood count (CBC), erythrocyte sedimentation rate (ESR), and C-reactive protein (CRP), are important, as these are markers for infection and can be performed serially to determine appropriate response to surgical debridement and antibiotic therapy. In cases where the diagnosis is unclear, advanced imaging, such as an elbow MRI, can be helpful and diagnostic. Early recognition and prompt initiation of treatment are vital to curtail disease progression, prevent joint destruction, and avert life-threatening complications, such as septicemia.

This review aims to provide a comprehensive analysis of the latest evidence on septic elbow diagnosis and treatment.

INFECTIOUS AGENTS

Septic arthritis can arise from various infectious agents, with S aureus being the predominant microorganism, accounting for 37% to 56% of all cases.[11] According to findings from a retrospective study, more than 70% of septic arthritis cases were caused by hematogenous spreading.[12]

Other potential causative infectious agents include gram-negative rods, Brucella, fungal organisms like sporotrichosis and blastomycoses, and Mycobacterium tuberculosis (tuberculosis [TB]).[7,11,13] In the setting of infection with TB, the infection can be indolent, and the diagnosis may be delayed as the organism is slow growing. One published case study is that of a 77-year-old woman with no underlying diseases who presented with indolent persistent elbow pain. She was eventually diagnosed with septic arthritis in the left elbow. The radiographs and MRI depicted severe destruction of the joint, a common finding in atypical TB infections. Laboratory tests were performed, and TB grew out of the synovial fluid.[14] In addition, Neisseria gonorrhoeae presents in young patients who are sexually active.[15] Two case studies reported N. gonorrhoeae septic elbow arthritis occurring in 85% of patients with disseminated gonococcal infections.[16,17]

Typically, treatment of septic arthritis involves surgical joint debridement followed by the administration of IV antibiotics followed by conversion to oral antibiotics. Involvement of the infectious disease team can be helpful in antibiotic targeting and duration of antibiotic treatment.

PATIENT EVALUATION OVERVIEW
Clinical Presentation and Symptoms
Obtaining an in-depth medical history plays a pivotal role in identifying potential causes and aiding in the diagnosis of septic arthritis of the elbow. A history of trauma should be ruled out. Septic arthritis of the elbow manifests with distinctive clinical features, commonly presenting as an acute onset of monoarticular joint pain, accompanied by redness, swelling, and tenderness upon joint palpation. There is often restricted joint movement with severe pain with both active and passive joint range of motion. Furthermore, there is severe pain with any axial compression load of the joint, such as trying to use the arms to adjust body position in bed or in assisting from a sitting to a standing position.[6] It is essential to acknowledge that fungal and mycobacterial infections may contribute to delayed presentations of septic arthritis of the elbow, underscoring the need for a comprehensive diagnostic approach.[18,19]

In cases of systemic infection owing to the infected elbow joint, patients may exhibit an ill appearance with complaints of fever, decreased appetite, and irritability. Early recognition of these clinical indicators is vital in facilitating prompt and accurate diagnosis, enabling timely initiation of appropriate interventions to avoid complications and ensure optimal patient outcomes.

Physical Examination
On physical examination, characteristic signs include warmth, erythema, and tender upon palpation of the affected elbow, accompanied by a joint effusion.[6] Abnormal vital signs, such as tachycardia, and fever are nonspecific findings, detected in approximately 40% to 60% of cases.[11] In addition, the examiner should carefully note any presence of overlying cellulitis or abscess, which on occasion can track down the forearm. A circumferential examination of the extremity should be performed, including the forearm and arm. Evidence of trauma should be assessed with careful evaluation of the skin for any disruption. The affected joint's range of motion may be substantially limited, with restriction in extension, flexion, and, in some cases,

supination and pronation owing to intense pain.[7] These clinical findings are essential clues and should lead to prompt intervention, including joint aspiration and the initiation of antibiotic treatment and surgical intervention when indicated.

DIAGNOSTIC PROCEDURE
Imaging Workup
The physical examination is the best tool for diagnosing septic elbow; however, the evaluation of septic arthritis of the elbow warrants a comprehensive imaging approach. It is helpful in ruling out other potential diagnoses.

A lateral view radiograph is important for ruling out fracture and for evaluating joint effusion[11] (Fig. 1). In the setting of trauma, a fracture must be ruled out, as a fracture can mimic infection. In cases where joint infection with effusion or abscess is suspected, ultrasound can serve as a valuable and immediately accessible diagnostic tool to confirm its presence.[20]

Ultrasound and computed tomography (CT) scans can be helpful in identifying a uid collection, such as abscess or hematoma (Fig. 2).

In addition, an MRI can be helpful and may be diagnostic, as it can detect nonspeci c synovial thickening and enhancement, effusion, periarticular myositis, soft tissue abscess, or bone marrow edema resulting from adjacent bone involvement.[21] The utilization of these imaging techniques allows for a more accurate and comprehensive assessment of the condition, aiding in timely diagnosis and guiding appropriate treatment especially with associated osteomyelitis.

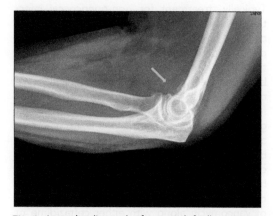

Fig. 1. Lateral radiograph of a septic left elbow joint in a patient who presented with a 24-hour history of worsening left elbow pain and swelling with painful motion. This radiograph shows degenerative arthritis and the presence of a large joint effusion indicated by the yellow arrow.

Laboratory Workup
In the diagnostic evaluation of septic elbow, the elbow joint should be aspirated. The synovial uid analysis guides treatment and remains the gold standard. The aspirate should undergo laboratory examination, including white blood cell (WBC) count with differential, gram-stain culture for both aerobic and anaerobic bacteria, fungal, crystal analysis, and acid-fast staining.[6] A purulent or cloudy aspirate with a total nucleated cell count greater than 50,000 to 80,000 and polymorphonuclear neutrophils (PMNs) greater than 75% indicate an infection. In patients with elbow prostheses, a WBC count greater than 1100 and PMNs greater than 65% serve as indicators of infection.[6,22] In addition, a study performed in 2019 indicated the sensitivity and specificity of D-lactate are valuable markers for recognizing infection in periprosthetic joint infection.[23,24]

The presence of crystals indicates gout or pseudogout, which is negative or positive in birefringence, respectively.[25] Gout is treated differently than septic elbow arthritis, as those with gout often improve with anti-inflammatories and empirical antibiotics and do not require operative joint irrigation and debridement. In crystalline arthropathies, the total nucleated cell count is often lower than in septic elbow. However, there are cases where crystalline arthropathy can become a septic arthropathy. In those cases of positive crystalline studies where the symptoms do not improve with anti-inflammatories, there should be a low threshold for operative joint debridement.

Blood tests should be obtained and include CBC, ESR, CRP, and uric acid levels. The blood uric acid level can be normal even in the setting of acute gouty are. Elevated WBC counts, particularly greater than 50,000 with 90% neutrophil predominance, strongly suggest a bacterial infection. Additional important in ammatory markers include ESR and CRP tests,[6,22] as these can be followed overtime to gauge resolution of infection.

ELBOW JOINT ASPIRATION

Given the importance of accurate diagnosis in septic elbow, synovial uid analysis stands as the most accurate way for diagnosis and necessitates the meticulous aspiration of the elbow joint synovial uid.

The technique for this critical procedure is outlined as follows (Note: The elbow joint is typically achieved through a lateral approach):

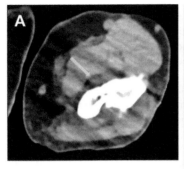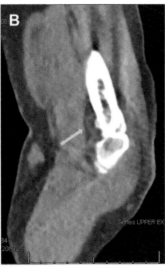

Fig. 2. CT scan of the septic left elbow joint. (*A*) Sagittal cut of the left elbow; (*B*) axial cut of the left elbow. The CT scan showed no fracture and confirmed joint effusion, indicated by the yellow arrows.

1. Place the patient in a supine position with the infected elbow at 45° of flexion ensuring the hand is in a neutral position.
2. Disinfect the skin along the lateral aspect of the elbow with alcohol and/or povidone-iodine.
3. Use an 18- or 20-gauge needle with a 3- or 10-mL syringe. Insert the needle into the lateral triangle of the elbow bordered by the lateral epicondyle, radial head, and olecranon process (as depicted by the "X" in Fig. 3).
4. Direct the needle toward the medial epicondyle and advance slowly until the needle is intra-articular.
5. Aspirate the synovial fluid and decant into sterile collection tubes.
6. Clean and apply dressings to the wound.
7. Send the synovial fluid to the laboratory for analysis immediately after the procedure. It is good practice to take the fluid to the laboratory yourself if the laboratory is located near you.

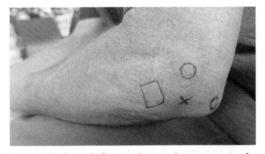

Fig. 3. The lateral elbow indicates the entry point for joint aspiration. The "square" indicates the radial head, and the "circles" denote the lateral epicondyle of the distal humerus and the olecranon. The "X" designates the soft spot, the entry point into the elbow joint for joint aspiration.

8. If available, ultrasound can be used for the elbow joint aspiration.

MEDICAL MANAGEMENT
First-Line Antibiotic and Antifungal Therapy

For the management of septic arthritis, the initial approach entails the administration of a broad-spectrum antibiotic.[11,26] To optimize therapeutic outcomes, the selection of antibiotics can be tailored and should be based on the specific pathogen sensitivities from cultures of the synovial. Table 1 presents a range of antibiotic treatment options for septic elbow. This targeted antibiotic regimen is the most effective way to achieve rapid and effective resolution of the infection.

Nongonococcal

Typically, treatment for *non-gonococcal* infections usually begins with IV antibiotics. The time of IV antibiotic administration is variable and can be administered for up to 6 weeks. Additional oral antibiotics may be indicated and is based on the pathogen and sensitivities.[11,27] Vancomycin is the most common treatment choice for gram-positive cocci infections, whereas, for gram-negative cocci, ceftriaxone is the preferred approach. In the case of gram-negative bacilli bacterium infection, ceftazidime is the prevailing option. If the Gram stain shows a negative result but there is a suspicion of bacterial arthritis, the optimal treatment strategy is the administration of vancomycin along with either ceftazidime or an aminoglycoside.[11,28]

The method of administration, dosages, and duration of antibiotic treatment should be tailored in accordance with the patient's clinical response and microbiology results. Typically,

Table 1
Antibiotic therapy options for treatment of septic arthritis of the elbow

Pathogen	Antibiotics
Methicillin-resistant *Staphylococcus aureus*	Linezolid, Trimethoprim-sulfamethoxazole, Clindamycin, Minocycline, or Doxycycline
Staphylococcus pneumoniae+	Vancomycin, Linezolid
Streptococci+	Penicillin
Gram-positive cocci	Vancomycin
Gam-negative cocci	Ceftriaxone
Gram-negative bacilli	Ceftazidime
Neisseriagonorrhoeae	Cipro oxacin, Ce xime
Mycobacterium tuberculosis	Rifampicin, Ethambutol, Isoniazid, Pyrazinamide
Fungal Organisms: Sporotrichosis or blastomycoses	Azole, Parenteral Amphotericin B

Note: This is a general guide on antibiotic and fungal treatment options. The appropriate dose and length of treatment should be considered on a case-by-case basis.
    Refs.[11,26–31]

the standard course of treatment for nongono-coccal infections extends up to 6 weeks.

Gonococcal
The primary approach for disseminated gonococcal of *N. gonorrhea* treatment typically involves antibiotic administration with vancomycin IV followed by administration of ceftriaxone for 24 to 48 hours until clinical signs of improvement. Continued oral administration of ciprofloxacin or cefixime is then indicated until symptom resolution.[29]

Streptococci
The most effective antibiotic for the treatment of *Streptococci* infection in the elbow joint is penicillin, which has shown to be highly effective.[6] Erythromycin offers a practical and efficient substitute when penicillin allergy is a concern. Following surgical intervention, a common protocol calls for the use of oral antibiotics for up to 6 weeks.[30]

Mycobacterium tuberculosis
The treatment approach for *M. tuberculosis* infection is the administration of antibiotics. There are several effective antibiotics available for combating TB, such as rifampicin, ethambutol, isoniazid, and pyrazinamide. The duration of treatment with these medications typically spans from 6 to 18 months.[31]

Fungus
Successful treatment of fungal infections in septic arthritis is targeted to the speci c fungal species. Generally, rst-line treatment includes the use of oral azole agents or parenteral amphotericin B.[32]

    We have included the most common organism that leads to septic elbow arthritis in addition to those that should be speci cally tested for with special media or pathology evaluation.

There are a myriad of organisms that can cause infection. The cultures and sensitivities should drive the antibiotic regiment.

SURGICAL TREATMENT OPTIONS
Indications for Surgical Intervention
In the most cases, barring patient factors that make surgical intervention a risk to the patient, the septic elbow is an orthopedic emergency necessitating swift surgical intervention. Typically, a joint aspiration is done before surgical intervention. If the diagnosis was clinical and no aspiration was done before the surgical procedure, the joint aspiration should be done in the operating room before joint debridement. Surgical treatment options encompass arthroscopic irrigation and debridement or arthrotomy with open irrigation and debridement.[11,26,28,33,34] Multiple intraoperative cultures should be obtained, and it may be good practice to send both fluid and soft tissue samples from the joint. If there is bone erosion, and bone is easily accessible, a bone sample for culture may be indicated. After surgical intervention, cultures should be closely followed for sensitivity, and antibiotic treatment should be tailored toward the specific organism isolated.

ARTHROSCOPIC IRRIGATION AND DEBRIDEMENT SURGICAL PROCEDURE OVERVIEW

The technique for arthroscopic irrigation and debridement is as follows(Note: The arthroscopy can be performed at the medial or lateral aspect of the elbow depending on the surgeon's preference):

1. The patient is positioned according to surgeons' preference.

- Shoulder is typically abducted to 90°.
- Elbow is typically flexed to 90°.
2. The arm is stabilized in an arm holder.
3. The entire arm is prepared and draped.[35]
4. A tourniquet is applied to the upper part of the arm in a sterile fashion and set to 250 mm Hg. The use of the tourniquet is surgeons' choice. If it is used, the arm is exsanguinated using gravity, and the tourniquet is elevated to 250 mm Hg.
5. For joint aspiration, the lateral soft spot is used. The soft spot is the region of the elbow that is bordered by the lateral epicondyle, radial head, and olecranon process (as depicted by the "X" in Fig. 3).
6. With the use of an 18- or 20-gauge needle with a 3- or 10-mL syringe, the elbow joint is first aspirated, and any joint fluid is sent to the pathology department and to the laboratory. It is then insufflated with 20 to 30 mL of sterile saline.
7. An anterolateral portal is created over the radiocapitellar joint 1 to 2 cm proximal to the distal humerus lateral epicondyle and 1 cm anterior to the distal humerus.
8. Create the anteromedial portal, 2 cm proximal to the medial epicondyle and one finger-breadth anterior to the intermuscular septum under direct visualization with the use of the inside-out approach.
9. With the use of a 4.0-mm 30° arthroscope and a 4.8-mm motorized shaver, debride the purulent and necrotic synovium and cartilage.
10. Collect intraoperative fluid and tissue samples.
11. Irrigate the anterior joint with 6 to 9 L of sterile saline.
12. After irrigation, establish the posterolateral portal for the arthroscope 3 cm proximal to the tip of the olecranon.
13. Create a direct posterior portal for the shaver also 3 cm proximal to the tip of the olecranon and medial to the posterolateral portal.
14. Debride the posterior aspect of the elbow joint.
15. Suture all portal sites.
16. Consider drain placement if indicated.

OPEN IRRIGATION AND DEBRIDEMENT SURGICAL PROCEDURE OVERVIEW

An anterolateral approach, the Kaplan type approach, to the elbow is typically performed. The intermuscular plane is between the brachialis and brachioradialis (proximally) and the pronator teres and brachioradialis (distally).

The technique for open irrigation and debridement is as follows:

1. The patient is placed in a supine position with the upper extremity on a radiolucent arm board.
2. Prepare the upper and lower extremities of the arm in the usual sterile fashion.
3. An incision is made over the radial head and extends from the lateral condyle of the distal humerus to the bicipital tuberosity.
4. Incise deep fascia in line with the extensor insertion.
5. Elevate the capsule off of the anterior and posterior aspect of the distal humerus.
6. Collect intraoperative fluid and tissue cultures for laboratory analysis.
7. Debride any necrotic tissue or abnormal-appearing tissue.
8. Profusely irrigate the joint with sterile saline.
9. Place drain if indicated.
10. Close annular ligament, joint capsule, fascia, and skin.

Postoperative Rehabilitation Options

For best patient outcomes during the immediate postoperative care, it is recommended that patients be placed in a long-arm posterior splint for soft tissue rest. Monitoring of WBC, ESR, and CRP levels is helpful to con rm trends toward normalization of in ammatory markers. This is an indicator of infection clearance.[26,28] The antibiotic chosen is tailored toward the organism sensitivies, and if cultures and Gram stain are negative, then broad-spectrum antibiotics are administered until resolution of symptoms and normalization of laboratory inflammatory markers.

Initiation of elbow range-of-motion exercises encompassing exion, extension, supination, and pronation is crucial to avoid stiffness of the elbow and should be initiated as soon as possible. Gradual introduction of light weight-bearing exercises, if tolerable, can also help with recovery and minimizes loss of muscle.[36]

Ef cient pain management can be achieved with the use of anti-in ammatories, and narcotics should be minimized to the immediate postoperative period.

SEPTIC ARTHRITIS OF THE ELBOW TREATMENT ALGORITHM
Complications
Common Complications and Management Strategies

Fig. 4 The most common complication after septic arthritis of a joint is joint damage from infection.

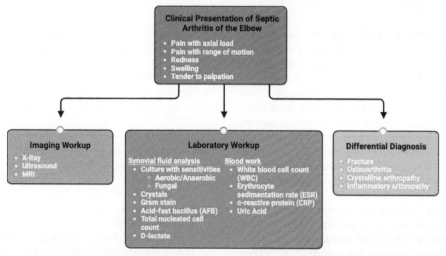

Fig. 4. Overview of the Management of Septic Arthritis of the Elbow Joint. The visual representation outlines the comprehensive management pathway for septic arthritis of the elbow joint. The flow chart offers a clear and systematic depiction of the steps involved in effectively addressing the septic elbow joint.

The cartilage is affected, and follow-up radiographs may show decreased joint space from articular cartilage loss owing to infection. This is especially true in cases of delayed presentation or delayed diagnosis of the joint infection. Multiple washouts may be indicated depending on the severity of the infection.[37,38] Another potential complication is injury to surrounding structures during the surgical procedures. Understanding of anatomy in this region is important, as the posterior interosseous nerve is within the surgical region. To safeguard against neurovascular injury, meticulous attention is directed toward protecting the neurovascular structures, particularly the radial nerve during surgical procedures.[39]

Pearls and pitfalls

- Once septic arthritis of the elbow is suspected, arthrocentesis of the joint should be performed immediately to ensure early diagnosis and the prompt administration of antibiotics. Basic blood work should be obtained immediately, including CBC, ESR, and CRP.
- Once synovial fluid is obtained, broad-spectrum antibiotics should be administered, and the fluid should be sent for total nucleated cell count, aerobic/anaerobic cultures with sensitivities.
- It is important to rule out other causes, such as fracture or inflammatory arthropathy, with the most common being gout.
- If septic arthritis is suspected, immediate surgical intervention is indicated. Depending on the surgeon's preference, they may opt for either an open or arthroscopic technique. In either case, it

is crucial to use copious irrigation and thorough debridement of the joint.
- A repeat irrigation and debridement may be indicated depending on the severity of the infection.
- A drain may be placed intra-articularly to allow efflux of intra-articular fluid for 24 to 48 hours and then removed.
- Antibiotic treatment is tailored toward the organism, and route and duration are based on presentation and Gram stain, cultures, and sensitivities. The antibiotics can be administered orally or IV and for up to 6 weeks. Infectious disease involvement may be indicated.

DISCUSSION

Septic arthritis of the elbow is a complex and challenging condition, necessitating a comprehensive approach to diagnosis and management. Septic arthritis affects both adults and children.[40] Risk factors, ranging from the presence of a joint prosthesis, immunocompromised states, to cutaneous ulcers and diabetes, highlight the diverse predisposing conditions that can contribute to septic arthritis of the elbow.[41] These factors underscore the significance of a comprehensive risk assessment to enable timely intervention and mitigate potential complications.

Septic arthritis of the elbow can be caused by a diverse range of microorganisms, with S aureus predominating as the causative pathogen.[8] However, an array of bacterial and fungal organisms can also be the cause of the infection. The involvement of atypical pathogens, such as M. tuberculosis and N. gonorrhoeae, highlights the importance of considering a variety of infectious causes, especially in cases with delayed presentation.[14,42] Tailoring treatment strategies to the precise pathogen identified is pivotal for optimizing therapeutic outcomes.

Early and accurate diagnosis of septic elbow is imperative to prevent irreversible joint damage. The clinical presentation, characterized by joint pain, swelling, redness, and limited range of motion, underscores the need for a multidimensional diagnostic approach.[6] Imaging techniques, including radiographs, ultrasound, and MRI, are helpful and may identify abscess or other cause. Laboratory assessments, encompassing blood tests and synovial fluid analysis, aid in confirming infection and sepsis.[20] Synovial fluid aspiration remains the standard, providing essential microbiological information to guide targeted therapy.[6] The early administration of antibiotics tailored to the identified pathogen in the synovial fluid and blood is foundational to reducing disease progression.[43,44]

Postoperative rehabilitation, including splinting and range-of-motion exercises, complements surgical interventions, ensuring optimal joint function and joint mobility.[36]

Despite the advancements in surgical intervention, complications can occur in septic elbow management. Complications can be mitigated through vigilant antibiotic selection, preservation of bone health, and careful attention to neurovascular structures. In addition, pain management, physical therapy, and diligent follow-up play pivotal roles in averting complications.

The multifaceted nature of septic arthritis of the elbow demands a comprehensive approach, uniting clinical acumen, diagnostic precision, and therapeutic innovation. By implementing a combination of medical and surgical strategies, septic elbow can be met with effective intervention and improved patient outcomes.

DISCLOSURE

The authors have nothing to disclose.

REFERENCES

1. Kennedy N, Chambers ST, Nolan I, et al. Native Joint Septic Arthritis: Epidemiology, Clinical Features, and Microbiological Causes in a New Zealand Population. J Rheumatol 2015;42(12):2392–7.
2. Weston VC, Jones AC, Bradbury N, et al. Clinical features and outcome of septic arthritis in a single UK Health District 1982-1991. Ann Rheum Dis 1999; 58(4):214–9.
3. Kaandorp CJ, Krijnen P, Moens HJ, et al. The outcome of bacterial arthritis: a prospective community-based study. Arthritis Rheum 1997; 40(5):884–92.
4. Mathews CJ, Weston VC, Jones A, et al. Bacterial septic arthritis in adults. Lancet 2010;375(9717): 846–55.
5. Esterhai JL Jr, Gelb I. Adult septic arthritis. Orthop Clin North Am. Jul 1991;22(3):503–14.
6. Earwood JS, Walker TR, Sue GJC. Septic Arthritis: Diagnosis and Treatment. Am Fam Physician 2021;104(6):589–97.
7. Goldenberg DL. Septic arthritis. Lancet 1998; 351(9097):197–202.
8. Goldenberg DL, Reed JI. Bacterial arthritis. N Engl J Med. Mar 21 1985;312(12):764–71.
9. Smith IDM, Milto KM, Doherty CJ, et al. A potential key role for alpha-haemolysin of Staphylococcus aureus in mediating chondrocyte death in septic arthritis. Bone Joint Res 2018;7(7):457–67.
10. Buckholz JM. The surgical management of osteomyelitis: with special reference to a surgical classification. J Foot Surg 1987;26(1 Suppl):S17–24.
11. Hassan AS, Rao A, Manadan AM, et al. Peripheral Bacterial Septic Arthritis: Review of Diagnosis and Management. J Clin Rheumatol 2017;23(8):435–42.
12. Morgan DS, Fisher D, Merianos A, et al. An 18 year clinical review of septic arthritis from tropical Australia. Epidemiol Infect 1996;117(3):423–8.
13. Hashemi SH, Keramat F, Ranjbar M, et al. Osteoarticular complications of brucellosis in Hamedan, an endemic area in the west of Iran. Int J Infect Dis 2007;11(6):496–500.
14. Tangadulrat P, Suwannaphisit S. Tuberculosis Septic Arthritis of the Elbow: A Case Report and Literature Review. Cureus 2021;13(3):e13765.
15. Tong KM, Huang KC, Chang WS, et al. Unmasking the silent invader: A rare encounter of Neisseria gonorrhoeae in joint fluid. Kaohsiung J Med Sci 2023. https://doi.org/10.1002/kjm2.12729.
16. Al-Suleiman SA, Grimes EM, Jonas HS. Disseminated gonococcal infections. Obstet Gynecol 1983;61(1):48–51.
17. O'Brien JP, Goldenberg DL, Rice PA. Disseminated gonococcal infection: a prospective analysis of 49 patients and a review of pathophysiology and immune mechanisms. Medicine (Baltim) 1983;62(6): 395–406.
18. Gupta MN, Sturrock RD, Field M. A prospective 2-year study of 75 patients with adult-onset septic arthritis. Rheumatology (Oxford) 2001;40(1):24–30.
19. Gupta MN, Sturrock RD, Field M. Prospective comparative study of patients with culture proven and high suspicion of adult onset septic arthritis. Ann Rheum Dis. Apr 2003;62(4):327–31.
20. Blanco P, Menendez MF, Figueroa L, et al. Ultrasound-aided diagnosis of septic arthritis of the

elbow in the emergency department. J Ultrasound 2022;25(2):315–8.

21. Karchevsky M, Schweitzer ME, Morrison WB, et al. MRI findings of septic arthritis and associated osteomyelitis in adults. AJR Am J Roentgenol 2004; 182(1):119–22.

22. Li SF, Henderson J, Dickman E, et al. Laboratory tests in adults with monoarticular arthritis: can they rule out a septic joint? Acad Emerg Med 2004;11(3):276–80.

23. Yermak K, Karbysheva S, Perka C, et al. Performance of synovial fluid D-lactate for the diagnosis of periprosthetic joint infection: A prospective observational study. J Infect 2019;79(2):123–9.

24. Li Z, Li C, Wang G, et al. Diagnostic accuracy of synovial fluid D-lactate for periprosthetic joint infection: a systematic review and meta-analysis. J Orthop Surg Res 2021;16(1):606.

25. Rosales-Alexander JL, Balsalobre Aznar J, Magro-Checa C. Calcium pyrophosphate crystal deposition disease: diagnosis and treatment. Open Access Rheumatol 2014;6:39–47.

26. van den Ende KI, Steinmann SP. Arthroscopic treatment of septic arthritis of the elbow. J Shoulder Elbow Surg 2012;21(8):1001–5.

27. Horowitz DL, Katzap E, Horowitz S, et al. Approach to septic arthritis. Am Fam Physician 2011;84(6): 653–60.

28. Sharff KA, Richards EP, Townes JM. Clinical management of septic arthritis. Curr Rheumatol Rep 2013;15(6):332.

29. Centers for Disease C, Prevention, Workowski KA, Berman SM. Sexually transmitted diseases treatment guidelines, 2006. MMWR Recomm Rep (Morb Mortal Wkly Rep) 2006;55(RR-11):1–94.

30. Haas T, Gaston MS, Rutz E, et al. Septic arthritis of the elbow with Streptococcus pneumoniae in a 9-month-old girl. BMJ Case Rep 2014;2014. https://doi.org/10.1136/bcr-2014-205204.

31. Sotgiu G, Centis R, D'Ambrosio L, et al. Tuberculosis treatment and drug regimens. Cold Spring Harb Perspect Med 2015;5(5):a017822.

32. Kohli R, Hadley S. Fungal arthritis and osteomyelitis. Infect Dis Clin North Am 2005;19(4):831–51.

33. Rupp M, Mika J, Biehl C, et al. Successful Total Elbow Replacement after Septic Arthritis with Staphylococcus aureus- a Case Report and Review of the Literature. Acta Chir Orthop Traumatol Cech 2018;85(1):70–4. Uspesna nahrada loketniho kloubu po septickem zanetu zpusobenem Staphylococcus aureus- kazuistika a prehled literatury.

34. Spaans AJ, Donders CML, Bessems J, et al. Aspiration or arthrotomy for paediatric septic arthritis of the shoulder and elbow: a systematic review. EFORT Open Rev 2021;6(8):651–7.

35. Dumville JC, McFarlane E, Edwards P, et al. Preoperative skin antiseptics for preventing surgical wound infections after clean surgery. Cochrane Database Syst Rev 2015;2015(4):CD003949.

36. Voss A, Pfeifer CG, Kerschbaum M, et al. Postoperative septic arthritis after arthroscopy: modern diagnostic and therapeutic concepts. Knee Surg Sports Traumatol Arthrosc 2021;29(10):3149–58.

37. Schmitt SK. Osteomyelitis. Infect Dis Clin North Am 2017;31(2):325–38.

38. Seamon J, Keller T, Saleh J, et al. The pathogenesis of nontraumatic osteonecrosis. Arthritis 2012;2012: 601763.

39. Finley ZJ, Savoie FH. Advanced elbow arthroscopy: Tips and tricks. J Clin Orthop Trauma 2021;20: 101476.

40. Garcia-De La Torre I. Advances in the management of septic arthritis. Infect Dis Clin North Am 2006; 20(4):773–88.

41. Kaandorp CJ, Van Schaardenburg D, Krijnen P, et al. Risk factors for septic arthritis in patients with joint disease. A prospective study. Arthritis Rheum 1995;38(12):1819–25.

42. Piazza MJ, Gonzales-Zamora JA. Acute septic elbow monoarthritis with associated Neisseria gonorrhoeae bacteraemia: an uncommon presentation of an old disease. Infez Med 2020;28(2): 253–7.

43. Sakiniene E, Bremell T, Tarkowski A. Addition of corticosteroids to antibiotic treatment ameliorates the course of experimental Staphylococcus aureus arthritis. Arthritis Rheum 1996;39(9):1596–605.

44. Verdrengh M, Carlsten H, Ohlsson C, et al. Addition of bisphosphonate to antibiotic and anti-inflammatory treatment reduces bone resorption in experimental Staphylococcus aureus-induced arthritis. J Orthop Res 2007;25(3):304–10.

Diagnostic Evaluation of Prosthetic Joint Infections of the Shoulder

What Does the Literature Say?

Jeffrey Klott, MD[1], Tyler J. Brolin, MD*

KEYWORDS

- Shoulder • Infection • Total shoulder arthroplasty • Prosthetic joint infection
- Arthroscopic biopsy

KEY POINTS

- Total number of shoulder joint replacement is increasing, so number of infections will also rise.
- *Cutibacterium acnes* is the most common pathogen in shoulder prosthetic joint infection (PJI), which has different characteristics than common total knee and hip pathogens.
- Diagnostic workup for shoulder PJI is more nuanced than total hip and knee evaluation.

INTRODUCTION

The yearly incidence of shoulder arthroplasty continues to increase at rates that outpace that of hip and knee arthroplasty. This, in conjunction, with an aging population, means that more patients each year will be living with a shoulder prosthesis. Recent projections have shown that 800,000 people within the United States have undergone a total shoulder replacement.[1] Given this, shoulder surgeons need to be aware of the workup and treatment of potential complications that can arise after shoulder arthroplasty.

One such complication is prosthetic joint infection (PJI). The rate of shoulder PJI is cited around 0.7% to 1.8% in primary procedures and 4% to 15.4% in revision procedures.[2,3] This places a significant burden on the patient and has negative implications on morbidity and mortality, mirroring that of PJI in lower-extremity arthroplasty. One recent study examined the difference between aseptic and septic revision surgery and found that at 2 years postoperatively, the mortality rate was double in the septic patients.[4] It has also been recognized that prosthetic shoulder infections present differently than those in the knee or hip, have different causative organisms, and may ultimately need a different treatment algorithm. Given the significant financial burden placed on society by PJI, accurate diagnosis and appropriate treatment of shoulder PJI are paramount. Much of the strategy for the diagnostic workup of prosthetic shoulder infections has been borrowed from algorithms developed for the diagnosis of PJI in total hips and knees. This article highlights some of the differences between infections in the upper extremity versus lower extremity and summarizes where the current literature stands on diagnostic workup for suspected prosthetic shoulder infections.

Musculoskeletal Infection Society Criteria for Prosthetic Joint Infections and the International Consensus Meeting on Orthopedic Infections

Total joint arthroplasty is a great operation for treating end stage degeneration in various joints. Total knee arthroplasty (TKA) and total

---

Department of Orthopaedic Surgery and Biomedical Engineering, University of Tennessee Health Science Center—Campbell Clinic, 1211 Union Avenue, Suite 520, Memphis, TN 38104, USA
[1] Present address: 1208 Markway Mills Ct, Jefferson City, MO 65101, USA.
* Corresponding author. 1211 Union Avenue, Suite 520, Memphis, TN 38104.
E-mail address: tbrolin@campbellclinic.com

hip arthroplasty (THA) have been common in the U.S. for many decades; this as well as the increased prevalence of TKA and THA has allowed surgeons to establish objective data for the diagnosis and treatment of PJI in the lower extremity. These surgeons and subspecialty societies have been continuously reevaluating and developing diagnostic algorithms for PJI, which has evolved into the Musculoskeletal Infection Society (MSIS) Criteria for PJIs. The most recent update to this algorithm came in 2018, which uses major and minor criteria which are assigned a numerical value. The provider then uses a cumulative points value to establish a diagnosis of PJI.[5] While these algorithms have been used in the past as a framework for evaluation of shoulder PJI, differences between the upper and lower extremity can make it difficult to apply the MSIS to shoulder PJI. Infections of the knee and hip tend to be caused by staphylococcus species, whereas *Cutibacterium. acnes* is the more common causative organism in the shoulder.[6] The patients' presenting complaints, as well as their immune responses to these different pathogens, can be quite different which makes the diagnosis of shoulder PJI challenging. Because of these differences, an attempt was made at the 2018 International Consensus Meeting (ICM) on Orthopedic Infections to develop a more specific algorithm for the diagnosis of shoulder PJIs. That group identified signs that demonstrate a definite infection; in addition, they published a scoring system for diagnosis of definite infection, probable infection, possible infection, and unlikely infection.[7] Criteria diagnostic of definitive periprosthetic shoulder infection include presence of deep sinus track, gross intraarticular pus, and two positive tissue cultures with phenotypically identical virulent organisms (Box 1). Other criteria, termed minor criteria, were assigned a point value that include unexpected wound drainage, single positive culture with virulent organism, single positive culture with low-virulence organism, second positive culture, humeral loosening,

positive frozen section, positive preoperative aspirate culture, elevated synovial white blood cell (WBC) count, elevate synovial alpha defensin level, elevated C-reactive protein (CRP), elevated erythrocyte sedimentation rate (ESR), and cloudy fluid (Table 1). If the cumulative point value of all positive minor criteria is 6 or higher, probable PJI is termed. The ICM criteria provide a framework for the workup of shoulder PJI. This article will review the information surrounding C. acnes, the current research around workup for PJI in the shoulder, and how new research may assist in the workup for shoulder PJI.

CUTIBACTERIUM ACNES AND PROSTHETIC SHOULDER INFECTIONS

Cutibacterium acnes is a lipophilic, grampositive, facultative, anaerobic bacillus that lives in the pilosebaceous glands in the deep dermal layer of the skin.[8,9] It has been shown to have a greater colonization in the shoulder and axillae than the hip or knee. Colonization is also greater in male patients compared with female patients, which may be linked to higher testosterone production and increased sebum production in

Box 1
International Consensus Meeting criteria of definitive periprosthetic joint infection
Presence of a sinus tract from the skin surface to the prosthesis
Gross intra-articular pus
2 positive tissue cultures with phenotypically identical virulent organisms

Table 1 Minor criteria for definition of shoulder periprosthetic joint infection, based on International Consensus Meeting criteria	
	Score
Unexpected wound drainage	4
Single positive tissue culture with virulent organism	3
Single positive tissue culture with low-virulent organism	1
Second positive tissue culture (identical low-virulence organism)	3
Humeral loosening	3
Positive frozen section (5 PMNs in $\geq$ 5 high-power fields)	3
Positive preoperative aspirate culture (low or high virulence)	3
Elevated synovial neutrophil percentage (>80%)	2
Elevated synovial WBC count (>3000 cells/µL)	2
Elevated ESR (>30 mm/h)	2
Elevated CRP level (>10 mg/L)	2
Elevated synovial α-defensin level	2
Cloudy fluid	2

CRP, XXX; ESR, XXX; WBC, white blood cell.

these areas in males.[10,11] It is currently understood to be the most common causative organism in infections present after rotator cuff repair and shoulder arthroplasty. However, culture positivity with *C acnes* does not necessarily denote a diagnosis of infection, given it is readily found as a commensal organism at the time of shoulder surgery. Although some physicians believe the incidence of infection caused by this organism is increasing, others have argued that the increase is most likely linked to greater awareness and newer techniques in detection of *C acnes* in cultures.[12] Isolation of *C acnes* in cultures is increased by holding the cultures for at least 14 days in a microbiology laboratory. Although *C acnes* generally demonstrates good susceptibility to the typical antibiotics used for musculoskeletal infections, particularly beta-lactams, rifampin, and quinolones, resistance to certain antibiotics like clindamycin is emerging, and even though it is an anaerobic bacterium, it shows natural resistance to metronidazole.[13] *C acnes* also forms a biofilm that can make eradication difficult in chronic infections.

Given the prevalence of *C acnes* and heightened awareness of *C acnes* PJIs, studies have investigated how to decrease the burden of *C acnes* on the skin and in surgery preoperatively and intraoperatively. A recent review article compared various prehospital treatments and surgical skin preparations, reporting preoperative home treatments with benzoyl peroxide showed a reduction of *C acnes* and an average cost between $8.50 to $10.[14] It also reviewed 6 studies looking at chlorhexidine gluconate in various concentrations and determined that it was not effective at reducing *C acnes* on the skin; however, 2 studies comparing chlorhexidine gluconate to hydrogen peroxide demonstrated that hydrogen peroxide lessened *C acnes*. Adding to the difficulty in eradicating *C acnes* preoperatively is the fact that it also resides in the dermal tissue and sebaceous glands. However, 1 group looked at the level of *C acnes* DNA in the soft tissues around the shoulder and found a low abundance of DNA in any tissue other than the skin. Therefore, the authors argued that most infections do come from skin contamination and not from opportunistic expansion of *C acnes* into the shoulder joint.[15] More studies are needed to evaluate preoperative and intraoperative techniques for decreasing *C acnes*. These may look into use of intraoperative antibiotic treatments, or other mechanisms to decrease infection rates.

RADIOGRAPHIC ANALYSIS OF A SHOULDER WITH POSSIBLE PROSTHETIC JOINT INFECTION

Routine monitoring is typical following total shoulder arthroplasty (TSA). These images, obtained by the treating doctor, can monitor for dislocation, loosening, soft tissue failures, and infection. The images are usually obtained at standard intervals to monitor the prosthesis and compare with previous imaging. These postoperative images can be the rst indicator of infection. One study demonstrated that radiographic evidence of humeral component loosening and humeral osteolysis on radiographs was linked with threefold and tenfold risk of positive *C acnes* cultures; glenoid loosening on imaging was also found to have a threefold risk of positive culture for other organisms in workup for shoulder infection.[16] Patient symptoms, physical examination, and radiographic evaluation can be the first indicators of infection.

SERUM WORKUP FOR SHOULDER PROSTHETIC JOINT INFECTION

Obtaining laboratory values has been standard practice in evaluating for signs of in ammation and infection. As described previously, the ICM criteria on PJI assigns a point value to elevated ESR (>30 mm/h) and CRP (>10 mg/L).[7] Most practitioners also get a complete blood cell count (CBC) as part of their workup to evaluate the serum white blood cell count. In addition, various other laboratory markers have been discussed, which can be incorporated in the evaluation for PJI. These serum markers can have differing effectiveness when comparing their merits to assessing infection in the upper or lower extremity. A shoulder infected with *C acnes* can present with normal laboratory values, adding to the difficulty in establishing an accurate diagnosis of infection.

One study compared preoperative CRP and ESR values of patients who underwent implant removal of the knee, hip, shoulder, and spine for either infectious or noninfectious causes and found a statistically signi cant difference in CRP values for hip, knee, shoulder, and spine patients that were deemed to be infected, but no difference in ESR values between aseptic and septic shoulder patients.[16,17] The authors found a significant difference in CRP between aseptic and septic shoulder patients and established a CRP cutoff of 4.6 mg/L to detect shoulder infection with a corresponding sensitivity and specificity of 63% and 73%, respectively. This was much lower than the sensitivities and specificities for diagnosis of hip, knee, and spine infections, leading the authors to caution against basing an infection decision on ESR and CRP data alone with shoulder PJI. Another study noted that ESR and CRP may be normal in PJI involving low-virulence organisms or in the setting of chronic infection; the researchers remarked that this may cause one to misdiagnose up to one-fourth of all PJIs if based solely on ESR and CRP workup.[18] Therefore, these laboratory tests should not be used alone but in conjunction to make decisions on shoulder PJI.

As ESR and CRP have been shown to not be highly predictive of shoulder PJI, researchers have looked at other serum laboratory tests to determine if those data could be more helpful. D-dimer has been studied for PJI in other joint infections in the past, and was recently evaluated in shoulder PJI. The researchers found D-dimer was elevated in patients with de nitive or probable shoulder infections based on the ICM criteria compared to those with possible or unlikely infection; however, when they ran a receiver operating characteristic curve analysis, they found that D-dimer had weak diagnostic value for shoulder PJI.[19] The same group found a higher specificity of detecting shoulder PJI when 3 positive serum markers (ESR, CRP, D-dimer) were required, but that was at the expense of sensitivity.

Another serum laboratory value that has been discussed is serum interleukin-6 (IL-6). IL-6 is a pro-in ammatory cytokine that is released by macrophages in response to speci c microbial molecules and is an important mediator of the acute phase response in infection.[20] One group performed a prospective cohort study looking at serum levels of IL-6 collected preoperatively, then compared those values to collected intraoperative cultures to determine if a link existed between IL-6 and positive intraoperative cultures. They failed to find a significant difference between IL-6 levels in patients who were either infected or not infected; with a normal serum IL-6 level of less than 10 pg/mL, the test had sensitivity, specificity, positive predictive value, negative predictive value, and accuracy of 0.14, 0.95, 0.67, 0.61, and 0.62, respectively.[21] Therefore, the researchers could not support using serum IL-6 as a diagnostic marker for infection in shoulder PJI.

These studies demonstrate that it can be dif - cult to accurately diagnose a shoulder PJI based on serum laboratory values alone. Given this, laboratory values are best used in conjunction with aspiration, microbiology, and radiographic data.

INTRA-ARTICULAR ASPIRATION AND TESTING OF ASPIRATE

As the workup for PJI is continued, many providers perform aspiration of the shoulder, which can allow for uid analysis and microbiology data. The ICM on shoulder PJI also weighed in on evaluation of shoulder synovial uid and assigned a numerical value to certain tests that can be obtained from this aspirate. These include a positive preoperative aspirate culture (with either high- or low-virulence organism), elevated synovial neutrophil percentage greater than 80%, elevated synovial WBC greater than 3000 cell/μL, elevated synovial α-defensin level, and cloudy uid seen in the aspirate[7] (see Table 1).

Defensins are antimicrobial peptides that represent a part of the innate immune system that help in neutralizing foreign pathogens.[22] They have been shown to have broad spectrum antimicrobial activities against both gram-positive and gram-negative organisms.[23] Because of their presence in PJI, α-defensin has been used in the workup for total knee and total hip infections, with some studies showing 100% sensitivity and specificity in diagnosing PJI in these joints.[24] Recently, more studies have evaluated the usefulness of α-defensin in the workup of shoulder PJI. One research group showed synovial α-defensin could be more effective than other diagnostic tests of detecting shoulder PJI with area under the curve of 0.78, sensitivity of 63%, specificity of 95%, positive likelihood ratio of 12.1, and negative likelihood ratio of 0.38.[25] Another study looked at 121 patients and evaluated the α-defensin test's ability to predict shoulder PJI, finding the overall accuracy of α-defensin to be 91%, sensitivity of 75%, specificity of 96%, negative predictive value of 93%, and positive predictive value of 86%.[26] These studies lend credence to the usefulness of the α-defensin test in shoulder PJI, and for its inclusion in the ICM algorithm.

Two other values that are included in the ICM algorithm are synovial WBC count and synovial neutrophil percentage. Although the ICM lists a cutoff value of synovial WBC greater than 3000 cells/μL and a synovial neutrophil percentage greater than 80%,[7] these are not recognized by all researchers as definitive cutoff values, and various studies cite different cutoffs based on the level of sensitivity and specificity they deem acceptable. One study argued a threshold of 2800 leukocytes/mm[3] demonstrated a sensitivity of 87% and specificity of 88%.[27] In another study by a Swiss group, leukocyte count and synovial neutrophil differential were evaluated. Those researchers found a leukocyte count greater than 12.2 g/L had a sensitivity of 92% and specificity of 100%; they also demonstrated a neutrophil differential of greater than 54% had a sensitivity of 100% and specificity of 75%.[28] Those studies show that even though no standard cutoff value exists, these tests can be helpful in the workup for shoulder PJI.

Synovial IL-6 and synovial leukocyte esterase are 2 other tests worth discussion, but they are not included in the ICM algorithm for workup of shoulder PJI. Serum IL-6 was already discussed, but some studies have also looked at synovial IL-6 levels as a way to help diagnose shoulder PJI. One study evaluated synovial fluid IL-6 levels and computed a receiver operator curve to determine the diagnostic utility of synovial fluid IL-6 analysis; it calculated an area under the curve of 0.891 with sensitivity, specificity, positive likelihood ratio, and negative likelihood ratio of 87%, 90%, 8.45, and 0.15, respectively.[29] The researchers inferred this test has a good diagnostic utility and could be an additional test for the provider trying to decide about shoulder PJI. Others have looked at synovial leukocyte esterase testing; 1 study noted that 17% to 30% of those tests can be nonreadable because of blood contamination of the aspirate.[30] Another study demonstrated that compared with other synovial tests, leukocyte esterase testing may not give information of as high a quality with an accuracy of 76%, sensitivity of 50%, specificity of 87%, positive predictive value of 60%, and negative predictive value of 81%.[23] Synovial leukocyte esterase's issues with contamination and lower predictive value in shoulder PJI may be why it is not used as commonly.

As a practitioner continues to work through the evaluation for shoulder PJI, an aspiration can give meaningful data on the workup for infection. However, compared with hip and knee PJI workup, aspiration results can still be inconclusive, and in many cases can result in an inability to retrieve fluid for analysis. Given this, some surgeons have sought other ways to achieve tissues for microbiology analysis.

ARTHROSCOPIC BIOPSY FOR THE EVALUATION OF SHOULDER PROSTHETIC JOINT INFECTION

Shoulder arthroscopy in the pre-revision setting of shoulder arthroplasty has been discussed as a method of evaluating a patient with a painful shoulder prosthesis. Compared with a shoulder aspiration, diagnostic shoulder arthroscopy has the added benefit of potentially detecting component loosening, allowing for synovial biopsy, evaluating and treating postoperative adhesions, and evaluation for potential rotator cuff tears following anatomic TSA.[31] Given the significant physical and financial burden that revision surgery for shoulder PJI imposes, arthroscopic biopsy may be a less invasive way to accurately diagnose PJI before revision shoulder arthroplasty.

It has been demonstrated that intraoperative frozen biopsies were only positive in 8% of cases; however, 60% of the patients went on to have positive intraoperative cultures that were taken at the same operation.[32] This can lead to misdiagnosis and inadequate treatment of patients if infection is missed at the time of revision. Preoperative biopsy and culture allow the provider the opportunity to review culture results before proceeding with revision surgery. Hsu recommended when proceeding with biopsy to get samples from 6 separate areas, including the synovium and capsule, the membrane between the humeral head prosthesis and the collar of the prosthetic stem, the periglenoid tissue, the glenoid cavity tissue, the membrane within the humeral canal, and the explanted prosthesis.[33] Some of these areas will not be available for arthroscopic biopsy, but the suggestion provides a framework for consistently performing intraoperative biopsies. Another factor that needs to be communicated to the treating surgeon's microbiology laboratory is that these cultures need to be held for up to 14 days to evaluate for less virulent pathogens, such as C acnes. One study demonstrated that with adequate laboratory technique, C acnes could be detected in 57% of the positive cultures, making it the most common pathogen in shoulder PJI, and when monitoring the patients with negative cultures long term, there was no incidence of missed periprosthetic infection.[34]

Many publications have examined the usefulness of pre-revision biopsy to demonstrate shoulder PJI, but those studies have had a fairly small number of patients.[35–38] Building on these publications, a recent systemic review and meta-analysis looked at the aggregate values of pre-revision tissue biopsy when combining previous studies to give a larger sample size; it demonstrated when 1 pre-revision biopsy-positive culture was used to calculate statistics, there was an aggregate sensitivity of 92%, specificity of 70%, aggregate positive predictive value of 65.7%, and aggregate negative predictive value of 93.3%.[39] Although a smaller sample size was used, the authors also calculated these values when 2 positive cultures were present at the time of pre-revision biopsy, and found aggregate sensitivity of 100%, aggregate specificity of 50%, aggregate positive predictive value of 33.3%, and aggregate negative predictive value of 100%.[39] One study also examined results of diagnostic arthroscopic biopsy for shoulder PJI, finding a sensitivity of 67% with a specificity of 95%. But when they performed a subgroup analysis of patients who underwent a diagnostic biopsy in addition to the standard diagnostic workup, that group had a sensitivity of 100% and a specificity of 83%.[40] Because of that, the authors concluded that a pre-revision biopsy should be considered in most cases, as it can help increase the predictive value of the diagnostic workup.

These findings demonstrate that a pre-revision arthroscopic biopsy can provide valuable information to a treating provider when other results are inconclusive. Not only can the practitioner evaluate the soft tissues and implants at the time of biopsy, but he or she can also obtain tissue for culture that has a better ability of identifying infection compared with aspiration alone.

SUMMARY

In summary, as demonstrated by the literature, the diagnosis of shoulder PJI can be much more difcult than that of the lower extremity. Given the indolent nature of shoulder PJIs, a delayed or missed diagnosis can occur if the provider does not have heightened awareness. The ICM gives practitioners a guideline by which to evaluate for infection in a TSA patient. However, there is still some ambiguity built into the ICM's scoring system with categories of denitive infection, probable infection, possible infection, and infection unlikely, which puts the onus on the treating provider to decide whether to pursue revision surgery. This article discussed other serum and synovial tests that have been suggested for diagnosis of infection. It also notes that while a diagnostic arthroscopic biopsy is not included in the ICM criteria, research has demonstrated it can be helpful in determining if there is a shoulder PJI. Although it is more invasive and has higher associated costs than serum blood tests or joint aspirations, the data can be helpful in coming to an accurate diagnosis of a septic or aseptic painful prosthesis. Future research is needed to aid surgeons in diagnosing shoulder PJI and decreasing the ambiguity of cases of probable and possible infection.

DISCLOSURE

The authors report no conflicts of interest.

REFERENCES

1. Farley KX, Wilson JM, Kumar A, et al. Prevalence of shoulder arthroplasty in the United States and the increasing burden of revision shoulder arthroplasty. JBJS Open Access 2021;6(3):e2000156. https://doi.org/10.2106/jbjs.oa.20.00156.
2. Padegimas EM, Maltenfort M, Ramsey ML, et al. Periprosthetic shoulder infection in the United States: incidence and economic burden. J Shoulder Elbow Surg 2015;24(5):741–6. https://doi.org/10.1016/j.jse.2014.11.044.
3. Singh JA, Sperling JW, Schleck C, et al. Periprosthetic infections after total shoulder arthroplasty: a 33-year perspective. J Shoulder Elbow Surg 2012;21(11):1534–41. https://doi.org/10.1016/j.jse.2012.01.006.
4. Austin DC, Townsley SH, Rogers TH, et al. Shoulder periprosthetic joint infection and all-cause mortality: a worrisome association. JBJS Open Access 2022;7(1):e2100118. https://doi.org/10.2106/jbjs.oa.21.00118.
5. Parvizi J, Tan TL, Goswami K, et al. The 2018 definition of periprosthetic hip and knee infection: an evidence-based and validated criteria. J Arthroplasty 2018;33(5):1309–14.e2. https://doi.org/10.1016/j.arth.2018.02.078.
6. Elston MJ, Dupaix JP, Opanova MI, et al. Cutibacterium acnes (formerly Proprionibacterium acnes) and shoulder surgery. Hawaii J Health Soc Welf 2019;78(11 Suppl 2):3–5.
7. Garrigues GE, Zmistowski B, Cooper AM, et al, ICM Shoulder Group. Proceedings from the 2018 International Consensus Meeting on Orthopedic Infections: the definition of periprosthetic shoulder infection. J Shoulder Elbow Surg 2019;28:S8–12.
8. Foster AL, Cutbush K, Ezure Y, et al. Cutibacterium acnes in shoulder surgery: a scoping review of strategies for prevention, diagnosis, and treatment. J Shoulder Elbow Surg 2021;30(6):1410–22. https://doi.org/10.1016/j.jse.2020.11.011.
9. Boisrenoult P. Cutibacterium acnes prosthetic joint infection: diagnosis and treatment. Orthop Traumatol Surg Res 2018;104(1):S19–24. https://doi.org/10.1016/j.otsr.2017.05.030.
10. Levy PY, Fenollar F, Stein A, et al. Propionibacterium acnes postoperative shoulder arthritis: an emerging clinical entity. Clin Infect Dis 2008;46(12):1884–6. https://doi.org/10.1086/588477.

11. Patel A, Calfee RP, Plante M, et al. Propionibacterium acnes colonization of the human shoulder. J Shoulder Elbow Surg 2009;18(6):897–902. https://doi.org/10.1016/j.jse.2009.01.023.

12. Trampuz A, Piper KE, Jacobson MJ, et al. Sonication of removed hip and knee prostheses for diagnosis of infection. N Engl J Med 2007;357(7):654–63. https://doi.org/10.1056/nejmoa061588.

13. Achermann Y, Goldstein EJ, Coenye T, et al. Propionibacterium acnes: from commensal to opportunistic biofilm-associated implant pathogen. Clin Microbiol Rev 2014;27(3):419–40. https://doi.org/10.1128/cmr.00092-13.

14. Sagkrioti M, Glass S, Arealis G. Evaluation of the effectiveness of skin preparation methods for the reduction of Cutibacterium acnes (formerly Propionibacterium acnes) in shoulder surgery: a systematic review. Shoulder Elbow 2021;14(6):583–97. https://doi.org/10.1177/17585732211032523.

15. Qiu B, Al K, Pena-Diaz AM, et al. Cutibacterium acnes and the shoulder microbiome. J Shoulder Elbow Surg 2018;27(10):1734–9.

16. Pottinger P, Butler-Wu S, Neradilek MB, et al. Prognostic factors for bacterial cultures positive for Propionibacterium acnes and other organisms in a large series of revision shoulder arthroplasties performed for stiffness, pain, or loosening. J Bone Joint Surg Am 2012;94(22):2075–83. https://doi.org/10.2106/jbjs.k.00861.

17. Piper KE, Fernandez-Sampedro M, Steckelberg KE, et al. C-reactive protein, erythrocyte sedimentation rate and orthopedic implant infection. PLoS One 2010;5(2):e9358. https://doi.org/10.1371/journal.pone.0009358.

18. Pérez-Prieto D, Portillo ME, Puig-Verdié L, et al. C-reactive protein may misdiagnose prosthetic joint infections, particularly chronic and low-grade infections. Int Orthop 2017;41(7):1315–9. https://doi.org/10.1007/s00264-017-3430-5.

19. Zmistowski B, Chang M, Shahi A, et al. Is D-dimer a reliable serum marker for shoulder periprosthetic joint infection? Clin Orthop Relat Res 2021;479(7):1447–54. https://doi.org/10.1097/corr.0000000000001774.

20. Tanaka T, Narazaki M, Kishimoto T. IL-6 in inflammation, immunity, and disease. Cold Spring Harb Perspect Biol 2014;6(10):a016295. https://doi.org/10.1101/cshperspect.a016295.

21. Villacis D, Merriman JA, Yalamanchili R, et al. Serum interleukin-6 as a marker of periprosthetic shoulder infection. J Bone Joint Surg Am 2014;96(1):41–5. https://doi.org/10.2106/jbjs.l.01634.

22. Hazlett L, Wu M. Defensins in innate immunity. Cell Tissue Res 2010;343(1):175–88. https://doi.org/10.1007/s00441-010-1022-4.

23. Ericksen B, Wu Z, Lu W, et al. Antibacterial activity and specificity of the six human α-defensins. Antimicrob Agents Chemother 2005;49(1):269–75. https://doi.org/10.1128/aac.49.1.269-275.2005.

24. Deirmengian C, Kardos K, Kilmartin P, et al. Diagnosing periprosthetic joint infection: has the era of the biomarker arrived? Clin Orthop Relat Res 2014;472(11):3254–62. https://doi.org/10.1007/s11999-014-3543-8.

25. Frangiamore SJ, Saleh A, Grosso MJ, et al. A-defensin as a predictor of periprosthetic shoulder infection. J Shoulder Elbow Surg 2015;24(7):1021–7. https://doi.org/10.1016/j.jse.2014.12.021.

26. Ecker NU, Koniker A, Gehrke T, et al. What is the diagnostic accuracy of alpha-defensin and leukocyte esterase test in periprosthetic shoulder infection? Clin Orthop Relat Res 2019;477(7):1712–8. https://doi.org/10.1097/corr.0000000000000762.

27. Streck LE, Gaal C, Forster J, et al. Defining a synovial fluid white blood cell count threshold to predict periprosthetic infection after shoulder arthroplasty. J Clin Med 2021;11(1):50. https://doi.org/10.3390/jcm11010050.

28. Strahm C, Zdravkovic V, Egidy C, et al. Accuracy of synovial leukocyte and polymorphonuclear cell count in patients with shoulder prosthetic joint infection. J Bone Jt Infect 2018;3(5):245–8. https://doi.org/10.7150/jbji.29289.

29. Frangiamore SJ, Saleh A, Grosso MJ, et al. Synovial fluid interleukin-6 as a predictor of periprosthetic shoulder infection. J Shoulder Elbow Surg 2015;24(4):E112–3. https://doi.org/10.1016/j.jse.2014.11.010.

30. Ruangsomboon P, Chinprasertsuk S, Khejonnit V, et al. Effect of depth of centrifuged synovial fluid on leukocyte esterase test for periprosthetic joint infection. J Orthop Res 2017;35(11):2545–50. https://doi.org/10.1002/jor.23561.

31. Parker DB, Smith AC, Fleckenstein CM, et al. Arthroscopic evaluation and treatment of complications that arise following prosthetic shoulder arthroplasty. JBJS Rev 2020;8(8):e200020–8. https://doi.org/10.2106/jbjs.rvw.20.00020.

32. Topolski MS, Chin PYK, Sperling JW, et al. Revision shoulder arthroplasty with positive intraoperative cultures: the value of preoperative studies and intraoperative histology. J Shoulder Elbow Surg 2006;15(4):402–6. https://doi.org/10.1016/j.jse.2005.10.001.

33. Hsu JE, Bumgarner RE, Matsen FA. Propionibacterium in shoulder arthroplasty: what we think we know today. J Bone Jt Surg 2016;98(7):597–606. https://doi.org/10.2106/jbjs.15.00568.

34. Ellsworth HS, Zhang L, Keener JD, et al. Ten-day culture incubation time can accurately detect bacterial infection in periprosthetic infection in shoulder arthroplasty. JSES Int 2020;4(2):372–6. https://doi.org/10.1016/j.jseint.2019.12.006.

35. Dilisio MF, Miller LR, Warner JJP, et al. Arthroscopic tissue culture for the evaluation of

periprosthetic shoulder infection. J Bone Jt Surg 2014;96(23):1952–8. https://doi.org/10.2106/jbjs.m.01512.

36. Tashjian RZ, Granger EK, Zhang Y. Utility of prerevision tissue biopsy sample to predict revision shoulder arthroplasty culture results in at-risk patients. J Shoulder Elbow Surg 2017;26(2):197–203. https://doi.org/10.1016/j.jse.2016.07.019.

37. Akgün D, Maziak N, Plachel F, et al. Diagnostic arthroscopy for detection of periprosthetic infection in painful shoulder arthroplasty. Arthroscopy 2019;35(9):2571–7. https://doi.org/10.1016/j.arthro.2019.03.058.

38. Guild T, Kuhn G, Rivers M, et al. The role of arthroscopy in painful shoulder arthroplasty: is revision always necessary? Arthroscopy 2020;36(6):1508–14. https://doi.org/10.1016/j.arthro.2020.01.045.

39. Cotter EJ, Winzenried AE, Polania-Gonzalez E, et al. Role of pre-revision tissue biopsy in evaluation of painful shoulder arthroplasty: A systematic review and meta-analysis. J Shoulder Elbow Surg 2021;30(6):1445–57. https://doi.org/10.1016/j.jse.2020.10.018.

40. Mederake M, Hofmann UK, Fink B. The significance of synovial biopsy in the diagnostic workup of the low-grade periprosthetic joint infection of shoulder arthroplasty. Arch Orthop Trauma Surg 2021;142(11):3157–64. https://doi.org/10.1007/s00402-021-03932-x.

Hand and Wrist

Fingertip Infections

James Barger, MD, Reed W. Hoyer, MD*

KEYWORDS

• Fingertip infections • Felon • Paronychia • Osteomyelitis

KEY POINTS

- *Staphylococcus aureus* is the most common cause of bacterial fingertip infections.
- Paronychia, or infections of the nailfold, are the most common infection of the hand, whereas felons, or pulp space infections, represent the second most common infection.
- Untreated paronychia and felons, particularly in the patient with diabetes, can develop into osteomyelitis, septic arthritis, or septic flexor tenosynovitis.
- There are a range of diagnoses that are mistaken for common fingertip infections, including calcific peritendonitis/arthritis, gout, and herpetic whitlow, among others.

INTRODUCTION

The fingertip is the interface between humans and the world, including the various thorns, dirty needles, and other hazards to be found there. It is therefore unsurprising that this is the site where hand infections most frequently occur.[1,2] Although they are commonly encountered by hand surgeons and other physicians, fingertip infections have several mimics and diagnosis and management is not always straightforward. Without exception, early diagnosis and treatment are key to success.[3] As with all infections, they are more common and are more aggressive in immunosuppressed patients.[1,3,4] This article reviews fingertip anatomy, common and uncommon fingertip infections and their mimics, and recommendations for management.

ANATOMY

The fingertip consists of the distal phalanx; the germinal and sterile matrix; the nail plate; the insertion of the terminal extensor and flexor digitorum profundus tendons; the volar pad; and the enveloping skin including the eponychium, hyponychium, and nail gutters. The fingertip pad is a fascial compartment that is separated from the finger proximally at the level of the distal interphalangeal joint (DIP) flexion crease. The skin of the fingertip and the pad of fat are stabilized by a web of thin fascial bands that extend from periosteum to the skin,[5] although it is unlikely that these bands envelop discrete subcompartments.[5]

The flexor digitorum profundus inserts onto the middle three-fifths of the distal phalanx volarly, whereas the terminal extensor inserts dorsally at the physeal scar. The flexor digitorum profundus is enveloped in its sheath, which provides a path of communication between the otherwise walled-off fingertip and the rest of the hand.

The fingernail shields the fingertip and provides counterpressure for the richly innervated sensory apparatus.[6] It also regulates temperature and, in some cases, is used as a weapon. It is generated by the underlying nailbed, which consists of the germinal matrix proximally and sterile matrix distally and is attached to the periosteum of the phalanx. The germinal matrix is appreciated in the intact fingertip as the white arc of the lunula and originates approximately 2 mm distal to the terminal extensor insertion. Ninety-five percent of nail growth comes from these cells and 5% from cells on the undersurface of the eponychial fold. They lose their white color as they lose their nuclei and migrate distally to become the sterile matrix. The nail plate is more firmly adherent to the sterile matrix than the germinal.[7] The skin folds on either side are the paronychium and the proximal skin fold

Indiana Hand to Shoulder Center, Indianapolis, IN, USA
* Corresponding author. 8501 Harcourt Road, Indianapolis, IN 46260.
E-mail address: rhoyer@ihtsc.com

Orthop Clin N Am 55 (2024) 265–272
https://doi.org/10.1016/j.ocl.2023.10.003
0030-5898/24/© 2023 Elsevier Inc. All rights reserved.

is the eponychium. The plug of keratinous material at the junction of the distal sterile matrix and the skin, the hyponychium, contains white blood cells and seals the subungal space.[6]

ACUTE PARONYCHIA
Background and Epidemiology
Fingertip infections are the most common hand infections and paronychia are the most common fingertip infections.[8] These are periungal infections that occur from inoculation of bacteria, often after minor trauma, which may not have been memorable to the patient.[9] They typically present with several days of painful swelling and erythema of the paronychium and/or eponychium[2,10] They are associated most commonly with onychophagia, and manicures, artificial nails, and hangnails (stripping of the paronychium).[2,4] If an aggressive infection is suspected or the infection has been present for more than a few days, radiographs may be obtained to rule out bony erosion; laboratory tests are usually unnecessary. Subungal infections are rare but can occur in those who engage in activities that disrupt the hyponychium, such as dishwashing.[6] The presence of an abscess is distinguished from an early paronychia without fluid collection using the Turkmen digital pressure test, where the skin overlying the abscess blanches after pinching the fingertip.[11] The history taker should query for exposure to oral secretions or labial lesions (raising suspicion for herpetic whitlow), medical diagnoses that can mimic or predispose to paronychia, and use of medications associated with paronychia (discussed later).[9]

Microbiology
Staphylococcus aureus is the most common cause of bacterial fingertip infections.[2,3,12] In a report of 1500 patients undergoing incision and drainage of hand infections in an urban center, 458 had positive cultures. Fifty-three percent had methicillin-resistant *S aureus* (MRSA), 23% methicillin-sensitive *S aureus*, and 19% polymicrobial infection (the latter was strongly associated with diabeted mellits (DM), intravenous drug use (IVDU), or human bites, suggesting that broad-spectrum coverage should be considered in these patients).[3]

Treatment
Nonoperative
If no abscess has formed, early paronychia may be treated with a trial of topical or oral antibiotics. Topical fusidic acid with betamethasone has been shown to be effective.[13] Oral antibiotics should offer gram-positive coverage, including for MRSA in communities with greater than 10% prevalence; patients with exposure to human or animal flora should receive antibiotics covering anaerobes (eg, amoxicillin/clavulanate).[3,9,14,15] Soaks with soapy water, saline, or antiseptic mixtures are advocated as an adjunct by several authors, although their marginal benefit is not clear.[1,9,16,17]

Operative
In cases in which an abscess is present, drainage is required. The abscess is often accessible through the eponychial fold, although a skin incision may be required for more distant spread. This space may be opened up with a blade; a blunt instrument, such as a Freer elevator; or a hypodermic needle with the bevel angling upward (no matter the instrument, care should be taken not to injure the nailbed (Fig. 1).[9,18,19] As with any abscess, adequate and sustained decompression is key. Communication between the abscess cavity and the outside world should be maintained by stenting it open with an iodoform wick or other packing. Nail plate elevation and removal are only required if the infection has dissected deep to this structure,[9] but removal of a small section of the nail can help maintain drainage. If a skin incision is required, it should not be immediately adjacent to the nailfold, to prevent skin necrosis.[18] If there is an extensive subeponychial abscess, the eponychium may be reflected proximally via longitudinal incisions on the radial and ulnar sides of the dorsal distal phalanx and sutured over gauze for 2 to 7 days to allow drainage, but the eponychium should not be excised because the cells on its deep surface provide growth and luster to the nail.[6,9,20] Furthermore, care should be taken not to damage the germinal matrix and terminal extensor

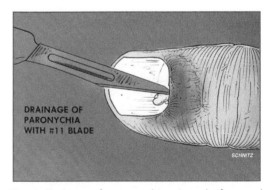

DRAINAGE OF
PARONYCHIA
WITH #11 BLADE

SCHNITZ

Fig. 1. Drainage of a paronychia using a knife turned flat and placed between the nailfold and the nail plate. An incision in the paronychium is to be avoided, because this results in a permanent deformity.

while reflecting the eponychium, although it presumably will have been dissected away from these structures by the abscess.

Antibiotics

Studies on fingertip infections and abscesses elsewhere in the body have demonstrated that adjuvant antibiotics are usually not necessary after adequate incision and drainage.[2,21,22] Our practice is to give antibiotics if there is substantial associated cellulitis; this requires some clinician judgment regarding the balance between the need for infection control versus antibiotic stewardship and morbidity.

Wound care

Comparative data on wound care are lacking. If a wick is required for a paronychia, we typically remove it the day following incision and drainage, followed by daily dry sterile dressing changes until resolution. Maintenance of a contaminated or saturated dressing can lead to skin maceration or infection persistence, although maintaining a large bulky dressing for a longer period may be considered in unreliable patients.

Soaks

Soaking the affected digit in water (with or without soap), saline, or antiseptic solutions, such as povidone-iodine, hydrogen peroxide, and chlorhexidine, is often used following irrigation and debridement (I&D). Typically soaks are performed once or twice daily for 10 to 15 minutes, and are recommended for 5 to 7 days or until symptom resolution.[1,8,14] However, Tosti and colleagues[17] recently performed a randomized, controlled trial of soaks with povidone-iodine solution after debridement of hand infections and found no benefits from the soaks as compared with daily dressing changes alone.

CHRONIC PARONYCHIA
Background and Epidemiology

Chronic paronychia is a condition characterized by inflammation of the nailfold that persists for 6 weeks or longer.[9] Erythema and swelling are typically less severe than in the acute form.[1] Chronic paronychia often occurs in people who repeatedly subject their fingers to mechanical and chemical stressors that damage the skin, such as dishwashers or hair stylists.[9,18,23] In these cases, there is typically involvement of multiple digits and transverse grooves in the nail plate (Beau lines) may be present.[24] People with diabetes and those who are immunosuppressed are at higher risk.[9] Additionally, some medications, such as epidermal growth factor receptor (EGFR) inhibitors, taxanes, antiretrovirals, retinoids, antiepileptics, and methotrexate, can cause chronic paronychia because of their toxicity to the epithelium. In some cases, the effects of these drugs may not manifest until several weeks after administration.[14,25–29]

Treatment

Although fungal infection was previously thought to be the causative organism in chronic paronychia, recent studies have shown that *Candida albicans* is present in about 40% to 95% of cases and that topical steroids are more effective than antifungal treatments in resolving the condition.[9,14,23,24,30] The presence of *Candida* is likely secondary to the underlying repetitive compromise of the skin barrier.[30] Therefore, the primary treatment of chronic paronychia is to avoid the repetitive irritants that caused the inflammation in the first place.[9,24] Topical steroids or calcineurin inhibitors are used to reduce inflammation and provide relief.[30] Antibacterial medications are typically not necessarily unless there is an acute-on-chronic presentation involving erythema and/or purulence.[24] In recalcitrant cases where nonsurgical treatments are ineffective, surgery may be required. This can involve marsupialization, which allows the proximal nailfold to communicate with the external environment and may include the reflection or excision of the eponychium, removal of the nail plate, or excision of a crescent of eponychium. However, the mechanism behind the success of these methods is not fully understood.[9,31–33] In patients whose symptoms persist despite surgery, ablation of the nailbed and full-thickness skin grafting may be required; in these cases the diseased tissue should be sent for pathology to rule out cancer (discussed later).

FELON
Overview

A felon is an infection of the volar pulp of the distal phalanx that presents with erythema, swelling, and pain. As the infection progresses within the closed compartment of the fingertip pad, it can lead to tissue necrosis and abscess formation.[34] Felons account for 15% to 20% of all hand infections and the cause is often unclear.[10,35] Kanavel,[36] in his classic 1912 description of hand infections, suggested that atraumatic felons may occur when pathogenic bacteria enter through the glands in the columns of fat. Penetrating causes, such as diabetic fingersticks and wood splinters, are also well documented.[37] The most common causative agent is *S aureus*, although felons may be polymicrobial in individuals who engage in intravenous drug use or farm work.[38] People with diabetes are higher risk for felon in general and for polymicrobial infections.[37]

There is limited evidence on the optimal treatment of felon, and the decision to pursue operative versus nonoperative management often depends on clinical judgment and experience. It has been proposed that felon has a cellulitic stage, amenable to medical management, and an abscess phase requiring drainage.[10] Others have suggested that incision is necessary once the skin of the distal phalanx becomes tense, regardless of whether an abscess has formed, to alleviate vascular congestion in the fingertip.[34] If nonoperative management is pursued, antibiotics should be selected to cover gram-positive cocci, with coverage for MRSA and other pathogens included if there is reasonable suspicion of their involvement. Close follow-up is necessary to determine if incision is eventually required. The authors tend to err on the side of surgical management for felons to stay ahead of a worsening infection.

Neglecting the treatment of felon can have severe consequences, including skin sloughing, necrosis of the fingertip because of a local compartment syndrome, septic arthritis, osteomyelitis, flexor tenosynovitis (**Fig. 2**), and flexor tendon rupture. These sequelae may require radical treatment including amputation.[35] The reason these occur is that felons are limited in their proximal spread through the subcutaneous tissues by the attachment of the deep fascia at the DIP joint. They therefore tend to decompress through several other routes, including a sinus tract to the skin, through the nailfold to form a paronychia, or through periosteum to bone, joint, and tendon sheath.[34] The presence of a sinus warrants radiographs to evaluate the possibility of osteomyelitis.[35] In some cases,

pus may decompress through the dermis but not the epidermis, creating a superficial abscess that may dissect proximally subepidermally.[10]

Once the decision for surgical intervention is made, the physician must choose an approach for incision and drainage. Some authors recommend a midlateral J incision on the noncontact side of the fingertip. This is designed to keep away from the volar pad and prevent devascularization of dorsal skin. It is our preference, if pus is present, to center a longitudinal incision directly over the area of maximum fluctuance given the potential for injury to digital nerve branches and ensuing causalgia in lateral incisions.[10,34,39] Fishmouth incisions are not recommended because of risk for devascularization.[39] In the presence of a sinus, it is essential to excise it with an ellipse of tissue. It is prudent to avoid aggressive proximal probing because inadvertent penetration of the tendon sheath can cause flexor tenosynovitis.[10] A wick should usually be placed at the conclusion of the procedure to ensure continued drainage, and may be serially replaced in subsequent days if necessary.[39] As with all hand infections, incisions should be closed loosely or left open entirely.

The conventional theory of felon anatomy suggests that the collagen bands of the volar pulp form microcompartments that make simple incision and drainage inadequate for infection control unless they are broken up.[40] This is not anatomically correct.[5] Therefore, the surgeon must endeavor to break up any loculations and enable egress of infection, but not feel obligated to traumatize every fibrous septation in the fingertip.[41]

DISTAL INTERPHALANGEAL JOINT SEPTIC ARTHRITIS

Septic arthritis of the DIP can occur as a result of spread of the infections discussed previously, or

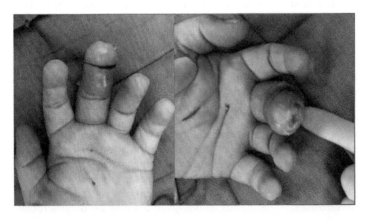

Fig. 2. A neglected felon from a burn to the tip of the middle finger in a patient with uncontrolled diabetes mellitus that caused osteomyelitis of the distal phalanx and then broke out into the flexor tendon sheath resulting in septic flexor tenosynovitis. This is best managed with an amputation of the distal phalanx and drainage of the flexor sheath, often closed in a staged fashion to allow drainage.

as a result of penetrating inoculation, such as attempted puncture of a mucous cyst.[42,43] It presents with erythema and swelling of the joint with restricted active and passive motion, with or without a draining wound. Radiographs should be obtained to assess for erosive changes, fracture, chondrocalcinosis, and foreign bodies; other imaging modalities may be obtained if indicated by the clinical scenario (eg, MRI to assess for osteomyelitis). Aspiration may be indicated for diagnosis or culture data, but often the clinical picture is clear and urgent arthrotomy, irrigation, and debridement is indicated. Any of the typical dorsal approaches to the DIP joint, such as the H-shaped, inverted Mercedes, hockey stick, or midaxial longitudinal incision, may be used, guided by the presence or absence of a wound and by surgeon preference. The capsule is excised, maintaining the terminal extensor tendon, and cultures taken, joint thoroughly irrigated and debrided, and skin loosely closed.[42] Saito and colleagues[44] reported on a novel technique of the use of a Masquelet technique with delayed DIP fusion for patients with osteomyelitis or preexisting joint destruction/arthritis, which may be considered in these scenarios. Broad-spectrum parenteral antibiotics should be given initially, followed by 2 to 3 weeks of culture-guided oral antibiotics.[45] Infectious disease consultation should be considered in complicated or established infections and in immunocompromised patients. Soaks may be considered in the setting of an open wound, as discussed previously for other infections.

OSTEOMYELITIS

Osteomyelitis (the infection of bone) can occur as a sequela of the infections mentioned previously; from trauma, such an open distal phalanx fracture; as a postoperative complication; or in the setting of vascular insufficiency and resulting ulcerations. Hematogenous spread to the fingertip or DIP is rare in immunocompetent adults, and less common than in larger joints in immunocompromised patients and children.[46] Diagnosis is made with an active or recurrent infection and erosive changes on radiographs. Given the generally favorable blood supply in the hand, osteomyelitis of the distal phalanx can often be treated with curettage/resection of infected bone, coverage of any soft tissue defects, and a less than 2-week course of culture-directed oral antibiotics after a response is noted to initial doses of parenteral antibiotics. Hardware removal is recommended if present. Persistent infections or vascularly compromised

digits often require amputation of the infected portion of the finger.[46,47]

ZOONOSES

Several less common fingertip infections fall under the umbrella of "farmyard pox." Orf disease is caused by parapoxvirus and usually affects those who care for sheep or goats. It causes a painful wheal on the fingertip with a clear exudate. It may cause systemic symptoms, particularly in the immunocompromised.[48] Orf disease is self-limiting, lasts 6 to 8 weeks, and should not be treated surgically.[49] Parapox virus can also be acquired from the teats of cows, in which case it is caused milker's nodule.[48]

The bacteria *Erysipelothrix rhusiopathiae* causes erysipeloid (of Rosenbach). This is found in patients who have handled lobsters, livestock, meat, and the like. It presents with an inflamed purple-red lesion and there may be vesicular eruptions. Most antibiotics are effective.[50]

Cat and dog bites are a frequent cause of infection in the hand and fingertips. Unlike dog bites, cat bites may inoculate bacteria deeply without disrupting the overlying soft tissues, and *Pasteurella multocida* is the most common pathogen in these bites.[51] Amoxicillin-clavulanate is effective in cases without deep fluid collections or tendon/joint involvement. However, if medical management is to be trialed, follow-up must be close because surgical management is frequently required.[51]

Sporothrix Schenkii

Sporothrix schenkii is a fungus that may cause hand and finger infections in gardeners. Sporotrichosis begins days to weeks after the fungus breaches the skin barrier, typically carried by a thorn. An ulcerative nodule develops and there is characteristically lymphatic streaking.[52] Sporotrichosis requires a 3- to 6-month course of itraconazole.[53]

MIMICS

There are a range of oncologic, rheumatologic, and infectious conditions that may be easily mistaken for the infections discussed previously, particularly paronychia. It is important to differentiate between these conditions because they require different management strategies, namely oncologic resection for malignancies and medical therapy for rheumatologic and infectious conditions. If a patient does not respond to antibiotics or drainage, it is important to consider these other diagnoses.

In a recent study from the dermatology literature, cytology was performed on 58 patients who had been diagnosed with paronychia but had not improved with antibiotics. Although bacterial infection was confirmed in 43% of patients, most received other diagnosis. Herpes and parapoxvirus (Orf) were most common, with other causes including fungal infections, drug reactions, and pemphigus vulgaris.[54] These findings highlight the importance of considering a wide differential diagnosis in cases that are nonresponsive to usual therapies.

Calcific Tendinitis/Periarthritis

Calcific tendinitis/periarthritis is a rare condition in the hand, characterized by the deposition of calcium hydroxyapatite in tendon or joint capsule. In the fingertip, it can present as acute onset of pain, edema, and erythema with elevated inflammatory markers, which can mimic a felon, DIP septic arthritis, or flexor tenosynovitis.[55,56] Findings of calcific deposition on radiographs can make the diagnosis, although superimposed infection should still be considered. Treatment with nonsteroidal anti-inflammatory drugs, oral steroids, and/or corticosteroid injection is effective.

Gout

Gout (the inflammatory response to deposition of monosodium urate in joints) can involve the DIP joints. Acute tophaceous gout can mimic felon, paronychia, and DIP septic arthritis, and liquid tophus can mimic purulent discharge.[57] Radiographs likely reveal erosive arthritic changes. Medical management with nonsteroidal anti-inflammatory drugs and/or colchicine is usually effective, although surgical resection of large tophi and synovectomy is certainly reasonable. Joint fusion may be considered in the setting of advanced and symptomatic arthritic changes.

Herpetic Whitlow

Herpetic whitlow refers to herpes simplex virus-1 and -2 infections that affect the distal phalanx, with the possibility of involving the rest of the hand. Traditionally, health care workers with occupational exposure to oral secretions were considered high risk, although this is no longer the case because of widespread use of gloves. Herpetic whitlow is common in children who suck their thumbs.[48] The condition is characterized by erythematous and vesicular eruptions that are painful and highly contagious during the initial 2 weeks (Fig. 3).[48] In the late stages of the infection, white blood cells may deposit in the lesion, but there is no purulence except in cases of bacterial superinfection.[48] The disease

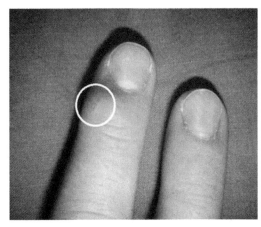

Fig. 3. Herpetic whitlow of the finger. Note the vesicles associated with the erythema and swelling, differentiating this from a paronychia or septic arthritis.

is self-limiting over a 3- to 4-week course and incision/unroofing is not recommended because of the risk of superinfection.[38,48,54,58] Instead, oral acyclovir should be prescribed in equivalent doses to oral or genital herpes infections.[48]

Cancer

Several cancers can mimic chronic paronychia when they occur in or adjacent to the nailbed. Reported examples include squamous cell carcinoma/Bowen disease, melanoma, Kaposi sarcoma, papillary adenocarcinoma, and amyloidosis.[59–64] The possibility of malignancy should be considered when what seems to be a chronic paronychia exists in the absence of occupational risk factors or other affected fingers, particularly if it is refractory to treatment.[14,24] Chronic immunosuppression is also a risk factor.[63] Treatment starts with tissue diagnosis and should be directed in collaboration with an oncologist.

Rheumatologic

Several immune-mediated conditions can cause nail changes. For example, psoriasis causes nail pitting and oil spots and pencil-in-cup arthritic changes, in association with purple skin plaques on extensor surfaces. Pemphigus vulgaris can also mimic fingertip infection and would be characterized by numerous blistering lesions on the skin and in the mouth.[65] Reactive arthritis (Reiter syndrome) causes inflamed joints and urethritis and conjunctivitis.

SUMMARY

The human fingertip is a common site of infections commonly encountered by hand surgeons.

Early diagnosis and treatment, most frequently with surgical drainage followed by tailored antibiotic therapy based on cultures, represents the key to a successful outcome. Comorbidities, such as diabetes mellitus and immunosuppression, may complicate management of these infections. It is also important for the hand surgeon to recognize the several mimics of fingertip infections, because their treatment differs greatly.

CLINICS CARE POINTS

- When draining a paronychia, place the blade flat between the nail plate and the eponychial fold. Do not incise the eponychial fold; doing so results in a permanent, unsightly scar.

- For chronic paronychia, the first line of treatment is to avoid repetitive irritants and to use topical steroids; surgery is indicated in recalcitrant cases.

- Incision sites for felons are usually approached laterally from a midlateral approach. Incise skin and then spread down to the distal phalanx to liberate any fluid collections.

DISCLOSURE

The authors have nothing to disclose.

REFERENCES

1. Jebson P. Infections of the fingertip. Paronychias and felons. Hand Clin 1998;14(4):547–55.
2. Rabarin F, Jeudy J, Cesari B, et al, Orthopedics and Traumatology Society of Western France SOO. Acute finger-tip infection: management and treatment. A 103-case series. Orthop Traumatol Surg Res 2017;103(6):933–6.
3. Fowler J, Ilyas A. Epidemiology of adult acute hand infections at an urban medical center. J Hand Surg Am 2013;38(6):1189–93.
4. Franko OI, Abrams RA. Hand infections. Orthop Clin North Am 2013;44(4):625–34.
5. Hauck R, Camp L, Ehrlich H, et al. Pulp nonfiction: microscopic anatomy of the digital pulp space. Plast Reconstr Surg 2004;113(2):536–9.
6. Zook EG. Anatomy and physiology of the perionychium. Clin Anat 2003;16(1):1–8.
7. Zook E. Anatomy and physiology of the perionychium. Hand Clin 1990;6(1):1–7.
8. Ritting AW, O'Malley MP, Rodner CM. Acute paronychia. J Hand Surg Am 2012;37(5):1068–70.
9. Shafritz A, Coppage J. Acute and chronic paronychia of the hand. J Am Acad Orthop Surg 2014; 22(3):165–74.
10. Bolton H, Fowler PJ, Jepson RP. Natural history and treatment of pulp space infection and osteomyelitis of the terminal phalanx. J Bone Joint Surg 1949; 31B:499–504.
11. Turkmen A, Warnter R, Page R. Digital pressure test for paronychia. Br J Plast Surg 2004;57(1):93–4.
12. Rockwell P. Acute and chronic paronychia. Am Fam Physician 2001;63:1113–36.
13. Wollina U. Acute paronychia: comparative treatment with topical antibiotic alone or in combination with corticosteroid. J Eur Acad Dermatol Venereol 2001;15(1):82–4.
14. Rigopoulos D, Larios G, Gregoriou S, et al. Acute and chronic paronychia. Am Fam Physician 2008; 77(3):339–46.
15. Tosti R, Ilyas A. Empiric antibiotics for acute infections of the hand. J Hand Surg Am 2010;35(1):125–8.
16. Daniel CI. Paronychia. Dermatol Clin. 1985;3(3): 461–4.
17. Tosti R, Iorio J, Fowler J, et al. Povidone-iodine soaks for hand abscesses: a prospective randomized trial. J Hand Surg Am 2014;39(5):962–5.
18. Canales F, Newmeyer WI, Kilgore EJ. The treatment of felons and paronychias. Hand Clin 1989; 5(4):515–23.
19. Ogunlusi J, Oginni L, Ogunlusi O. DAREJD simple technique of draining acute paronychia. Tech Hand Up Extrem Surg 2005;9(2):120–1.
20. Pabari A, Iyer S, Khoo C. Swiss roll technique for treatment of paronychia. Tech Hand Up Extrem Surg 2011;15(2):75–7.
21. Pierrart J, Delgrande D, Mamane W, et al. Acute felon and paronychia: antibiotics not necessary after surgical treatment. Prospective study of 46 patients. Hand Surg Rehabil 2016;35(1):40–3.
22. Singer A, Thode HJ. Systemic antibiotics after incision and drainage of simple abscesses: a meta-analysis. Emerg Med J 2014;31(4):576–8.
23. Daniel CI, Daniel M, Daniel C, et al. Chronic paronychia and onycholysis: a thirteen-year experience. Cutis 1996;58(6):397–401.
24. Leggit JC. Acute and chronic paronychia. Am Fam Physician 2017;96(1):44–51.
25. Tosti A, Piraccini B, D'Antuono A, et al. Paronychia associated with antiretroviral therapy. Br J Dermatol 1999;140(6):1165–8.
26. Daudén E, Pascual-López M, Martinez-García C, et al. Paronychia and excess granulation tissue of the toes and finger in a patient treated with indinavir. Br J Dermatol 2000;142(5):1063–4.
27. Sass JO, Jakob-Sölder B, Heitger A, et al. Paronychia with pyogenic granuloma in a child treated with indinavir: the retinoid-mediated side effect theory revisited. Dermatology 2000;200(1):40–2.
28. Dianichi T, Tanaka M, Tsuruta N, et al. Development of multiple paronychia and periungual granulation in patients treated with gefitinib, an inhibitor

of epidermal growth factor receptor. Dermatology 2003;207(3):324–5.

29. Hardin J, Haber R. Onychomadesis: literature review. Br J Dermatol 2015;172(3):592–6.

30. Tosti A, Piraccini B, Ghetti E, et al. Topical steroids versus systemic antifungals in the treatment of chronic paronychia: an open, randomized double-blind and double dummy study. J Am Acad Dermatol 2002;47(1):73–6.

31. Bednar M, Lane L. Eponychial marsupialization and nail removal for surgical treatment of chronic paronychia. J Hand Surg Am 1991;16(2):314–7.

32. Grover C, Bansal S, Nanda S, et al. En bloc excision of proximal nail fold for treatment of chronic paronychia. Dermatol Surg 2006;32(3):393–9.

33. Keyser J, Eaton R. Surgical cure of chronic paronychia by eponychial marsupialization. Plast Reconstr Surg 1976;58(1):66–70.

34. Kilgore EJ, Brown L, Newmeyer W, et al. Treatment of felons. Am J Surg 1975;130(2).

35. Watson PA, Jebson PJ. The natural history of the neglected felon. Iowa Orthop J 1996;16:164–6.

36. Kanavel A. Infection of the hand. New York: The Classics of Surgery Library, division of Gryphon Editions; 1992.

37. Tannan SC, Deal DN. Diagnosis and management of the acute felon: evidence-based review. J Hand Surg Am 2012;37(12):2603–4.

38. Abrams RA, Botte MJ. Hand infections: treatment recommendations for specific types. J Am Acad Orthop Surg 1996;4(4):219–30.

39. Stevanovic MV, Sharpe F. Acute infections of the hand. In: Wolfe SW, Hotchkiss RN, Pederson WC, et al, editors. Green's operative hand surgery. 7th edition. Philadelphia, PA: Elsevier; 2017.

40. Koch SL. Felons: acute lymphangitis and tendon sheath infections. JAMA 1929;92(14):1171–3.

41. Meislin H, McGehee M, Rosen P. Management and microbiology of cutaneous abscesses. JACEP 1978; 7(5):186–91.

42. Chenoweth B. Septic joints: finger and wrist. Hand Clin 2020;36(3):331–8.

43. Rangarathnam CS, Linscheid RL. Infected mucous cyst of the finger. J Hand Surg Am 1984;9(2):245–7.

44. Saito T, Noda T, Kondo H, et al. The masquelet technique for septic arthritis of the small joint in the hands: case reports. Trauma Case Rep 2020;25:100268.

45. Kowalski TJ, Thompson LA, Gundrum JD. Antimicrobial management of septic arthritis of the hand and wrist. Infection 2014;42(2):379–84.

46. Sendi P, Kaempfen A, Uçkay I, et al. Bone and joint infections of the hand. Clin Microbiol Infect 2020; 26(7):848–56.

47. Honda HM JR, McDonald JR. Current recommendations in the management of osteomyelitis of the hand and wrist. J Hand Surg Am 2009;34(6): 1135–6.

48. Adisen E, Onder M. Acral manifestations of viral infections. Clin Dermatol 2017;35(1):40–9.

49. Arnaud J, Bernard P, Souyri N, et al. Human ORF disease localized in the hand: a "false felon". A study of eight cases. Ann Chir Main 1986;5(2): 129–32.

50. Veraldi S, Girgenti V, Dassoni F, et al. Erysipeloid: a review. Clin Exp Dermatoal 2009;34(8):859–62.

51. Babovic N, Cayci C, Carlsen B. Cat bite infections of the hand: assessment of morbidity and predictors of severe infection. J Hand Surg Am 2014; 39(2):286–90.

52. Barros M, Paes RdA, Schubach A. *Sporothrix schenckii* and sporotrichosis. Clin Microbiol Rev 2011;24(4):633–54.

53. Sharkey-Mathis P, Kauffman C, Graybill J, et al. Treatment of sporotrichosis with itraconazole. NIAID Mycoses Study Group. Am J Med 1993; 95(3):279–85.

54. Durdu M, Ruocco V. Clinical and cytologic features of antibiotic-resistant acute paronychia. J Am Acad Dermatol 2014;70(1):120–6.

55. Kim J, Lee J, Park J, et al. Acute calcific tendinitis in the distal interphalangeal joint. Arch Plast Surg 2016;43(3):301–3.

56. Munjal A, Munjal P, Mahajan A. Diagnostic dilemma: acute calcific tendinitis of flexor digitorum profundus. Hand (NY) 2013;8(3):352–3.

57. Fitzgerald B, Setty A, Mudgal C. Gout affecting the hand and wrist. J Am Acad Orthop Surg 2007; 15(10):625–35.

58. Szinnai G, Schaad U, Heininger U. Multiple herpetic whitlow lesions in a 4-year-old girl: case report and review of the literature. Eur J Pediatr 2001;160:528–33.

59. Gorva A, Mohil R, Srinivasan M. Aggressive digital papillary adenocarcinoma presenting as a paronychia of the finger. J Hand Surg Br 2005;30(5):534.

60. Keith J, Wilgis E. Kaposi's sarcoma in the hand of an AIDS patient. J Hand Surg Am 1986;11(3):410–3.

61. Ahmed I, Cronk J, Crutchfield CI, et al. Myeloma-associated systemic amyloidosis presenting as chronic paronychia and palmodigital erythematous swelling and induration of the hands. J Am Acad Dermatol 2000;42(2):339–42.

62. Ware J. Sub-ungal malignant melanoma presenting as sub-acute paronychia following trauma. Hand 2010;9(1):49–51.

63. Fung V, Sainsbury D, Seukeran D, et al. Squamous cell carcinoma of the finger masquerading as paronychia. J Plast Reconstr Aesthet Surg 2010;63(2): e191–2.

64. Bryant J, Gardner P, Yousif M, et al. Aggressive digital papillary adenocarcinoma of the hand presenting as a felon. Case Rep Ortho 2017;2017:6456342.

65. Engineer L, Norton L, Ahmed A. Nail involvement in pemphigus vulgaris. J Am Acad Dermatol 2000; 43(3):529–35.

Management of the Septic Wrist
A Systematic Review of Etiology and Therapeutic Strategies

Heather L. Mercer, PhD[a], Diego Rodriguez, BS[b],
Rhiana Rivas, BS[b], Elizabeth Rivenbark, BS[b],
Elizabeth Mikola, MD[b], Deana Mercer, MD[b,*]

KEYWORDS

- Wrist joint • Septic joint • Septic wrist • Infection • Arthrotomy • Arthroscopy • Antibiotic

KEY POINTS

- For accurate and expedited diagnoses of septic arthritis of the wrist joint, it is important to conduct a careful physical examination, obtain appropriate imaging when indicated, and perform a joint arthrocentesis.
- Analysis of the joint fluid obtained from the arthrocentesis includes aerobic and anaerobic cultures, a white blood cell count with differential, acid-fast bacillus, fungal culture, and assessment for crystalline arthropathies.
- Bloodwork obtained should include complete blood count, erythrocyte sedimentation rate, and C-reactive protein. This provides a baseline which can be followed over time to assess infection resolution.
- Timely initiation of broad-spectrum antibiotics, followed by targeted antibiotic treatment tailored to the offending pathogen is crucial in the treatment of septic wrist.
- In the treatment of septic arthritis of the wrist joint, effective surgical interventions include arthroscopic or open surgical debridement of the wrist joint.

INTRODUCTION

Intra-articular radiocarpal infections or septic arthritis of the wrist are uncommon but may lead to destructive arthropathy of the wrist joint if not diagnosed expediently and treated appropriately. Septic arthritis can be monoarticular involving only the wrist joint, or polyarticular, with polyarticular cases accounting for up to 10% to 20% of cases and carrying a mortality rate of 50%.[1] Wrist sepsis accounts for approximately 5% of all septic arthritis cases and can manifest in various wrist regions, including the radiocarpal joint, midcarpal, and distal radioulnar joints.[2]

The diagnosis is confirmed if any one of the following is present: (I) aspiration or intraoperative identification of pus in the joint, (II) evidence of leukocytes in laboratory analysis of obtained samples with elevated total nucleated cell count, or (III) growth of microorganisms in culture.[3]

Several risk factors that predispose individuals to septic arthritis of the wrist include age older than 80 years, diabetes mellitus, immunocompromised status due to medical condition or medications, inflammatory arthropathies, skin fragility, and joint trauma.[4–6] One common mechanism of infection is direct inoculation into the joint, resulting from penetration of the

[a] Institute of Microbiology and Infection, School of Biosciences, Univeristy of Birmingham, Edgbaston, B15 2TT, England; [b] UNMHSC Department of Orthopedics and Rehabilitation, 1 University of New Mexico, MSC 10-5600, Albuquerque, NM 87131, USA
* Corresponding author. 1 University of New Mexico, MSC 10-5600, Albuquerque, NM 87131, USA
E-mail address: dmercer@salud.unm.edu

skin over the joint such as is seen in animal bites. However, any trauma that leads to disruption of the skin can lead to inoculation of the wrist joint such as lacerations, penetrating injuries, or crush injuries.[7] The potential pathogens include viral, bacterial, or fungal agents that infiltrate the joint space causing an acute inflammatory response that can, within a short period of time, lead to severe post infectious arthritic changes.[8,9] *Staphylococcus aureus* is the most common infecting organism in septic arthritis and osteomyelitis cases.[10,11] Failure to promptly diagnose septic arthritis of the wrist can lead to permanent and irreversible joint damage, and in advanced cases can lead to sepsis, and death.[4]

To optimize patient outcomes, prompt diagnosis and intervention are paramount with low threshold for diagnostic wrist aspiration. Suspicion of wrist joint infection necessitates a comprehensive patient history and physical examination. Radiographs should be taken to rule out trauma and fracture. Radiographs are also helpful in diagnosis advanced disease with osteomyelitis. Clinical diagnostic criteria include swelling, redness, and severe pain particularly with range of motion and axial compression load across the wrist joint.[12] Immediate joint aspiration for diagnosis, surgical debridement when indicated, and the administration of broad-spectrum antibiotics are imperative to minimize joint destruction.

Joint fluid aspiration sent for laboratory analysis is crucial and should include gram stain culture for aerobic and anaerobic bacteria, fungal species, crystal analysis, Gram stain, acid-fast bacillus (AFB), and total nucleated cell count. A total nucleated cell count exceeding 50,000 to 80,000 with polymorphonuclear neutrophils (PMNs) >75% is diagnostic for septic joint.[13] Blood work, including a complete blood count (CBC) with differential, erythrocyte sedimentation rate (ESR), and C-reactive protein (CRP) aid in the diagnosis of wrist infection.

This review aims to provide a treatment algorithm for the optimal management of septic arthritis of the wrist. The authors provide an up-to-date review of the literature and overview of patient assessment, clinical manifestations, diagnostic methodologies, treatment options, and potential complications associated with septic wrist joint infections, with the ultimate goal of improving patient outcomes.

PATIENT EVALUATION OVERVIEW
Clinical Presentation and Symptoms
Patients afflicted with septic arthritis of the wrist commonly manifest with clinical symptoms, including erythema, increased temperature, redness, tenderness, and severe pain with active or passive range of motion of the wrist and severe pain with axial compressive loading of the wrist.[13] The axial compression of the wrist joint in septic arthritis is not tolerated. Recognizing these clinical indicators plays a crucial role in the timely management of septic wrist.

Physical Examination
The first step in achieving an accurate diagnosis of septic arthritis of the wrist hinges on a careful, thorough physical examination. A careful examination of the entire extremity is important as there may be other factors contributing to the infection. The presence of streaking erythema can indicate more severe infection. Other clues to infectious etiologies include evidence of skin wounds proximal to the wrist from IV injection, or other trauma. Examination of the axilla may reveal lymphadenopathy indicative of longer infection duration. If risk factors for infection are present including advanced age, immunosuppression, penetrating trauma, or preexisting joint disease, then the suspicion for septic joint should be heightened.

DIAGNOSTIC PROCEDURES

The diagnostic procedure should include imaging (X-ray, MRI, and computed tomograhy [CT] scan if MRI is contraindicated) and blood work. Expedited procedures are critical to confirm the presence of septic wrist joint infection.

Imaging
Septic arthritis of the wrist necessitates a comprehensive imaging approach to diagnose the severity of infection and deterioration of the joint. Posteroanterior (PA) and lateral views radiographs of the affected wrist should be taken as they may show joint effusion, bone changes including juxta articular osteopenia and erosion, and joint space narrowing[14,15] (Fig. 1A and B). MRI, CT scans, and ultrasound can be helpful to elucidate bone changes consistent with osteomyelitis and fluid collections or abscesses[10,15] (Fig. 2A and B). In this case, a CT scan was obtained as an MRI was contraindicated due to the patient having a pacemaker.

Prompt imaging allows for an accurate and broad assessment of the infected wrist aiding in timely diagnosis and guiding appropriate treatment.

Laboratory Testing
In the diagnostic process for septic arthritis of the wrist, a critical step involves joint aspiration of the affected wrist joint. A retrospective study

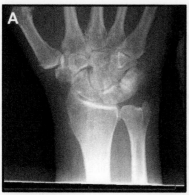 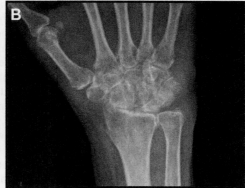

Fig. 1. Posterior anterior (PA) view X-rays of a septic wrist joint (A) PA view of the wrist before infection (B) PA view of the wrist after delayed diagnosis of right septic wrist arthritis showing severe joint and bony destruction.

which sought to determine the most effective initial treatment approach, conducted a comparative analysis between needle aspiration and surgical joint drainage. The findings strongly favor needle aspiration as the preferred fist-line treatment strategy in cases of septic arthritis of the wrist.[16]

The joint fluid collected during arthrocentesis should be sent for laboratory analysis including white blood cell count (WBC) with differential analysis, Gram stain targeting both anaerobic and aerobic bacteria, fungal examination, uric acid crystal analysis, and acid-fast staining. A WBC count of greater than 50,000 cells/mL is considered a substantial indicator of infection.[13]

However, there is not an absolute number and the clinical examination should guide treatment. The presence of an organism confirmed through a positive Gram stain is regarded as conclusive evidence of infection within the wrist joint, providing insights for precise diagnosis and appropriate intervention.

If crystals are present in the joint aspirate, this is an indication of gout or pseudogout.[17] Gout or pseudogout should be treated with anti-inflammatories, and empirical antibiotics when indicated. If the symptoms subside with anti-inflammatory treatment, this confirms the diagnosis of crystalline arthropathy and may not warrant a wash out in the operating room. In the

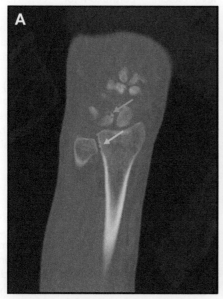 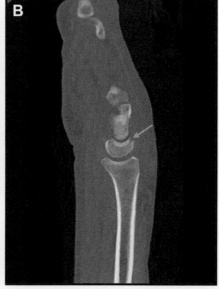

Fig. 2. Computed tomography (CT) scan of the septic wrist joint (A) Evidence of bony erosions of the distal radial ulnar joint, indicated by the yellow arrow. Lunate erosion due to infection marked by the orange arrow (B) Bony erosions of the dorsal lunate shown by the orange arrow.

rare cases where crystalline arthropathy has evolved into septic arthropathy where symptoms do not improve with anti-inflammatories, there should be a low threshold for operative joint debridement.

A comprehensive blood culture analysis is essential in the diagnosis of septic arthritis of the wrist and should include WBC, ESR, CRP, and crystal assessment. In diagnosing bacterial infection, critical markers must be observed including, WBC count exceeding 50,000 cells/mL, with a preponderance (at least 90%) of polymorphonuclear cells.[15,18,19] Other indicators of infection that can be relied upon include ESR levels exceeding 10 mm/h and CRP levels surpassing >1.5 mg/dL.[20–22] Fig. 5 presents a comprehensive overview of the management protocol for septic arthritis of the wrist.

INFECTIOUS AGENTS

The most common pathogen responsible for septic wrist joint infections is *Staphylococcus aureus (S aureus)* accounting for up to 40% of the cases.[4,8] Notably, a retrospective study has shown *S aureus* is responsible for more than 70% of all septic arthritis cases.[23]

An 11-year review has identified several other causative agents of septic arthritis of the wrist, in addition to *S aureus*. These include methicillin-sensitive and methicillin-resistant *S aureus* (MSSA, MRSA), *Streptococcus*, *Escherichia coli*, *Pasteurella multocida*, *Pseudomonas aeruginosa*, *Mycobacteria (M. tuberculosis and M. intacellulare)*, and *Neisseria gonorrhea*.[24–27] In those with advanced age, *Escherichia coli* has been implicated as the primary causative agent, contributing to 23% to 30% of septic arthritis in the wrist among this group.[28] *Pasturella multocida* is responsible for 6% to 11% of cases in the hand due to animal bites.[29] *Pasteurella* species are isolated in as much as 35% of reported cases involving animal bite wounds.[30] While *Pseudomonas aeruginosa*, a gram-negative organism, is a rare cause of septic arthritis, it is more common among young individuals who experience puncture wound injuries or engage in intravenous drug use.[31] Septic wrist infection caused by *Mycobacterium avium intracellulare* is infrequent; however, several case reports and case series have highlighted *M. avium intacellulare* as the causative pathogen in the wrist joint.[32,33]

NN. gonorrhoeae is the second most prevalent sexually transmitted pathogen in North America, warranting consideration in sexually active individuals under 40 years of age.[34] Disseminated gonococcal infection (DGI),

attributable to gram-negative diplococci *N. gonorrhoeae*, occurs in approximately 0.5% to 3% of patients with *N gonorrhoeae* infections, with skin involvement observed in 40% of these cases.[35] DGI predominantly presents as distal joint arthritis affecting, the wrists, knees, and ankles.[36]

In exceedingly rare cases, *Borrelia burgdorferi*, the spirochete responsible for Lyme disease, may be associated with septic arthritis of the wrist, particularly in younger patients living in endemic regions like the North-eastern, Mid-Atlantic, and Mid-western regions of the United States.[37] Lyme disease follows a well-documented progression of symptoms, with knee joint pain being a characteristic feature in advanced stages of infection, although wrist involvement can also occur. It is very difficult to culture *B burgdorferi* from the joint fluid, so polymerase chain reaction testing is the recommended test.[38,39]

MEDICAL MANAGEMENT
First-Line Antibiotics
Timely and appropriate antibiotic therapy is a cornerstone of treatment. Less severe cases of septic arthritis of the wrist should be addressed through non-surgical medical management involving close monitoring, rest, effective pain control, immobilization, and antibiotic therapy.

To arrest the further progression of infection, immediate intra-venous (IV) administration of broad-spectrum antibiotics such as vancomycin, levofloxacin, ceftriaxone,or ceftazidime is crucial.[40,41] Delaying the initiation of appropriate antibiotic therapy within the initial 24 to 48 hours of onset can result in subchondral bone loss and permanent joint dysfunction.[31,42] Wrist joint arthrocentesis (as outlined in the arthrocentesis of the wrist joint section) should be performed to analyze the joint aspirate in the laboratory. Once culture results are available, antibiotic therapy should be tailored to combat the specific pathogen responsible for infection.

Staphylococcus aureus and Methicillin-Resistant Staphylococcus aureus
The primary approach for treatment of *Staphylococcus aureus* infection, a gram-positive cocci, in the wrist begins with the immediate administration of intravenous antibiotics. The length of treatment with IV antibiotics is variable, depending on the severity of the case. Typically, penicillin is administered IV for 2 weeks followed by 1 to 2 weeks of oral antibiotic therapy. In cases where MRSA is present, vancomycin or

daptomycin should be administered intravenously followed by a course of oral antibiotics for 2 to 4 weeks.[10,43]

Streptococcus

To treat Streptococcus in the wrist, it is recommended penicillin be administered IV. If penicillin allergy is a concern, erythromycin can be given as a substitute. Oral antibiotics should be administered for up to 6 weeks post operation.

Escherichia coli

The antibiotics typically used to treat Escherichia coli are ciprofloxacin, amikacin, and nalidixic acid, which should be given intravenously.[44] Sensitivity testing should be performed to ensure the pathogen is not resistant to the drugs prescribed. Appropriate antibiotics should be prescribed after surgery and should be chosen based on sensitivity testing.[21]

Pasteurella

To effectively treat Pasteurella species infections, intravenous ampicillin-sulbactam should be initiated. Additionally, a prescription of oral amoxicillin-clavulanic acid should be continued after surgical treatment. If sensitivity testing indicates resistance to ampicillin, penicillin, and amoxicillin-clavulanic acid, the antibiotic should be promptly switched to an alternative antibiotic, such as levofloxacin, to which the pathogen is susceptible.[30,45]

Pseudomonas aeruginosa

To treat Pseudomonas aeruginosa infection, piperacillin-tazobactam, amoxicillin-clavulanate should be given IV followed by oral antibiotics of gentamicin or tobramycin for 4 to 6 weeks.[40,46] Effective alternative antibiotics that can be given include aztreonam and meropenem. For the treatment of multidrug resistant strains, a combination of ceftolozane-tazobactam, ceftazidime-avibactam, imipenem-cilastatin relebactam, or polymyxin drugs such as polymyxin B and colistin can be administered.[47,48]

Mycobacteria

The primary treatment approach for wrist Mycobacteria infection typically involves an initial course of rifampin, ethambutol, isoniazid, and pyrazinamide. This is followed by a secondary antibiotic usually consisting of isoniazid and rifampin.[26] The duration of treatment spans from 6 to 18 months depending on the susceptibility of the isolated strain.[49]

Neisseria gonorrhea

The treatment approach for disseminated gonococcal infection typically involves initial 1-week course of intravenous ceftriaxone, supplemented with doxycycline to address potential Chlamydia trachomatis co-infection risk.[35,36] Subsequent to the initial ceftriaxone treatment, a prescription of ciprofloxacin or cefixime should be administered orally until symptoms resolve.[50]

Borrelia burgdorferi

In general, patients exhibiting neurologic symptoms should receive treatment for Borrelia burgdorferi with a course of IV ceftriaxone or penicillin G, followed by a regimen of doxycycline, amoxicillin, or cefuroxime axetil. For pediatric patients, amoxicillin or cefuroxime may be the preferred option. In the case of adults who do not exhibit neurologic symptoms, oral doxycycline to be taken for a duration of 28 days is generally recommended.[37]

Fungal species

To achieve successful treatment of fungal infections in septic arthritis, a tailored approach is crucial, with the choice of treatment contingent on the specific fungal species cultured from the joint aspirate. Typically, as a first-line therapeutic option, physicians opt for the administration of oral azole agents or parenteral amphotericin B.[51]

Determining the appropriate dosages and duration of antibiotics for treatment of septic arthritis of the wrist infections should be tailored to each individual case. Moreover, while antibiotics serve as the primary treatment strategy and have demonstrated success in many instances of septic arthritis, it is essential to acknowledge the potential benefits of combining medical and surgical interventions. A comparative study evaluating the initial treatment of septic arthritis showed that 30% of patients initially treated with antibiotics eventually required surgical intervention as part of their treatment plan.[52]

CONSULTATION

The infectious disease team should be consulted in cases of joint infection. They can guide appropriate antibiotic selection, duration, and route of administration. Additionally, they can offer recommendations for supplementary tests, such as blood cultures and cardiac evaluation for endocarditis or other such indicated tests.

SURGICAL TREATMENT OPTIONS FOR SEPTIC WRIST JOINT

Indications for Surgical Intervention

Confirmed wrist joint infection warrants surgical debridement in most cases. The only contraindication would be inability of the patient to go to the operating room due to instability. The

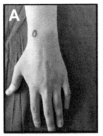 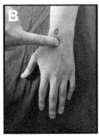 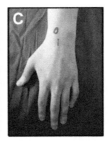 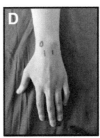 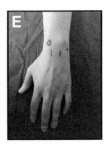

Fig. 3. Image of the wrist indicating the entry point for wrist aspiration and arthroscopy.(*A*) The "O" indicates the Lister's tubercle, bony landmark which guides identification of 3 to 4 portal (*B*) Identification of the soft spot, 3 to 4 portal, where the needle is inserted for aspiration (*C*) Marking of the 3 to 4 portal indicates the site for incision (*D*) The second line denotes the incision location for the 4 to 5 portal (*E*) Marking of the 6U portal, as indicated by the dot (".")

spectrum of surgical procedures available for consideration includes open surgical drainage, and arthroscopic surgical debridement.

Prior to performing any surgical procedure, it is advisable to perform joint aspiration. The aspirate should be sent to the laboratory for analysis.

It is important to obtain intra-operative tissue and joint fluid cultures for subsequent laboratory analysis. In cases where there is bone degradation, collecting a bone sample for culture may be indicated.

After the surgical procedure, the collected samples should be sent to the laboratory for comprehensive testing. The antibiotic treatment regimen should be tailored to the specific organism isolated through culture, ensuring effective therapeutic targeting.

ARTHROCENTESIS OF THE WRIST JOINT

It is crucial to aspirate the joint fluid from the wrist joint to accurately diagnose septic arthritis of the wrist (**Fig. 3**). Wrist arthrocentesis should be conducted under sterile conditions by those familiar with the technique and with specimen handling. The following steps outline the procedure.

1. Place the patient in a supine position with the palm down and forearm pronated. The wrist is placed in neutral position and deviated ulnaly.
2. Clean the affected area with alcohol, betadine, or chlorhexidine.
3. Palpate Lister's tubercle and mark the location (as depicted by the "O" in **Fig. 3**A)
4. Identify the soft spot just distal to Lister's tubercle which corresponds to the 3-4 portal or the area between the third and fourth extensor compartments (shown in **Fig. 3**B and indicated by the line in 3C)
5. Using an 18 or 22-gauge sterile needle the joint is entered, and the joint fluid is

aspirated. An 18-gauge needle may be preferred as it allows aspiration of thick fluid.
6. Using the dorsal approach, advance the needle at about a 10-degree angle to follow the volar tilt of the distal radius.
7. Upon entering the joint space, aspirate the joint fluid. Some resistance may be present due to the viscosity of the fluid, amount of fluid, and presence of fibrin clots. Rotating the needle or a slight withdraw of the needle may be helpful.
8. Place the aspirated joint fluid in sterile specimen tubes for laboratory analysis. It is good practice to take the sample to the laboratory immediately after the procedure has been completed.
9. Clean the puncture site and dress the wound.
10. Some cases may present with a large amount of inflammation, in these cases ultrasound may be helpful in performing arthrocentesis of the wrist.

OPEN SURGICAL DRAINAGE OF THE WRIST JOINT

The radiocarpal joint is accessible by a standard dorsal approach beginning with a dorsal incision centered between the third and fourth extensor compartment and slightly ulnar to Lister's tubercle. The arthrotomy of the wrist joint is created between the third and fourth extensor compartment (as depicted by the line in **Fig. 3**C).

1. Place the patient in a supine position. Anesthesia is administered. Either general and/or regional anesthesia is appropriate.
2. The affected extremity is prepped and draped.
3. Elevation exsanguination is used, as an esmark should not be used in the setting of infection.

4. Prior to incision, the joint may be aspirated by entering the joint 1 cm distal to Lister's tubercle following the distal radius volar tilt (as indicated in **Fig.** 3B and denoted by the line in 3C). An 18-gauge needle with a 3-cc syringe can be used to obtain a sample of fluid from the wrist joint prior to the arthrotomy.
5. Make a longitudinal midline incision over the dorsum of the wrist just ulnar to Lister's Tubercle (as depicted by the line in **Fig.** 4).
6. The extensor pollicis longus is identified and protected. The extensor pollicis longus is the tendon most at risk for injury during this procedure.
7. The tendons are retracted, and the dorsal capsule of the wrist joint is visualized.
8. A linear dorsal capsulotomy is performed, and the joint is entered. The ligaments are preserved during the exposure.
9. Fluid and tissue may be collected at this point to send to the laboratory and to pathology (as outlined in the Laboratory Testing section).
10. Synovitic tissue can be sent to pathology and for culture as a separate specimen.
11. The joint is then copiously irrigated.
12. A drain is placed. The joint arthrotomy is not closed as it will allow drainage.

13. A volar splint is applied for soft tissue rest. The skin is loosely closed around the drain.
14. Immobilize the wrist in a plaster splint.
15. If there is gross infection with frank pus in the joint, a repeat irrigation and debridement may be indicated 24 to 48 hours later.
16. If the clinical examination does not improve after the first wash out, a repeat wash out may be indicated.
17. Follow cultures sent intra operatively and tailor antibiotic treatment to the organism.
18. Remove drains after 24 to 48 hours

Post Operative Care

Post operatively, the clinical examination is most indicative of resolving infection. If the clinical examination does not improve, repeat debridement in the operating room may be necessary. If the clinical examination improves, then supportive care is initiated. The wrist is splinted but motion is encouraged when the patient is comfortable enough to do so. Finger motion therapy is very important and should be emphasized as much as wrist range of motion. Elbow and shoulder range of motion should also be encouraged. An occupational therapist fabricated removable volar wrist-based orthoses can be used to facilitate easy removal and encourage frequent motion. Blood work can be followed for resolution of abnormalities in inflammatory markers. The splint should be discontinued as soon as possible to minimize stiffness of the fingers and the wrist.[7] Cultures should be followed until final for all organisms and antibiotics can be tailored to sensitivities. Typically, broad spectrum antibiotics are utilized initially followed by more targeted antibiotics.

ARTHROSCOPIC DRAINAGE AND DEBRIDEMENT OF THE WRIST JOINT

Arthroscopic drainage and debridement is also effective in the treatment of septic wrist arthritis.[46]

The procedural steps are outlined as follows.

1. The patient is positioned supine. Either general and/or regional anesthesia is appropriate for administration.
2. The affected extremity is prepped and draped.
3. Place the extremity in an arthroscopy wrist tower and suspend the hand in finger traps with about 10 to 12 lb (4.5–5.4 kg) of traction.
4. The joint is aspirated by entering the joint 1 cm distal to Lister's tubercle following the distal radius volar tilt through the 3 to 4 portal with an 18-gauge needle and a 3-

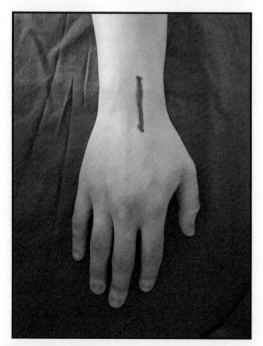

Fig. 4. Entry point for open surgical drainage of the wrist joint. The demarcated line denotes the precise location for the incision during dorsal wrist arthrotomy for open procedure.

cc syringe to collect a fluid sample from the wrist joint. This fluid sample should be sent to the laboratory for culture (as indicated by the line in **Fig. 3**C).

5. Establish a 3 to 4 portal for visualization (as indicated by the line in **Fig. 3**C).
6. Under direct visualization through the 3 to 4 portal, the 4 to 5 radiocarpal portal is first localized with a needle (as indicated by the 2nd line in **Fig. 3**D). A shaver is then introduced into the 4 to 5 portal. The 6U is established under direct visualization by placing an 18-gauge needle into the joint as an outflow portal (as indicated by the "dot" in **Fig. 3**E).
7. The 30° 2.7-mm arthroscope is introduced into the 3 to 4 portal and the wrist is evaluated.
8. The shaver irrigator is introduced into the 4 to 5 portal and the joint is debrided of inflammatory tissue and abnormal fluid.
9. Synovity or consolidated infected tissue can be captured with a biter through the 4 to 5 portal and sent to pathology.
10. The joint is then copiously irrigated with normal saline solution.
11. If there are clinical signs of infection within the midcarpal or distal radioulnar joint, these joints should also be irrigated.
12. Place a drain in the 3 to 4 portal and loosely close the incisions to allow drainage.
13. Remove drains after 24 to 48 hours.

SEPTIC ARTHRITIS OF THE WRIST TREATMENT ALGORITHM

The flow chart delineates the management pathway for septic arthritis of the wrist, offering a visual representation of the systematic and most optimal approach to its treatment (**Fig. 5**).

COMPLICATIONS

Potential complications that can arise with surgical treatment for septic wrist cases encompass various challenges, including damage to adjacent structures like nerve injury, local tendon rupture, hemarthrosis, wrist stiffness, and infection.[53] To mitigate these complications, stringent measures must be taken. Safeguarding nerves and tendons is paramount to prevent rupture. Moreover, precise needle insertion into the joint can prevent hemarthrosis. Prescribed antibiotics must be administered diligently to stave off further infections. Furthermore, it is essential to commence wrist physical therapy as soon as the wrist heals enough to tolerate it.

POSTOPERATIVE CARE

Postoperative care should encompass a comprehensive approach to wrist joint recovery. Passive mobilization of the wrist joint is recommended ensuring some movement of the wrist.[15] As the joint condition improves, active mobilization exercises may be initiated. Additionally, the administration of antibiotics, tailored to the specific culture results, should be continued for the prescribed duration.

PEARLS AND PITFALLS

- In the setting of septic wrist joint, expedient administration of broad-spectrum antibiotics is crucial to minimize the spread of infection.
- Prompt diagnosis of infection of the wrist is accomplished by careful physical examination and arthrocentesis of the infected joint.

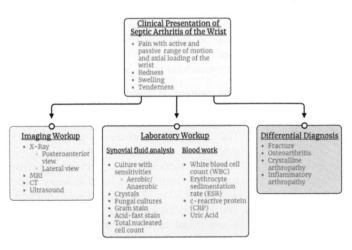

Fig. 5. A concise overview of the management of septic arthritis of the wrist.

- For timely and comprehensive diagnostic assessment of septic wrist, it is imperative to send joint aspirate samples and bloodwork including CBC, ESR, and CRP analysis.
- When septic arthritis of the wrist is strongly suspected or confirmed, surgical debridement should be done expediently. Irrigation or debridement can be done either open or arthroscopically.
- During open surgical drainage of the wrist joint, it is essential to protect the extensor tendon. The extensor pollicis longus is the most susceptible to injury during this procedure.
- After obtaining the joint aspirate sample, antibiotic treatment should initially be broad and then tailored to the cultured organism. The route of administration and treatment duration should be based upon the Gram stain, cultures, and sensitivities.

DISCUSSION

Septic arthritis of the wrist is a condition which requires swift and accurate diagnosis as well as the application of appropriate treatment strategies to prevent the onset of long-term disability and complications. The collaborative efforts between various professionals, including orthopedic surgeons, infectious disease specialists, and primary care providers are of paramount importance in ensuring the most favorable outcomes for patients facing this challenging condition.

Several risk factors can predispose individuals to septic arthritis of the wrist, including advanced age, immunocompromised states, skin fragility, weakened immune systems, and a history of joint trauma.[4–6]

In the initial diagnosis, a comprehensive approach should be used, starting with a thorough physical examination supplemented by imaging techniques. X-rays, CT scans, MRI scans, and ultrasonography can be helpful in the initial diagnosis of septic arthritis of the wrist.[10,14,15] Additionally, analysis of the blood, focusing on WBC, ESR, CRP, and uric acid is indispensable in the diagnostic process.

The causative agents responsible for septic arthritis of the wrist encompass a spectrum of pathogens, with *Staphylococcus aureus*, emerging as the predominant offender, followed by *Streptococcus, Escherichia coli, Pasteurella, Pseudomonas, Mycobacteria, Neisseria gonorrhea, Borrelia burgdorferi*, and some fungal species.[10,11] To establish an accurate diagnosis, the gold standard involves the aspiration of wrist joint fluid for subsequent analysis to identify the offending pathogen. Initial treatment primarily revolves around the administration of antibiotics tailored to combat the specific causative agent. However, in certain instances, surgical intervention may be deemed necessary.

In cases where antibiotic therapy alone proves insufficient to clear the infection, surgical intervention may be indicated. Two surgical options can be of use: open surgical drainage of the wrist joint and arthroscopic drainage and debridement of the wrist joint.[46] These surgical techniques are very useful in ensuring prompt healing and restoring full functionality of the wrist joint.

Although there have been notable advancements in surgical intervention, it is important to acknowledge that the management of septic wrist remains susceptible to complications. These complications, however, can be effectively mitigated through a systematic approach characterized by meticulous antibiotic selection, safeguarding nerves and tendons during surgery, and precise needle insertion into the joint.[53] Furthermore, pain management and the structured application of physical therapy is paramount in averting the occurrence of complications in septic arthritis of the wrist cases.

Septic arthritis of the wrist joint demands a multidisciplinary approach, early diagnosis, and tailored treatment plans to mitigate the potential for long-term sequelae. Timely intervention, guided by a comprehensive evaluation, remains pivotal in ensuring best patient outcomes.

DISCLOSURE

The authors have nothing to disclose.

REFERENCES

1. Kelly PJ. Bacterial arthritis in the adult. Orthop Clin North Am 1975;6(4):973–81.
2. Skeete K, Hess EP, Clark T, et al. Epidemiology of suspected wrist joint infection versus inflammation. J Hand Surg Am 2011;36(3):469–74.
3. Meier R, Wirth T, Hahn F, et al. Pyogenic arthritis of the fingers and the wrist: can we shorten antimicrobial treatment duration? Open Forum Infect Dis. Spring 2017;4(2):ofx058.
4. Jennings JD, Ilyas AM. Septic arthritis of the wrist. J Am Acad Orthop Surg 2018;26(4):109–15.
5. Triki MA, Naouar N, Benzarti S, et al. Septic arthritis of the wrist: about six cases. Pan Afr Med J 2019;33: 237.

6. Wu CJ, Huang CC, Weng SF, et al. Septic arthritis significantly increased the long-term mortality in geriatric patients. BMC Geriatr 2017;17(1):178.

7. Chenoweth B. Septic joints: finger and wrist. Hand Clin 2020;36(3):331–8.

8. Mehta P, Schnall SB, Zalavras CG. Septic arthritis of the shoulder, elbow, and wrist. Clin Orthop Relat Res 2006;451:42–5.

9. Hugenberg S, Brandt KD. Septic arthritis. an acute bacterial joint infection. Indiana Med 1987;80(6):521–5.

10. Horowitz DL, Katzap E, Horowitz S, et al. Approach to septic arthritis. Am Fam Physician 2011;84(6):653–60.

11. Goldenberg DL, Reed JI. Bacterial arthritis. N Engl J Med 1985;312(12):764–71.

12. Sammer DM, Shin AY. Arthroscopic management of septic arthritis of the wrist. Hand Clin 2011;27(3):331–4.

13. Sammer DM, Shin AY. Comparison of arthroscopic and open treatment of septic arthritis of the wrist. Surgical technique. J Bone Joint Surg Am 2010;92(Suppl 1 Pt 1):107–13.

14. Sommer OJ, Kladosek A, Weiler V, et al. Rheumatoid arthritis: a practical guide to state-of-the-art imaging, image interpretation, and clinical implications. Radiographics 2005;25(2):381–98.

15. Voss A, Pfeifer CG, Kerschbaum M, et al. Postoperative septic arthritis after arthroscopy: modern diagnostic and therapeutic concepts. Knee Surg Sports Traumatol Arthrosc 2021;29(10):3149–58.

16. Manadan AM, Block JA. Daily needle aspiration versus surgical lavage for the treatment of bacterial septic arthritis in adults. Am J Therapeut Sep-Oct 2004;11(5):412–5.

17. Rosales-Alexander JL, Balsalobre Aznar J, Magro-Checa C. Calcium pyrophosphate crystal deposition disease: diagnosis and treatment. Open Access Rheumatol 2014;6:39–47.

18. Schlesinger N. Diagnosis of gout: clinical, laboratory, and radiologic findings. Am J Manag Care 2005;11(15 Suppl):S443–50. quiz S465-8.

19. Smith JW, Piercy EA. Infectious arthritis. Clin Infect Dis 1995;20(2):225–30. quiz 231.

20. Li SF, Henderson J, Dickman E, et al. Laboratory tests in adults with monoarticular arthritis: can they rule out a septic joint? Acad Emerg Med 2004;11(3):276–80.

21. Earwood JS, Walker TR, Sue GJC. Septic arthritis: diagnosis and treatment. Am Fam Physician 2021;104(6):589–97.

22. Yu MM, Xu Y, Zhang JH, et al. Total cholesterol content of erythrocyte membranes levels are associated with the presence of acute coronary syndrome and high sensitivity C-reactive protein. Int J Cardiol 2010;145(1):57–8.

23. Morgan DS, Fisher D, Merianos A, et al. An 18 year clinical review of septic arthritis from tropical Australia. Epidemiol Infect 1996;117(3):423–8.

24. Yap RT, Tay SC. Wrist Septic arthritis: an 11 year review. Hand Surg 2015;20(3):391–5.

25. Sharff KA, Richards EP, Townes JM. Clinical management of septic arthritis. Curr Rheumatol Rep 2013;15(6):332.

26. McDermott DG, Hill SM, Desai K, et al. Septic mycobacterium avium intracellulare extensor tenosynovitis of the wrist. J Wrist Surg 2023;12(3):273–9.

27. Kawamura K, Yajima H, Omokawa S, et al. Septic arthritis of the wrist caused by Mycobacterium intracellulare: a case report. Case Reports Plast Surg Hand Surg 2016;3(1):79–82.

28. Lieber SB, Fowler ML, Zhu C, et al. Clinical characteristics and outcomes in polyarticular septic arthritis. Joint Bone Spine 2018;85(4):469–73.

29. Lipatov KV, Asatryan A, Melkonyan G, et al. Septic arthritis of the hand: From etiopathogenesis to surgical treatment. World J Orthop 2022;13(11):993–1005.

30. Malizos KN, Papadopoulou ZK, Ziogkou AN, et al. Infections of deep hand and wrist compartments. Microorganisms 2020;8(6). https://doi.org/10.3390/microorganisms8060838.

31. Goldenberg DL. Septic arthritis. Lancet 1998;351(9097):197–202.

32. Rolfe B, Sowa DT. Mixed gonococcal and mycobacterial sepsis of the wrist. Clin Orthop Relat Res 1990;257:100–3.

33. Whitaker MD, Jelinek JS, Kransdorf MJ, et al. Case report 653: Arthritis of the wrist due to Mycobacterium avium-intracellulare. Skeletal Radiol 1991;20(4):291–3.

34. Al-Suleiman SA, Grimes EM, Jonas HS. Disseminated gonococcal infections. Obstet Gynecol 1983;61(1):48–51.

35. Burns JE, Graf EH. The brief case: disseminated neisseria gonorrhoeae in an 18-year-old female. J Clin Microbiol 2018;56(4). https://doi.org/10.1128/JCM.00932-17.

36. Douedi S, Dattadeen J, Akoluk A, et al. Disseminated Neisseria gonorrhea of the wrist. IDCases 2020;20:e00763.

37. Smith BG, Cruz AI Jr, Milewski MD, et al. Lyme disease and the orthopaedic implications of lyme arthritis. J Am Acad Orthop Surg 2011;19(2):91–100.

38. Nocton JJ, Dressler F, Rutledge BJ, et al. Detection of Borrelia burgdorferi DNA by polymerase chain reaction in synovial fluid from patients with Lyme arthritis. N Engl J Med 1994;330(4):229–34.

39. Li X, McHugh GA, Damle N, et al. Burden and viability of Borrelia burgdorferi in skin and joints of patients with erythema migrans or lyme arthritis. Arthritis Rheum 2011;63(8):2238–47.

40. Clerc O, Prod'hom G, Greub G, et al. Adult native septic arthritis: a review of 10 years of experience and lessons for empirical antibiotic therapy. J Antimicrob Chemother 2011;66(5):1168–73.

41. Turker T, Capdarest-Arest N, Bertoch ST, et al. Hand infections: a retrospective analysis. PeerJ 2014;2:e513.

42. Mathews CJ, Weston VC, Jones A, et al. Bacterial septic arthritis in adults. Lancet 2010;375(9717):846–55.

43. Kowalski TJ, Thompson LA, Gundrum JD. Antimicrobial management of septic arthritis of the hand and wrist. Infection 2014;42(2):379–84.

44. Shariati A, Arshadi M, Khosrojerdi MA, et al. The resistance mechanisms of bacteria against ciprofloxacin and new approaches for enhancing the efficacy of this antibiotic. Front Public Health 2022;10:1025633.

45. Wei A, Dhaduk N, Taha B. Wrist abscess due to drug-resistant Pasteurella multocida. IDCases 2021;26:e01277.

46. Hassan AS, Rao A, Manadan AM, et al. Peripheral bacterial septic arthritis: review of diagnosis and management. J Clin Rheumatol 2017;23(8):435–42.

47. Kanj SS, Kanafani ZA. Current concepts in antimicrobial therapy against resistant gram-negative organisms: extended-spectrum beta-lactamase-producing Enterobacteriaceae, carbapenem-resistant Enterobacteriaceae, and multidrug-resistant Pseudomonas aeruginosa. Mayo Clin Proc 2011;86(3):250–9.

48. Magiorakos AP, Srinivasan A, Carey RB, et al. Multidrug-resistant, extensively drug-resistant and pandrug-resistant bacteria: an international expert proposal for interim standard definitions for acquired resistance. Clin Microbiol Infect 2012;18(3): 268–81.

49. Sotgiu G, Centis R, D'Ambrosio L, et al. Tuberculosis treatment and drug regimens. Cold Spring Harb Perspect Med 2015;5(5):a017822.

50. Centers for Disease C, Prevention, Work, Owski KA, Berman SM. Sexually transmitted diseases treatment guidelines, 2006. MMWR Recomm Rep (Morb Mortal Wkly Rep) 2006;55(RR-11):1–94.

51. Kohli R, Hadley S. Fungal arthritis and osteomyelitis. Infect Dis Clin North Am 2005;19(4):831–51.

52. Flores-Robles BJ, Jimenez Palop M, Sanabria Sanchinel AA, et al. Medical versus surgical approach to initial treatment in septic arthritis: a single spanish center's 8-year experience. J Clin Rheumatol 2019;25(1):4–8.

53. McBride S, Mowbray J, Caughey W, et al. Epidemiology, management, and outcomes of large and small native joint septic arthritis in adults. Clin Infect Dis 2020;70(2):271–9.

Foot and Ankle

Diagnosis and Management of Infected Total Ankle Replacements

Benjamin D. Umbel, DO[a],*,
Brandon A. Haghverdian, MD[a], Karl M. Schweitzer, MD[b],
Samuel B. Adams, MD[a]

KEYWORDS

- Total ankle arthroplasty • Total ankle replacement • Periprosthetic joint infection

---

KEY POINTS

- Periprosthetic joint infection (PJI) following total ankle arthroplasty is a significant and complex complication, reportedly occurring in up to 5% of cases.
- Diagnostic criteria specific to total ankle PJI is limited, and general guidelines for diagnosis have been extrapolated from hip and knee arthroplasty literature.
- Patient history, physical examination, imaging, screening blood tests, and joint aspiration should all be carefully assessed when attempting to diagnose infection following ankle arthroplasty.
- The surgical treatment of infection following ankle arthroplasty is complex and requires shared decision making between the patient and the treating surgeon.
- Surgical management is typically divided into 2 main options: limb salvage (total ankle revision and conversion to arthrodesis) and limb amputation.

INTRODUCTION

In the last few decades, the surgical treatment of end stage ankle arthritis has evolved. From 2009 to 2019, there has been a 120% increase in the incidence of total ankle arthroplasty (TAA) in the United States.[1] With this exponential rise in primary TAA cases, orthopedic foot and ankle surgeons should expect to see an increase in the number of patients requiring revision TAA.[2] Although TAA has the potential to fail for several reasons, with aseptic loosening being the most common, periprosthetic joint infection also remains a devastating cause of failure.

With a reported rate of 0% to 5%, periprosthetic joint infection (PJI) following TAA can be challenging to diagnosis and subsequently manage.[3–6] Early diagnosis from the onset of symptoms is critical and may help dictate treatment. A high level of suspicion is required, and diagnosis is usually made by a combination of clinical examination findings, imaging, and laboratory and microbiological workup.

The goal of treatment is to identify causative organisms, eliminate the infection with surgical and antibiotic treatment, and, if possible, salvage the limb while preventing future complications. Surgical intervention is typically in the form of revision limb salvage procedures or amputation. If limb salvage is undertaken, this is often done in a staged manner to ensure eradication of infection.

There are few data examining diagnosis and management of PJI in TAA. Most of the guidelines used for TAA have been defined for PJI of the hip and knee. This article discusses the current diagnostic and treatment options used when managing PJI in TAA.

---

[a] Department of Orthopedic Surgery, Duke University Medical Center, 200 Trent Drive, Durham, NC 27710, USA;
[b] Duke Orthopaedics of Raleigh, 3480 Wake Forest Road, Suite 204, Raleigh, NC 27609, USA
* Corresponding author. Duke University Medical Center, 200 Trent Drive, Durham, NC 27710.
E-mail address: benumbel@gmail.com

Orthop Clin N Am 55 (2024) 285–297
https://doi.org/10.1016/j.ocl.2023.08.001

PATIENT RISK FACTORS

As there continues to be an increase in primary TAA procedures performed for patients with end-stage ankle arthritis, the number of TAA failures will also continue to rise. PJI data following TAA have been described and studied less often than the hip and knee arthroplasty literature. However, over the last decade, more information has become available to surgeons regarding the incidence of PJI following TAA and potential risk factors.[7–10]

In 2012, Kessler and colleagues discussed the prevalence of TAA infection and reported a rate of 4.7%.[7] They found that most cases (85%) resulted in infection from an exogenous source, rather than hematogenous. *Staphylococcus aureus* was the most common organism identified. They suggested that previous foot and ankle surgery, lower preoperative American Orthopedic Foot and Ankle Score (AOFAS) hindfoot scores, longer duration of surgery, persistent wound dehiscence, and secondary drainage were associated with an increased risk of infection.[7] Patton and colleagues reported on 966 patients who had undergone TAA. For primary TAA and revision TAA, the incidence of infection was 2.6% and 4%, respectively. They identified diabetes, previous surgery, and wound complications greater than 14 days following surgery as risk factors for infection.[8] Notably, smoking and operative time were not related to increased infection risk. Gross and colleagues examined soft tissue wound complications in 762 consecutive TAAs.[9] Major wound complications occurred in 26 patients (3.4%), which required irrigation and debridement, split thickness skin grafting, or additional soft tissue reconstruction. They found that longer operating room time (214 minutes versus 189 minutes) was significantly associated with higher risk of wound issues. Also, longer tourniquet time (151 minutes versus 141 minutes) trended toward an increased risk for wound complications. TAA in primary osteoarthritis was associated with higher rates of wound complications compared with post-traumatic arthritis. Interestingly, the authors did not find any correlation with wound complications and diabetes, smoking, age or body mass index (BMI).[9]

More often discussed in the hip and knee replacement literature, transient bacteremia following dental procedures may be a potential risk factor for PJI following TAA. Although not extensively researched, case reports have been described.[11] Regarding the utilization of dental procedure antibiotic prophylaxis following foot and ankle surgery, Noori and colleagues recommend applying similar precautions and decision-making principles extrapolated from the hip and knee PJI literature.[12] Guidelines for appropriate use of dental procedure prophylaxis in preventing PJI have been formulated by the American Academy of Orthopedic Surgeons (AAOS). The decision tree takes several factors into consideration. If a patient is undergoing an invasive dental procedure, is immunocompromised, has a history of PJI, and is within 1 year of his or her index surgery, prophylactic antibiotic treatment is generally recommended. Even without a history of PJI or more than 1 year from surgery, prophylactic antibiotics are recommended when Hb A1C is greater than 8.[13]

DIAGNOSIS

Clinical Presentation

When evaluating the patient for PJI, it is important to consider all factors that may have contributed to infection. A thorough past medical history is critical in determining which of the previously mentioned risk factors may have played a role in the patient's infectious process. Modiable risk factors such as smoking, diabetes, and immunosuppressive medication use should be identied to limit further complications that may arise if revision surgeries are needed. A detailed past surgical history is also important when considering whether a painful total ankle may be related to infection. Documenting any previous postoperative infections or delayed wound healing issues should be part of the initial patient assessment.

Patients with PJI following TAA may present with various signs and symptoms. Often, the acuity of the infectious process can dictate the clinical presentation. In general, infections are considered either acute or chronic.[14] The timing that determines whether infection is acute versus chronic is also variable within the arthroplasty literature. For hip and knee arthroplasty data, acute PJI has been described as being less than 90 days from the time of the index procedure, whereas chronic PJI include those presenting more than 90 days from surgery.[14] Infections may also be considered acute in the setting of remote hematogenous spread from another area of infection in the body and new onset of ankle symptoms, even if the patient is outside of the 90-day window from his or her index procedure. Nonetheless, while timing of acute versus chronic infection may be more agreed upon in the hip and knee arthroplasty literature, there does not appear to be a consensus for PJI following TAA.[15] More recent consensus statements suggest that PJI less than 4 weeks from surgery places patients into an acute category.[16,17] Although other factors must be considered when determining the ultimate management of PJI following TAA, the acuity of the infectious process is often a major factor to consider when deciding between a single-stage versus 2-stage revision procedure, should ankle salvage be chosen.[17,18]

Acute infections may manifest with more abrupt increase in pain and swelling. Patients often have an acute effusion of the ankle joint with diffuse ankle pain, swelling, erythema, and increased warmth.[19] In the acute postoperative setting, wounds may show dehiscence and drainage. Systemically, patients may also present more acutely ill than in the chronic setting with fevers, chills, or night sweats.

In chronic PJI, symptoms may be more nonspeci c and mirror pain patterns similar to patients with aseptic loosening. An accurate description and characterization of the pain is crucial. Start-up pain, mechanical symptoms, pressure from underlying edema, pain at rest, and timing of the onset of pain following surgery may help to differentiate the underlying etiology. Chronic skin changes to the healed surgical wound may be present. A draining sinus tract or stula with or without gross purulence may be present and typically diagnosis a PJI until proven otherwise (Fig. 1A, B).

Severity of patient presentation may also be impacted by the virulence level of the infectious organism, which is an important factor when considering single- versus 2-stage surgical revision options.[18]

Inspection and examination or the ankle and foot should be undertaken, and the asymptomatic contralateral side should be compared. Assessing for ankle effusion, swelling, increased warmth, skin changes, and surgical wound abnormalities are mandatory. A thorough neurovascular examination should be performed to gain an understanding of the baseline neurologic and vascular status to the operative extremity. Location of pain around the ankle may clue the surgeon in to other potential sources of pain when determining if an infectious process is present of not. More diffuse or anterior pain may be related to PJI or aseptic loosening, whereas focal medial or lateral pain may be related to impingement or adjacent subtalar joint pathology. Ankle range of motion of the surgical ankle should be recorded and compared with the contralateral side. It is important to note whether pain is present throughout motion, at the extremes of motion, or even with micromotion of the ankle.

PREOPERATIVE WORK-UP
Imaging
The initial radiographic work-up for patients presenting with a painful total ankle begins with standard weight-bearing radiographs. Anteroposterior (AP) views of the foot and ankle, lateral view of the foot, and Saltzman hindfoot alignment views should be part of the initial assessment. Although an infectious process cannot de nitively be diagnosed by this imaging modality, some ndings may be evident that are concerning. Images should be inspected for acute periprosthetic fracture or stress fracture, implant malposition, subsidence, or periprosthetic osteolysis. These ndings may be seen more commonly with aseptic loosening of TAA implants, although in combination with concerning examination and laboratory ndings, PJI may be higher on the list of differential diagnosis possibilities. Importantly, comparison with past radiographs helps to evaluate for progressive implant subsidence or osteolysis. Radiographs are a critical part of the initial work-up for the painful TAA; however, more bony detail may be appreciated using computed tomography (CT). For example, osteolytic lesion size is often underestimated on conventional radiographs when compared with CT imaging. If possible, metal subtraction with CT imaging may help to decrease the amount of artifact scatter from the metal components to better evaluate bony detail. MRI is limited in evaluating painful TAA for underlying infection caused by implant artifacts. It is possible to identify a more super cial soft tissue abscess or sinus tract, although implant-associated artifact makes interpretation of the soft tissue structures more dif cult. Single photon emission CT (SPECT) may be helpful in the work-up of painful TAA by identifying areas that may be related to TAA-related pain. However, there does not appear to be a de nitive role for SPECT when speci cally diagnosing a TAA-related PJI.

LABORATORY TESTING
Blood Testing
In the setting of a painful TAA, once establishing whether the onset of symptoms is considered acute versus chronic, preoperative laboratory assessment is an important component when discerning whether an infectious etiology is the source of pain. This usually begins with a standard panel of blood tests, which include white blood count (WBC) with cell differential, erythrocyte sedimentation rate (ESR), and C-reactive protein (CRP). These may be used as a screening tool when trying to rule out PJI.

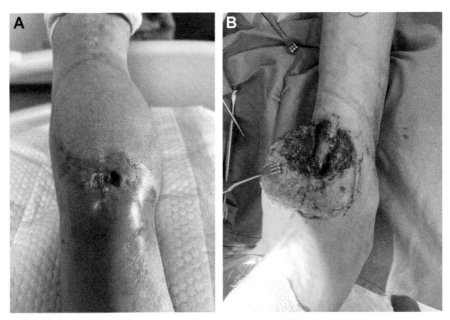

Fig. 1. (*A*) Clinical photograph of deep sinus tract communicating with ankle joint following revision total ankle arthroplasty and muscle flap coverage. (*B*) Intraoperative clinical photograph following muscle flap elevation demonstrating deep sinus tract communicating with ankle joint through extensor retinaculum defect.

Interpretation of serum CRP and ESR levels need to be done carefully, as these may remain elevated if obtained shortly after an elective surgical procedure.[20–22] CRP typically will peak in 1 to 2 days and return to normal by 3 weeks. However, ESR may remain elevated. Nonetheless, these are important screening tools that can easily be performed and have been shown to have a high negative predictive value when ruling out PJI.[23,24]

The utility of serum WBC with differential is more controversial and value as a screening tool, other than providing additional information to CRP and ESR, has been questioned in the literature pertaining to PJI.[19,25,26]

Synovial Fluid Aspiration and Analysis

Elevated systemic serum inflammatory markers should prompt consideration for joint aspiration and synovial fluid analysis, as interpretation of these results is an important component for diagnosis of PJI based on the Musculoskeletal Infection Society (MSIS) minor criteria.[14,16] Unfortunately, it can be difficult to successfully obtain any joint aspirate, even in the setting of infection. At the time of aspiration, gross inspection of the synovial fluid may be possible and may raise suspicion for infection (purulent fluid) or crystal arthropathy (chalky white deposits or straw-colored fluid). The use of a larger 18-gauge needle may allow for thicker joint fluid to be obtained. Typically, synovial fluid aspirate is sent for gram

staining, fluid analysis (total WBC with differential) and crystal analysis. While there is no current published literature regarding crystalline arthropathy following TAA, the authors anecdotally have discovered this association following TAA with significant osteolysis and concern for infection. Additionally, synovial fluid samples should be sent for microbiological assessment (aerobic, anaerobic, and fungal cultures). Importantly, if patients have taken antibiotics around the time of aspiration, this may falsely result in negative cultures. An antibiotic holiday of at least 2 weeks before aspiration has been suggested previously, although this delay is not always feasible in the work-up of PJI.[27]

More recently in the hip and knee PJI literature, synovial fluid assessment of CRP and alpha-defensin has been used. Alpha-defensin is an important synovial fluid microbial biomarker and has proven to demonstrate high sensitivity and specificity for PJI.[28,29] However, it has not been tested with regard to ankle PJI.

Intraoperative Assessment

Gross inspection of the ankle joint will be performed at the time of surgical intervention. Gross purulence or the presence of a deep communicating sinus tract is typically diagnostic for PJI.[14] In the situation where preoperative work-up for suspected infected TAA is inconclusive, intraoperative microbiological work-up remains the gold standard. Even with a high level of suspicion for infected TAA preoperatively, intraoperative microbiological assessment should be performed.

Frozen sections of synovial biopsies from the ankle joint should be obtained at the time of surgery, which may help in the decision for single-versus 2-stage revision surgery. This test is quantitative and looks for the presence of leukocytes per high power field under 400x microscopic evaluation.[19] This test is also controversial in the foot and ankle literature, as there is variation as to what leukocyte threshold indicates infection.[7,30,31] Generally, more than 5 leukocytes per high power field on synovial biopsy have been accepted as the definition of PJI; however, some authors suggest more than 10 leukocytes are indicative of infection[30]

As mentioned, microbiological diagnosis is crucial when treating PJI in TAA. The presence of 2 positive cultures by the same microorganism is considered a major criterion for definitively diagnosing a PJI.[14,16] Treatment considerations may be dictated by organism virulence and antibiotic sensitivity.[18] Arguably the most important reason for identification of the microorganism relates to the importance of targeted culture-specific antibiotic therapy following surgery. Various microorganisms may be causative agents in PJI following TAA depending on the route and underlying patient risk factors, however, Kessler and colleagues identified Staphylococcus aureus and coagulase-negative staphylococci as the most common.[7]

Alrashidi and colleagues published a review for diagnosing and treating PJI in TAA.[19] Although the authors sought to define specific examination, imaging, and laboratory findings that would suggest PJI in TAA, their approach appeared to be derived from criteria provided by the Musculoskeletal Infection Society and International Consensus Group for Periprosthetic Joint Infections, which has most often been applied to diagnosing PJI following hip and knee arthroplasty.[14,19,32] Parvizi and colleagues updated the diagnostic definition for PJI in 2018, which includes major and minor criteria and criteria for an inconclusive preoperative work-up.[16] There are 2 major criteria: sinus tract with communication to the joint, and 2 positive cultures for the same organism. Minor criteria are scored based on elevated or positive serum CRP or D-Dimer, serum ESR, synovial WBC or positive leukocyte esterase, synovial CRP, synovial polymorphonuclear (PMN) cell percentage, and positive alpha defensin.[16] In cases where preoperative work-up is inconclusive, the authors suggest using intraoperative criteria that include positive histology, 1 positive culture, and presence of purulence.[16]

Although these diagnostic criteria have been described for hip and knee PJI, their use has often been applied for diagnosing PJI following TAA.[7,8,19,31,33–35] In addition to the work by Alrashidi and colleagues, other reviews in the literature have offered definitions for PJI following TAA based on physical examination and laboratory and imaging studies.[7,8,31,33,36] There have been limited data on laboratory thresholds for these tests specific to TAA.[19] Therefore, the diagnostic criteria often used for work-up of TAA PJI have been extrapolated from validated and evidence-based research from the hip and knee arthroplasty literature.[16]

In 2019, Heidari and colleagues published their recommended algorithm for diagnosis of infection following TAA.[35] The authors' approach used similar diagnostic modalities described by the MSIS. However, they acknowledge that MSIS guidelines for diagnosis and treatment of PJI in the hip and knee may not be completely applicable to TAA because of anatomic differences in the soft tissue envelope of the ankle.[35] Additionally, the authors recognize that more research is needed examining these established diagnostic criteria in order to validate their use in TAA.

Management

Decision making surrounding PJI of the ankle is complex, and incorporates multiple factors including duration of infection, virulence of the pathogen, host type, and the integrity of the adjacent soft tissue. Moreover, high-quality studies, with the aim of comparing the various treatment options in PJI, are lacking. Although treatment success has improved over the recent decade, patients with ankle PJI should be cautioned regarding the guarded prognosis of limb salvage, particularly with virulent infection. Multiple operative visits may be required to adequately clear the offending organism, and the ability to re-implant a total ankle prosthesis depends on the residual bone stock and local soft tissue coverage. This section will explore the available treatment options and their reported success, thereby empowering the surgeon to provide appropriate counsel to patients with ankle PJI.

History

Early generations of total ankle replacement surgery were accompanied by high rates of PJI. In a systematic review including 827 total ankle replacements, Gougoulias found a rate of superficial wound healing complications to be as high as 8%, and deep infections ranging from 0% to 4.6% in the available studies.[37] In 2014, Myerson and colleagues reported a deep infection rate of 2.4% in their report of 613 replacements.[31] The relatively high rate of deep infection relative to the reported rates in hip and knee arthroplasty has been attributed to multiple hypotheses. First, the anterior approach to the ankle, which is the most popular method of insertion, represents a vascular watershed area with tenuous healing. Early instrumentation was unrefined, and surgeon experience was limited, leading to high operative time, extensive use of tourniquet, and prolonged employment of self-retraction. These factors led to the development of modified approaches to ankle replacement surgery, including anteromedial, anterolateral, and lateral transfibular approaches.[38–42]

At an average follow-up of 49 months, Myerson reported successful repeat implantation following 2-stage revision in only three of 19 patients with latent infection, whereas 6 patients ultimately underwent arthrodesis; 7 patients were left with a permanent antibiotic spacer, and 3 patients required a transtibial amputation.[31] Their conclusion was that only a select number of patients with a deep infection may expect to undergo successful revision arthroplasty. With recent advancements in technique and early diagnosis, outcomes following 2-stage revision may be expected to improve.

Management of Postoperative Cellulitis

The literature surrounding treatment of super - cial postoperative cellulitis following TAA is limited, and largely borrowed from scienti c reports total hip and knee literature. In an analysis of different postoperative immobilization techniques, Schipper reported a relatively high incidence of wounds with cellulitis requiring antibiotics (oral or intravenous), ranging between 16.7% and 22% depending on the immobilization method.[43] Cellulitic infections are frequently polymicrobial, although most commonly attributable to streptococcal or staphylococcal pathogens. Because of the limited distance and soft tissue separation between the prosthesis and subcutaneous planes, early and aggressive treatment with antibiotics with close monitoring is encouraged to prevent local spread to the prosthetic elements. In severe cases with a delay In presentation, a 2- to 6-day course of intravenous antibiotics may be required. Common antibiotic choices for initial treatment include cefalexin, vancomycin, cefuroxime, ampicillin, and gentamicin. Following the initial treatment response (as evidenced by a reduction in pain, swelling,

warmth, and erythema), transition to alternative agents such as doxycycline, trimethroprim-sulfamethoxazole, dicloxacillin, or clindamycin for a minimum of 2 weeks is beneficial. Although clinical evaluation is most prudent, serial monitoring of acute-phase reactants such as ESR and CRP may offer quantifiable evidence of the initial infection and treatment response or failure.[44]

A strong consensus of expert opinion agrees that patients with postoperative cellulitis should be evaluated to rule out deep PJI, and isolated cellulitis may be treated with conservative measures including antibiotics and close monitoring.[45] An aspiration of the ankle may be considered to obtain an intra-articular fluid sample. Ideally, areas affected by cellulitis should be avoided so as to prevent inadvertent inoculation; however, the concept of iatrogenic inoculation due to arthrocentesis through an area of cellulitis has been debated.[46]

Debridement, Antibiotics, and Implant Retention

Irrigation and debridement with modular component exchange is a well-accepted treatment for acute hematogenous infection in hip and knee arthroplasty.[47,48] Although a classic criterion for the DAIR (debridement, antibiotics, and implant retention) procedure was onset of symptoms within 2 to 4 weeks, the exact timing that would contraindicate the procedure has been recently disputed.[49,50] Nevertheless, presence of a sinus tract and infection with high-virulence organisms (most commonly, methicillin-resistant *S aureus* [MRSA]) are notable risk factors that portend poor outcomes following DAIR.[51] DAIR may therefore be considered for immunocompetent patients with acute postoperative infections (infection within 4 to 12 weeks of the index surgery) or acute hematogenous infection (acute onset of symptoms in a previously well-functioning joint), in whom there is no sinus tract or extensive wound breakdown.[18,52]

In comparison to hip and knee arthroplasty, there is a dearth of literature surrounding DAIR in total ankle arthroplasty. Initial reports were grim. Myerson reported 4 cases of DAIR, 3 cases in early postoperative infections (within 3–7 weeks of surgery) and 1 case with acute hematogenous infection.[31] Recurrent infection developed in all 4 patients, requiring revision to either arthroplasty, fusion, or definitive antibiotic spacer. By comparison, Patton and colleagues reported 2 patients following acute onset of symptoms who underwent DAIR and encountered no recurrent infection.[8] In a larger cohort of 14 patients, Lachman and colleagues reported the results of DAIR for acute hematogenous PJI. The long-term failure rate was 54%, and patients with failure were most likely to harbor MRSA. Moreover, patients with failure tended toward a longer duration of time from symptom onset to surgery (13 days compared with 8.2 days in successful cases), although no statistical comparison was performed.[10]

A key component of the DAIR procedure is appropriate postoperative antibiotic therapy.[53] Although the precise duration of antibiotic therapy has been contested, 2 consensus guidelines are available to direct treatment. The International Consensus on Periprosthetic Joint Infection, whose proceedings were reported in 2013, encouraged antibiotic therapy for 2 to 6 weeks after surgery.[54] By comparison, the Infectious Diseases Society of America (IDSA) Guidelines for the Diagnosis and Management of Prosthetic Joint Infection advised 4 to 6 weeks of pathogen-specific intravenous or highly bioavailable oral antimicrobial therapy, with consideration of chronic oral antimicrobial suppression thereafter.[55] In cases of staphylococcal PJI, the addition of rifampin 300 to 450 mg orally twice daily should followed by rifampin plus a companion oral drug for 3 months. Although these guidelines were designed for total hip and knee arthroplasty infections, total ankle infections may be managed similarly.

The employment of chronic suppressive antibiotics in patients who have undergone surgical treatment for ankle PJI has been proposed, as in the hip and knee literature.[56] Although appealing, this concept may add to the risk of adverse drug events, antimicrobial resistance, and cost. Ultimately, it is recommended that surgeons coordinate antibiotic therapy with an infectious disease (ID) specialist with consideration of infection characteristics, host factors, pathogen virulence, and prior infections.[53] Many antimicrobial agents require clinical and laboratory monitoring for efficacy and toxicity, so close ID follow-up is required.

Two-Stage Revision
Two-stage exchange of arthroplasty implants is considered the gold standard treatment of chronic PJI in the United States. Its success in eradicating PJI in hip and knee arthroplasty has been well documented.[57] Although early reports were mired by poor outcomes, more recent publications have found satisfactory long-term survival rates of revised prostheses and improvements in patient-reported outcomes. Conti reported on a cohort of eleven patients who underwent two-stage exchange arthroplasty.[58]

At a median follow-up of 3 years, ten of the eleven patients retained their total ankle arthroplasty; three patients had recurrent infections or wound complications requiring revision surgery. Two underwent repeat irrigation and debridement with polyethylene exchange, and one patient elected to undergo transtibial amputation. Clinical outcomes were found to be lower than after primary ankle arthroplasty, and all but one patient reported their level of function to be less than normal.

Taken together, the functional results of 2-stage revision following ankle PJI are worse than hip and knee PJI. Nevertheless, there is a strong consensus that deep chronic infection after ankle arthroplasty requires implant removal unless otherwise contraindicated.[59] Several possible risk factors for treatment failure have been proposed, including compromised soft tissues, significant bone involvement and osteomyelitis, and inadequate antibiotic therapy before repeat implantation.[60] A coordinated effort between the treating orthopedic surgeon, ID specialist, and plastic surgeon is therefore encouraged to optimize the likelihood of success. Key technical components of the surgery include complete synovectomy and debridement of necrotic/nonviable tissue, removal of all articular prosthetic material, and implantation of an antibiotic-laden cement spacer. When a complete debridement is performed and with appropriate antibiotic therapy, patients can be counseled to expect infection eradication and limb salvage, but with limited function compared with a primary ankle arthroplasty.

Several antimicrobial options are available for use in cement spacers, including gentamicin, tobramycin, vancomycin, clindamycin, ampicillin, and meropenem. Considerations for antibiotic selection include thermostability, patient allergy, and availability as a soluble powder.[61] Ideally, a preoperative aspiration with identification would be obtained to allow for pathogen-tailored therapy. In the absence of such data, creation of a spacer with broad-spectrum antimicrobial profile may be selected. A combination of 2 g of vancomycin with 2 g of gentamicin and 2 g of cefotaxime per 40 g packet of cement has been suggested.[62] These agents have empiric efficacy against MRSA, gram-negative bacteria, and gentamicin-resistant organisms.[63] Other additives include tobramycin and daptomycin (activity against gram-negative bacteria), amikacin (activity against gram-negative bacteria and *Staphylococcus*), clindamycin (activity against gram-positive cocci and anaerobes), imipenem/cilastin (broad-spectrum against gram-positive and gram-negative), and ceftazidime (against gram-negative bacteria).[64–69] Fungal PJI represents approximately 1% of cases, and may be addressed with the addition of amphotericin (200–420 mg per each pack of cement) to promote infection eradication.[70] In these instances, the addition of oral fluconazole for at least 6 months following 2-stage exchange arthroplasty has been proposed.[71,72]

The optimal timing for repeat implantation following prosthesis removal and cement spacer depends on several factors. Borrowing from literature in hip and knee arthroplasties, repeat implantation may be performed when there is: completion of antibiotic therapy (as detailed previously), absence of clinical signs of infection (including erythema, wound drainage, or constitutional symptoms), and a significant reduction of inflammatory marker values (including ESR, CRP, and possible D-Dimer and interleukin-6).[73–75] An antibiotic-free period of at least 2 weeks has traditionally been used to evaluate the existence of persistent infection; however, recent publications have contested the utility of such an antibiotic holiday.[76,77] This practice introduces the risk of failed treatment during the antibiotic-free period without necessarily improving PJI treatment, and thus several authors and consensus meetings have argued against routine antibiotic holidays.[78,79] An aspiration of an ankle with an antibiotic spacer may also be considered before repeat implantation to rule out persistent infection. Although no studies have been done to evaluate the utility of routine aspirations in ankle PJI, the procedure is low-cost, simple to perform, and low-risk.[80] Studies in infected knee arthroplasty have demonstrated higher specificity than sensitivity, and thus a positive aspirate is likely to indicate residual infection, whereas a negative aspirate should be interpreted with relative caution.[80]

Salvage following ankle PJI may include revision to ankle arthroplasty (classic 2-stage exchange arthroplasty), but also revision to ankle arthrodesis or tibiotalocalcaneal (TTC) fusion. A careful assessment of radiographs and advanced imaging should be performed to evaluate if there is sufficient bone stock to support ankle arthroplasty implants. At the time of this writing, 2 revision ankle prosthetic systems are available for use in the setting of bone loss (INVISION, Wright Medical, Memphis, Tennessee; Salto Talaris XT, Integra Life Sciences, Princeton, New Jersey). These systems use components with broad footprints to maximize cortical coverage, as well as extra-large polyethylene liner sizing to restore the native joint line

(Fig. 2A–F). In the setting of large talar bone loss, a subtalar arthrodesis may be performed at the time of cement spacer application to provide a stable base for future talar component fixation.

Pfahl and colleagues performed a retrospective study of 111 cases of revision procedures of failed ankle arthroplasty, of which 12 were for PJI.[81] There were lower failure rates, increased short-term survival, and improved clinical outcomes of revision arthroplasty and TTC fusion than ankle arthrodesis. Shared decision-making with the patient is critical in determining which of these options is most suitable, and should include a discussion regarding the adequacy of the soft tissue envelope, residual bone stock, preoperative range of motion, and patient expectations.

Soft Tissue Considerations

Soft tissue management during DAIR or 2-stage exchange arthroplasty is critical. The treating orthopedic surgeon is encouraged to consult with a plastic surgeon experienced in microsurgical procedures at the time of the initial presentation. A variety of local tissue flaps are available to offer coverage in the setting of wound breakdown and soft tissue loss. These are restricted to small or narrow defects, but are relatively easy to perform and may provide supple coverage of all tissue composites.[82] Namely, the reverse sural flap, perforator-based propeller flap, reverse peroneus brevis, and reverse hemi-soleus flaps are available and described for coverage of the anterior ankle.[82] When local tissues are unavailable, free tissue transfer is required. These may be drawn from muscle flaps originating from the latissimus dorsi, serratus anterior, rectus abdominis, or gracilis muscles. Alternatively, the anterolateral thigh (ALT) free flap is a fasciocutaneous free skin perforator flap provides full defect coverage and has become a workhorse in the management of large soft tissue defects.

In recurrent cases of ankle PJI following 2-stage exchange arthroplasty, patients may elect to undergo repeat 2-stage revision, definitive cement spacer application, or below-knee amputation. Outcomes for repeat 2-stage revision are lacking for ankle PJI; however, rates of success following the procedure in hip and knee PJI are decidedly poor, with a high chance of repeat infection.[83,84] Alternatively, definitive treatment with cement spacer application may be considered in low-demand patients with significant comorbidities. In a small case series of 9 patients, Ferrao found that only 1 patient treated with a definitive cement spacer for ankle

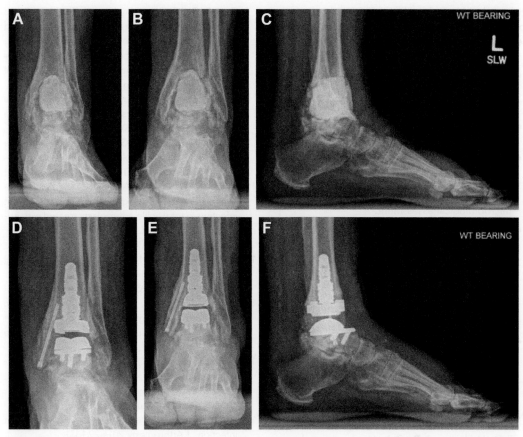

Fig. 2. (*A–F*) Successful repeat implantation in setting of severe tibial bone loss following implant removal and cement spacer application.

PJI developed recurrent infection.[36] Seven of the 9 patients had a functional result, were mobile, and were able to perform basic activities with minimal discomfort.[36] This treatment method has been criticized by some based on the limited time for antibiotic elution (generally, 6 to 8 weeks) and thus relatively high rates of bacterial colonization of the spacer (approximately 50% at the time of repeat implantation in 2-stage exchange arthroplasty).[85] For many patients, however, surgical amputation of the foot and ankle offers the best opportunity for an expeditious recovery and return to infection-free living. Amputation should not be viewed as a failure on the part of the treating surgeon or patient, but rather an opportunity to cure the patient of a challenging disease and relieve him or her of a substantial burden.

SUMMARY

The diagnosis and surgical treatment of ankle PJI is complex and requires shared decision making between the patient and the treating surgeon. Diagnosis can be challenging but begins with a careful history and physical examination in conjunction with a high clinical suspicion. Imaging, laboratory tests, and microbiological assessment are critical to further investigate ankle PJI and may guide management. Historically, outcomes following DAIR and 2-stage exchange arthroplasty have been fraught with poor outcomes and repeat infection. More recent studies suggest that ankle PJI may be successfully treated with a combination of surgery and culture-directed antimicrobial therapy. Nevertheless, patients should be alerted regarding the seriousness of the deep prosthetic infection and the possible need for implant removal, salvage reconstruction, and possibly amputation. Further work is needed to guide surgeons on the best management of ankle PJI, including technical improvements in diagnosis, surgical selection (DAIR vs 2-stage revision), salvage reconstruction, and development of antimicrobial regimens. Although much can be borrowed from the literature on hip and knee PJI, the unique features of the ankle joint and total ankle arthroplasty dictate that ankle-speci c studies may offer the best guidance on treatment efforts.

CLINICS CARE POINTS

- Periprosthetic infections following total ankle arthroplasty (TAA) ranges from 0-5%.
- Diagnosis takes in to consideration patient risk factors, history and physical exam, imaging, blood and synovial fluid testing and intra-operative tissue sampling with microbiological assessment.
- Several surgical treatment options exist depending on the acuity of the infection and virulence of the causative pathogen. Options include Irrigation and debridement with modular component exchange, 2-stage revision TAA, 2- revision ankle or tibiotalocalcaneal (TTC) arthrodesis, definitive cement spacer placement and amputation.
- Following limb salvage efforts, soft tissue coverage may be required and include local soft tissue flaps or free tissue transfers.

DISCLOSURE

Dr B.D. Umbel and Dr B.A. Haghverdian have nothing to disclose. Dr K.M. Schweitzer is a consultant for Arthrex and Stryker; Dr S.B. Adams is a consultant for Stryker, Enovis, Exactech, and Conventus.

REFERENCES

1. Karzon AL, Kadakia RJ, Coleman MM, et al. The rise of total ankle arthroplasty use: a database analysis describing case volumes and incidence trends in the United States between 2009 and 2019. Foot Ankle Int 2022;43(11):1501–10.
2. Shah JA, Schwartz AM, Farley KX, et al. Projections and epidemiology of total ankle and revision total ankle arthroplasty in the United States to 2030. Foot Ankle Spec 2022. https://doi.org/10.1177/19386400221109420. 19386400221109420.
3. Affatato S, Taddei P, Leardini A, et al. Wear behaviour in total ankle replacement: a comparison between an in vitro simulation and retrieved prostheses. Clin Biomech 2009;24:661–9.
4. Gougoulias N, Khanna A, Maffulli N. How successful are current ankle replacements? A systematic review of the literature. Clin Orthop Relat Res 2010;468:199–208.
5. Reuver JM, Dayerizadeh N, Burger B, et al. Total ankle replacement outcome in low volume centers: short-term followup. Foot Ankle Int 2010;31(12):1064–8.
6. Zaidi R, Cro S, Gurusamy K, et al. The outcome of total ankle replacement: a systematic review and meta-analysis. Bone Joint Lett J 2013;95-B:1500–7.
7. Kessler B, Sendi P, Graber P, et al. Risk factors for periprosthetic ankle joint infection: a case-control study. J Bone Joint Surg Am 2012;94:1871–6.
8. Patton D, Kiewiet N, Brage M. Infected total ankle arthroplasty: risk factors and treatment options. Foot Ankle Int 2015;36(6):626–34.
9. Gross CE, Hamid KS, Green C, et al. Operative wound complications following total ankle arthroplasty. Foot Ankle Int 2017;38(4):360–6.
10. Lachman JR, Ramos JA, DeOrio JK, et al. Outcomes of acute hematogenous periprosthetic joint infection in total ankle arthroplasty treated with irrigation, debridement, and polyethylene exchange. Foot Ankle Int 2018;39(11):1266–71.
11. Young JL, May MM, Haddad SL. Infected total ankle arthroplasty following routine dental procedure. Foot Ankle Int 2009;30(3):252–7.
12. Noori N, Myerson C, Charlton T, et al. Is antibiotic prophylaxis necessary before dental procedures in patients post total ankle arthroplasty? Foot Ankle Int 2019;40(2):237–41.
13. Available at: https://www.aaos.org/globalassets/quality-and-practice-resources/dental/dental-prophylaxis-auc-decision-tree-v2_condensed_1.29.20-003.pdf. Accessed August 4, 2023.
14. Parvizi J, Gehrke T. Definition of periprosthetic joint infection. J Arthroplasty 2014;29:1331.
15. Aynardi MC, Plöger MM, Walley KC, et al. What is the definition of acute and chronic periprosthetic joint infection (Pji) of total ankle arthroplasty (Taa)? Foot Ankle Int 2019;40(1_Suppl):19S–21S.
16. Parvizi J, Tan TL, Goswami K, et al. The 2018 definition of periprosthetic hip and knee infection: an evidence-based and validated criteria. J Arthroplasty 2018;33:1309–14.e2.
17. Raikin S, Parekh S, McDonald E. What is the treatment "algorithm" for an infected total ankle arthroplasty (TAA)? Foot Ankle Int 2019;40(1_Suppl):43S–6S.
18. Ellington K, Bemenderfer TB. What are the indications for one-stage versus two-stage exchange arthroplasty in management of the infected total ankle arthroplasty (TAA)? Foot Ankle Int 2019;40(1_suppl):55S–8S.
19. Alrashidi Y, Galhoum AE, Wiewiorski M, et al. How to diagnose and treat infection in total ankle arthroplasty. Foot Ankle Clin 2017;22(2):405–23.
20. Kim TW, Kim DH, Oh WS, et al. Analysis of the causes of elevated C-reactive protein level in the early postoperative period after primary total knee arthroplasty. J Arthroplasty 2016;31(9):1990–6.
21. Larsson S, Thelander U, Friberg S. C-reactive protein (CRP) levels after elective orthopedic surgery. Clin Orthop Relat Res 1992;275:237–42.

22. White J, Kelly M, Dunsmuir R. C-reactive protein level after total hip and total knee replacement. J Bone Joint Surg Br 1998;80(5):909–11.

23. Greidanus NV, Masri BA, Garbuz DS, et al. Use of erythrocyte sedimentation rate and C-reactive protein level to diagnose infection before revision total knee arthroplasty. A prospective evaluation. J Bone Joint Surg Am 2007;89(7):1409–16.

24. Spangehl MJ, Masri BA, O'connell JX, et al. Prospective analysis of preoperative and intraoperative investigations for the diagnosis of infection at the sites of two hundred and two revision total hip arthroplasties. J Bone Joint Surg Am 1999;81(5): 672–83.

25. Toossi N, Adeli B, Rasouli MR, et al. Serum white blood cell count and differential do not have a role in the diagnosis of periprosthetic joint infection. J Arthroplasty 2012;27(8 Suppl):51–4.

26. Zmistowski B, Restrepo C, Huang R, et al. Periprosthetic joint infection diagnosis: a complete understanding of white blood cell count and differential. J Arthroplasty 2012;27(9):1589–93.

27. Preininger B, Janz V, vonRoth P, et al. Inadequacy of joint aspiration for detection of persistent periprosthetic infection during two-stage septic revision knee surgery. Orthopedics 2017;40(4):231–4.

28. Wyatt MC, Beswick AD, Kunutsor SK, et al. The alpha-defensin immunoassay and leukocyte esterase colorimetric strip test for the diagnosis of periprosthetic infection: a systematic review and meta-analysis. J Bone Joint Surg Am 2016;98:992–1000.

29. Deirmengian C, Kardos K, Kilmartin P, et al. The alpha-defensin test for periprosthetic joint infection outperforms the leukocyte esterase test strip. Clin Orthop Relat Res 2015;473(1):198–203.

30. Hsu AR, Haddad SL, Myerson MS. Evaluation and management of the painful total ankle arthroplasty. J Am Acad Orthop Surg 2015;23:272–82.

31. Myerson MS, Shariff R, Zonno AJ. The management of infection following total ankle replacement: demographics and treatment. Foot Ankle Int 2014; 35(9):855–62.

32. Springer BD. The diagnosis of periprosthetic joint infection. J Arthroplasty 2015;30:908–11.

33. Kessler B, Knupp M, Graber P, et al. The treatment and outcome of peri-prosthetic infection of the ankle: a single cohor tcentre experience of 34 cases. Bone Joint Lett J 2014;96:772–7.

34. Usuelli FG, Indino C, Maccario C, et al. Infections in primary total ankle replacement: anterior approach versus lateral transfibular approach. Foot Ankle Surg 2019;25:19–23.

35. Heidari N, Oh I, Malagelada F. What is the diagnostic "algorithm" for infected total ankle arthroplasty (TAA)? Foot Ankle Int 2019;40(1_Suppl):21S–2S.

36. Ferrao P, Myerson MS, Schuberth JM, et al. Cement spacer as definitive management for postoperative ankle infection. Foot Ankle Int 2012;33(2):173–8.

37. Gougoulias N, Khanna A, Maffulli N. How successful are current ankle replacements?: a systematic review of the literature. Clin Orthop Relat Res 2010;468(1):199–208.

38. Bibbo C. A modified anterior approach to the ankle. J Foot Ankle Surg 2013;52(1):136–7.

39. Halai MM, Pinsker E, Daniels TR. Effect of novel anteromedial approach on wound complications following ankle arthroplasty. Foot Ankle Int 2020; 41(10):1198–205.

40. Clugston E, Ektas N, Scholes C, et al. Early clinical outcomes and complications of transfibular total ankle arthroplasty: the australian experience. Foot Ankle Int 2023;44(1):40–7.

41. Tiusanen H, Kormi S, Kohonen I, et al. Results of trabecular-metal total ankle arthroplasties with transfibular approach. Foot Ankle Int 2020;41(4): 411–8.

42. Usuelli FG, Maccario C, Granata F, et al. Clinical and radiological outcomes of transfibular total ankle arthroplasty. Foot Ankle Int 2019;40(1):24–33.

43. Schipper ON, Hsu AR, Haddad SL. Reduction in wound complications after total ankle arthroplasty using a compression wrap protocol. Foot Ankle Int 2015;36(12):1448–54.

44. Markanday A. Acute phase reactants in infections: evidence-based review and a guide for clinicians. Open Forum Infect Dis 2015;2(3):ofv098.

45. Plöger MM, Murawski CD. How should postoperative cellulitis be treated in patients with total ankle arthroplasty (TAA) in place? Foot Ankle Int 2019; 40(1_Suppl):61S–2S.

46. Dooley DP. Aspiration of the possibly septic joint through potential cellulitis: just do it. J Emerg Med 2002;23(2):210.

47. Boyle KK, Kapadia M, Landy DC, et al. Utilization of debridement, antibiotics, and implant retention for infection after total joint arthroplasty over a decade in the united states. J Arthroplasty 2020; 35(8):2210–6.

48. Grammatopoulos G, Kendrick B, McNally M, et al. Outcome following debridement, antibiotics, and implant retention in hip periprosthetic joint infection-an 18-year experience. J Arthroplasty 2017;32(7):2248–55.

49. Tarity TD, Gkiatas I, Nocon AA, et al. Irrigation and debridement with implant retention: does chronicity of symptoms matter? J Arthroplasty 2021; 36(11):3741–9.

50. van der Ende B, van Oldenrijk J, Reijman M, et al. Timing of debridement, antibiotics, and implant retention (DAIR) for early post-surgical hip and knee prosthetic joint infection (Pji) does not affect 1-year re-revision rates: data from the Dutch Arthroplasty Register. J Bone Jt Infect 2021;6(8):329–36.

51. Qasim SN, Swann A, Ashford R. The DAIR (Debridement, antibiotics and implant retention) procedure for infected total knee replacement - a literature review. SICOT J 2017;3:2.

52. Chan JJ, Mohamadi A, Walsh S, et al. What are the indications and contraindications for irrigation and debridement and retention of prosthesis (Dair) in patients with infected total ankle arthroplasty (TAA)? Foot Ankle Int 2019;40(1_Suppl):52S–3S.

53. Embil JM, O'Neil JT. What is the optimal (type, dose and route of administration) antibiotic treatment for patients with infected total ankle arthroplasty (TAA)? Foot Ankle Int 2019;40(1_suppl):46S–7S.

54. Parvizi J, Gehrke T, Chen AF. Proceedings of the international consensus on periprosthetic joint infection. Bone Joint Lett J 2013;95-B(11):1450–2.

55. Osmon DR, Berbari EF, Berendt AR, et al. Executive summary: diagnosis and management of prosthetic joint infection: clinical practice guidelines by the Infectious Diseases Society of America. Clin Infect Dis 2013;56(1):1–10.

56. Parekh S. Is there a role for suppressive antibiotics in patients with periprosthetic joint infection (PJI) of total ankle arthroplasty (TAA) who have undergone surgical treatment? Foot Ankle Int 2019;40(1_suppl):48S.

57. Charette RS, Melnic CM. Two-stage revision arthroplasty for the treatment of prosthetic joint infection. Curr Rev Musculoskelet Med 2018;11(3):332–40.

58. Conti MS, Irwin TA, Ford SE, et al. Complications, reoperations, and patient-reported outcomes following a 2-stage revision total ankle arthroplasty for chronic periprosthetic joint infections. Foot Ankle Int 2022;43(12):1614–21.

59. Kaplan J, Raikin S. Does deep chronic infection after total ankle arthroplasty (TAA) require implant removal? Foot Ankle Int 2019;40(1_Suppl):62S–3S.

60. McDonald E. What are the predictors of treatment failure in patients who have undergone two-stage exchange for infected total ankle arthroplasty (TAA)? Foot Ankle Int 2019;40(1_suppl):60S–1S.

61. Shakked R, Da Rin de Lorenzo F. What determines the type and dose of antibiotic that is needed to be added to the cement spacer in patients with infected total ankle arthroplasty (Taa)? Foot Ankle Int 2019;40(1_Suppl):48S–52S.

62. Koo KH, Yang JW, Cho SH, et al. Impregnation of vancomycin, gentamicin, and cefotaxime in a cement spacer for two-stage cementless reconstruction in infected total hip arthroplasty. J Arthroplasty 2001;16(7):882–92.

63. Cui Q, Mihalko WM, Shields JS, et al. Antibiotic-impregnated cement spacers for the treatment of infection associated with total hip or knee arthroplasty. J Bone Joint Surg Am 2007;89(4):871–82.

64. Adams K, Couch L, Cierny G, et al. In vitro and in vivo evaluation of antibiotic diffusion from antibiotic-impregnated polymethylmethacrylate beads. Clin Orthop Relat Res 1992;278:244–52.

65. Klekamp J, Dawson JM, Haas DW, et al. The use of vancomycin and tobramycin in acrylic bone cement: biomechanical effects and elution kinetics for use in joint arthroplasty. J Arthroplasty 1999;14(3):339–46.

66. Kuechle DK, Landon GC, Musher DM, et al. Elution of vancomycin, daptomycin, and amikacin from acrylic bone cement. Clin Orthop Relat Res 1991;264:302–8.

67. Hofmann AA, Goldberg T, Tanner AM, et al. Treatment of infected total knee arthroplasty using an articulating spacer: 2- to 12-year experience. Clin Orthop Relat Res 2005;430:125–31.

68. Penner MJ, Duncan CP, Masri BA. The in vitro elution characteristics of antibiotic-loaded CMW and Palacos-R bone cements. J Arthroplasty 1999;14(2):209–14.

69. Hsu YH, Hu CC, Hsieh PH, et al. Vancomycin and ceftazidime in bone cement as a potentially effective treatment for knee periprosthetic joint infection. J Bone Joint Surg Am 2017;99(3):223–31.

70. Kim JK, Lee DY, Kang DW, et al. Efficacy of antifungal-impregnated cement spacer against chronic fungal periprosthetic joint infections after total knee arthroplasty. Knee 2018;25(4):631–7.

71. Azzam K, Parvizi J, Jungkind D, et al. Microbiological, clinical, and surgical features of fungal prosthetic joint infections: a multi-institutional experience. J Bone Joint Surg Am 2009;91(Suppl 6):142–9.

72. Hwang BH, Yoon JY, Nam CH, et al. Fungal periprosthetic joint infection after primary total knee replacement. J Bone Joint Surg Br 2012;94(5):656–9.

73. Shahi A, Kheir MM, Tarabichi M, et al. Serum d-dimer test is promising for the diagnosis of periprosthetic joint infection and timing of reimplantation. J Bone Joint Surg Am 2017;99(17):1419–27.

74. Deirmengian C, Kardos K, Kilmartin P, et al. Diagnosing periprosthetic joint infection: has the era of the biomarker arrived? Clin Orthop Relat Res 2014;472(11):3254–62.

75. Senneville E, Lopez V, Slullitel G. What metrics can be used to determine the optimal timing of reimplantation in patients who have undergone resection arthroplasty as part of a two-stage exchange for infected total ankle arthroplasty (TAA)? Foot Ankle Int 2019;40(1_Suppl):58S–60S.

76. Tan TL, Kheir MM, Rondon AJ, et al. Determining the role and duration of the "antibiotic holiday" period in periprosthetic joint infection. J Arthroplasty 2018;33(9):2976–80.

77. Ascione T, Balato G, Mariconda M, et al. Continuous antibiotic therapy can reduce recurrence of prosthetic joint infection in patients undergoing 2-stage exchange. J Arthroplasty 2019;34(4):704–9.

78. Bejon P, Berendt A, Atkins BL, et al. Two-stage revision for prosthetic joint infection: predictors of outcome and the role of reimplantation microbiology. J Antimicrob Chemother 2010;65(3):569–75.

79. Ghanem E, Azzam K, Seeley M, et al. Staged revision for knee arthroplasty infection: what is the role of serologic tests before reimplantation? Clin Orthop Relat Res 2009;467(7):1699–705.

80. Fuchs D, Parekh SG. Should aspiration of the ankle with an antibiotic spacer be performed prior to reimplantation? Foot Ankle Int 2019;40(1_Suppl): 26S–7S.

81. Pfahl K, Röser A, Eder J, et al. Outcomes of salvage procedures for failed total ankle arthroplasty. Foot Ankle Int 2023;44(4):262–9.

82. Roukis T. Primary and revision total ankle replacement. 2nd edition. Cham, Switzerland: Springer; 2021.

83. Steinicke AC, Schwarze J, Gosheger G, et al. Repeat two-stage exchange arthroplasty for recurrent periprosthetic hip or knee infection: what are the chances for success? Arch Orthop Trauma Surg 2023;143(4):1731–40.

84. Brown TS, Fehring KA, Ollivier M, et al. Repeat two-stage exchange arthroplasty for prosthetic hip reinfection. Bone Joint Lett J 2018;100-B(9):1157–61.

85. Nelson CL, Jones RB, Wingert NC, et al. Sonication of antibiotic spacers predicts failure during two-stage revision for prosthetic knee and hip infections. Clin Orthop Relat Res 2014;472(7):2208–14.

The Differentiation Between Infection and Acute Charcot

Ryan G. Rogero, MD[a], Samhita Swamy, BS[b],
Clayton C. Bettin, MD[a,*]

KEYWORDS

- Charcot neuroarthropathy • Osteomyelitis • Diabetic foot • Diagnosis • Current concepts

KEY POINTS

- Acute Charcot neuroarthropathy and infection in the foot and ankle present with many shared characteristics that make differentiation of these conditions difficult for clinicians.
- History and physical examination are essential in differentiating infection and acute Charcot neuroarthropathy.
- Imaging, laboratory studies, and bone cultures with histopathological analysis should be used to aid in unclear diagnoses, and all have support in the current literature.
- Incorrect or delayed diagnosis can cause devastating effects to patients and can have negative determinants on the entire health care system.

INTRODUCTION/BACKGROUND

Differentiating infections of the foot and ankle and Charcot neuroarthropathy(CN) has become a progressively important topic due to their shared increasing prevalence.[1] What we today know as CN was first described by the French neuropathologist Jean-Martin Charcot in the late nineteenth century.[2] First described by Charcot in tertiary syphilis patients, it has since been described in a variety of conditions, including those with diabetes mellitus, spinal cord and peripheral nerve injuries, cerebral palsy, alcoholic peripheral neuropathy, and Charcot-Marie-Tooth disease.[2,3] Today, CN is most described in those with long-standing diabetes.[4] With the continued increase in the prevalence of diabetes in the modern world, the identification and understanding of this noninfectious destructive inflammatory process of the foot and ankle will be essential.

Infections of the foot and ankle, both soft tissue and bony, are a pathology more prevalent than CN but share many characteristics. They are also commonly seen in patients with neuropathy, particularly diabetics, due to the loss of sensation in the foot and ankle region combined with immune system deficits and microvascular changes.[5]

The differentiation between acute Charcot and acute infection in the foot and ankle region is important to clinicians, as treatment may differ, and both present risks of amputation and mortality if not managed in a correct and timely manner.[1] This article provides the current diagnostic methodology used to differentiate these 2 clinical entities.

NATURE OF THE PROBLEM

The cause of CN is multifactorial, with 2 accepted theories of its development: the neurotraumatic and neurovascular theories.[4]

The neurotraumatic theory of development is based on the principle that when a neuropathic limb has a loss of protective sensation, repetitive

---

[a] Department of Orthopaedic Surgery and Biomedical Engineering, University of Tennessee Health Science Center-Campbell Clinic, 1211 Union Avenue, Suite #510, Memphis, TN 38104, USA; [b] University of Tennessee Health Science Center College of Medicine, 847 E Parkway S, Memphis, TN 38104, USA
* Corresponding author.
E-mail address: cbettin@campbellclinic.com

Orthop Clin N Am 55 (2024) 299–309
https://doi.org/10.1016/j.ocl.2023.08.002

microtrauma activates an inflammatory process that leads to overproduction of osteoclasts and excessive bone turnover.[4,6] Soft tissues are also affected, as this increased inflammatory response to microtrauma weakens tendons and ligaments. This further destabilizes the foot and ankle via fractures, subluxations, and dislocations.[2,7]

The neurovascular theory of CN development is based on the alterations in the sympathetic nervous system leading to a state of hyperemia which in turn leads to increases in venous pressure.[2,4,8] This increased venous pressure leads to elevated compartmental pressures and deep tissue ischemia, which subsequently alter tendons and ligaments, leading to foot and ankle collapse. Hyperemia is also thought to directly increase the delivery of osteoclasts and monocytes, leading to bone resorption.[9]

Infections of the foot and ankle region also often present in a similar patient population, particularly those with diabetes mellitus. Uncontrolled hyperglycemia is the primary driving force for infection development in these individuals, leading to oxidative stress, a pro-inflammatory response, and immune system dysfunction.[10,11] A poorly regulated immune system combined with microvascular changes and loss of protective sensation from neuropathic changes leads to the development of diabetic foot ulcers. In addition, microvascular changes cause impaired healing and antibiotic penetration, causing ulcers to become secondarily infected.[5,12]

CONSIDERATIONS

The 2 entities are not exclusive, with osteomyelitis superimposed on CN being rare but possible. This situation makes diagnosis even more challenging.[13] Treatment is also a difficult predicament, as it involves the dual challenge of treating both bone infection and underlying structural changes.[14] Several studies have been reported looking at optimal management of this very rare clinical scenario,[14–17] but for the majority of our discussion, we will treat the 2 as separate clinical conditions.

PREVALENCE/INCIDENCE

Though the true prevalence of CN is difficult to estimate, studies have reported an incidence of 0.1% to 2.5% in the general diabetic population to 13% in high-risk diabetic patients,[2,3,18–20] though these values may still be underreported due to the uncertain diagnostic criteria. CN occurs most commonly in the fifth decade of life, though often varied between types of diabetes, with patients with type 1 diabetes occurring most frequently in the third and fourth decade, while those with type 2 diabetes suffer from the disease in the sixth and seventh decades of life.[21] Regardless of the diabetic type, patients presenting with CN have generally had long-standing diabetes for more than 10 years.[2] Around a tenth of patients will have bilateral disease.[20]

Infections are also a prevalent issue in diabetic patients. Diabetes is estimated to be prevalent in over 10% of the US population, now estimated to be in over 34 million individuals, with a continued increase expected.[22] In a large retrospective study of more than 2.2 million individuals with skin and soft tissue infections, over 10% had diabetes. Diabetic patients had a significantly high rate of hospitalization (4.9% vs 1.1%), a higher complication rate (4.9% vs 0.8%), and a higher rate of complications when hospitalized (25% vs 16%).[23] Up to 60% of diabetic patients with ulcers will become infected, with around 80% of infections being soft tissue infections and 20% bone infections.[5,12]

EVALUATION
History
One of the most vital evaluation tools in differentiating between acute CN and acute infection, whether soft tissue or bony, is the patient history. Pain may or may not be present in these individuals due to underlying neuropathy.[1,4] Patients with CN may report a slowly progressing alteration of gait and may report that their footwear no longer fits them.[4] A large percentage of patients may also report an instigating event when questioned,[3] though most will not recall a specific traumatic event.[24] Recent foot surgery has also been reported as an instigator for the development of acute CN, theorized to be associated with local inflammation following surgery.[25]

Past medical history should be reviewed to identify relevant diagnoses including but not limited to diabetes, spinal cord injuries, alcoholism, human immunodeficiency virus, and other genetic neurologic disorders, including Charcot-Marie-Tooth disease.[3,4,20] However, the presence of these diseases is not a prerequisite, as CN has also been shown to occur in those with idiopathic neuropathy.[26] Other conditions that commonly mimic infection and CN are gout and acute deep vein thrombosis; thus, any history of gout or hyper-thrombotic conditions should be asked as well.[27]

Patient factors like age, length of diabetes, hemoglobin A1c 7% or more, body mass index, and renal failure or transplantation are vital factors to obtain that have both been known risk factors for CN.[2,21,28,29] Patients with osteomyelitis and CN are also often afebrile, whereas those with acute soft tissue infections may present with a fever. Obesity has been demonstrated to increase the likelihood of CN by 59%, while those with combined obesity and neuropathy were 21 times more likely to develop CN.[29]

A detailed history of neuropathy and sensory changes in the lower extremities should be obtained. If there is any question of whether neuropathy is present, the clinician should perform the 3-site Semmes-Weinstein monofilament testing and examine the Achilles tendon reflex.[20,30]

Physical Examination

Physical examination features of the lower extremity can also help differentiate between the 2 disease processes, though there are many similarities. Infection and acute CN both present with erythema and edematous changes in the distal lower extremity (Fig. 1). When looking at the foot in CN, a skin thermometer can reveal an increased temperature of 2 to 6°C compared to the contralateral foot,[31] though this may also be present in soft tissue infections.

A useful and easy differentiating factor between infection and acute CN is the resolution of erythema and edema when elevating the lower extremity above the level of the heart for 5 to 10 minutes with the patient in a supine position, also referred to as the "dependent rubor" test. This is a characteristic of CN but not of acute infection, in which swelling and erythema will not resolve with elevation.[1,13,32] This is a test that is very easy to perform and is clinically informative, and thus recommended to be performed by all clinicians. Though skin changes such as erythema are often present, CN often lacks associated skin breakage present in skin and soft tissue infections. The presence of streaking erythema tracking proximally up the leg is also more likely to be associated with lymphangitis associated with infections.[4] Though deformity is often not present in the acute Charcot foot, those with advanced Charcot can have instability or a fixed deformity with a flatfoot and/or rocker bottom deformity.[4]

Regarding anatomic location, osteomyelitis and cellulitis are commonly found in the forefoot and are accompanied by soft tissue infection and/or ulceration.[10] A "sausage toe" may also be present in forefoot infections.[13] CN typically affects the midfoot, so erythema and swelling may be focused in this region. Though CN may present with ulcerations, especially in later states, they do not show signs of infection. Clinical signs of an infected ulcer or wound include the presence of purulent drainage and macerated tissue surrounding the wound,[10] though chronic osteomyelitis may not show any signs of local inflammation.[13] Deeper signs of infection include abscess, gangrene, and necrotizing fasciitis. Ulcer size should be taken into consideration. Wound size greater than 4.5 cm^2 has been shown to have a significantly greater chance of developing underlying osteomyelitis.[33] Others have also reported that diabetic patients with ulcers measuring greater than 2 cm^2 or a depth greater than 3 mm have a significantly higher likelihood of having lower extremity osteomyelitis.[34]

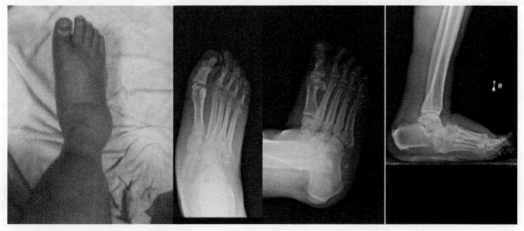

Fig. 1. Clinical and radiographic imaging of a patient presenting with acute Charcot neuropathy demonstrating longitudinal collapse of the medial column of the foot.

Another useful physical examination aid in diagnosis is the ability to palpate bone, generally through the "probe-to-bone" test, which examines whether the underlying bone can be palpated via a metal probe inserted into a wound.[35] The theory of this is if a metal probe can be inserted into a bone, thus bacteria can track there as well.[27] Sensitivity in this test has ranged from 38% to 95%, specificity from 84% to 98%, and a positive predictive value from 53% to 97% for the diagnosis of osteomyelitis.[27] A meta-analysis of 3 studies looking at the diagnostic applicability of the probe-to-bone test has demonstrated that a positive result increased the likelihood of osteomyelitis by more than 6-fold, while a negative probe-to-bone test result had a negative likelihood ratio of 0.39.[34]

IMAGING

Diagnostic imaging can assist in the differentiation between infection and acute CN when combined with clinical examination. Obtaining weight-bearing bilateral plain radiographs (anteroposterior and lateral) of the foot and ankle region is always recommended in those presenting with possible infection or CN, though often this is not helpful in early diagnosis. In detecting acute CN, plain radiography has a very low sensitivity and specificity, both less than 50%.[31,36] It may be useful to repeat weight-bearing radiographs after 2 weeks, at which point radiograph signs of acute CN may be more observable (see Fig. 1).[37]

The most widely recognized system for classifying radiographic changes in CN is the Eichenholtz classification, first described in 1966,[38] now modified to include a stage 0 representing clinical findings but no changes on plain radiographs (Table 1).[39] Often, acute CN presents with stage 0 findings. However, in early CN, Eichenholtz stage 1 findings such as focal bone demineralization, subtle subluxations or fractures, and ligamentous avulsions may be seen, particularly around multiple midfoot joints.[38] Flattening of the first metatarsal head may also be seen.[4,31]

Similarly, signs of bony infection present in radiographs often do not appear for 2 to 3 weeks after the onset of symptoms and require 40% to 50% loss of bone mass to identify.[40] Demineralization, cortical destruction, and periosteal reaction can all be seen in infections after some time.[1] The accuracy of plain radiography for early diagnosis of osteomyelitis has been reported at only 50% to 60%, with a sensitivity ranging from 22% to 75% and a specificity of 33% to 100%.[41]

Advanced imaging should therefore be utilized to aid in the diagnosis process, especially in early presentation.

Computed Tomography

Computed tomography (CT) imaging can be obtained, which can identify early intra-articular fractures and other bony pathology, including new periosteal bone formation and small foci of gas within bone, even better than MRI.[38] The use of contrast in CT imaging can also be used to detect abscess formation,[4] though differentiation between CN and osteomyelitis is less reliable in CT compared to MRI.[38] It can

Table 1 Modified Eichenholtz classification	
Stages	**Findings**
0 (Inflammatory)	Clinical: localized warmth, edema, erythema
	Plain radiography: minimal, if any abnormalities; MRI: subchondral bone marrow edema ± non-displaced pathologic fracture
1 (Development)	Clinical: localized warmth, marked edema, erythema
	Plain radiography: focal bone demineralization (early), debris formation at the articular margins, fragmentation of the subchondral bone, subluxation, dislocation, and periarticular fractures
2 (Coalescence)	Clinical: continued but decreased warmth, edema, erythema
	Plain radiography: absorption of fine debris, fusion of large fragments of adjacent bones, new periosteal bone formation
3 (Remodeling)	Clinical: decreased or absence of warmth, edema, erythema
	Plain radiography: remodeled and new bone formation, decreased osteosclerosis, possible gross residual deformity

Adapted from Mautone and Naidoo.[38]

be used when MRI is contraindicated in patients, such as those with pacemakers and aneurysmal clips.

MRI

MRI is the most used diagnostic imaging modality for differentiating acute CN and infection (Table 2). Both acute osteomyelitis and acute CN show increased bone and soft tissue edema, characterized by low signal on T1-weighted images and hyperintensity on T2-weighted images with contrast.[1,42] However, osteomyelitis nearly always comes after surrounding soft tissue infection, thus signs of abscesses, fistulas, adjacent ulcers, soft tissue swelling (ie, cellulitis), and sinus tracts on imaging would suggest infection.[42,43] Changes suggestive of osteomyelitis include focal bone involvement, often away from joints. Location is also a differentiating factor, with osteomyelitis often presenting in the weight-bearing surfaces of phalanges, metatarsal heads, calcaneus, and malleoli.[31,38]

In contrast, MRI of acute CN does not have soft tissue changes but usually demonstrates changes in periarticular and subchondral regions, with subchondral edema with or without microfracture being a common finding.[38] MRI signal in multiple joints, particularly in the midfoot tarsometatarsal and metatarsophalangeal joints, should be suggestive of CN.[44] MRI can also help identify early collapse of the longitudinal arch of the foot with increased T2 hyperintensity at the Lisfranc ligament as well as subtle abnormalities of subchondral bone at the subtalar joint, suggesting early structural changes present in CN.[4,42] MRI can help identify changes not present on standard x-rays (Eichenholtz stage 0).[45]

MRI is also the most useful imaging tool that can be used for the rare presentation of osteomyelitis superimposed on CN. Infected CN can present with large periarticular fluid collections and adjacent fluid collections, eroded bone cortices, and the "ghost sign", which is the presence of poor definition of bone margins on T1-weighted images which become clear after contrast administration.[31,38]

The importance of early MRI was demonstrated in a retrospective study of 71 patients with acute CN, demonstrating those who received early MRI diagnosing stage 0 CN had betting healing of midfoot lesions than those who had progressed to stage 1 CN due to delay in MRI and thus diagnosis of CN.[46]

A recently published meta-analysis on the accuracy of diagnostic imaging techniques in diabetic patients with pre-existing foot ulcers revealed MRI to have a sensitivity of 95% and specificity of 81% in diagnosing osteomyelitis, versus x-rays, which only had a sensitivity of 68% and a specificity of 77% in diagnosing osteomyelitis.[47] A previous meta-analysis demonstrated MRI to have a sensitivity of 77% to 100% and specificity ranging from 40% to 100% in diagnosing osteomyelitis.[41] A recent study also demonstrated that MRI had 87% to 90% sensitivity and 37% to 74% specificity when diagnosing osteomyelitis.[48]

Nuclear Imaging

Nuclear imaging techniques targeting biological activity have become more popular in facilitating the differentiation of CN and bony infection, though these are not commonplace in the everyday diagnostic arsenal. Scintigraphy using

Table 2		
MRI findings in acute osteomyelitis and noninfected Charcot neuroarthropathy		
MRI Feature	Acute Osteomyelitis	Charcot Neuroarthropathy
Signal	Low focal signal intensity on T1-weighted images, high focal signal on T2-weighted images	Low signal intensity in the subchondral bone on T1-weighted images, high signal intensity on T2-weighted images
Location	Phalanges, metatarsal heads, calcaneus, malleolus	Predominantly midfoot (tarsometatarsal, metatarsophalangeal joints)
Distribution	Focal involvement	Several joints/bones involved
Bone Marrow Signal Changes	Around ulcers, fistula tracts	Periarticular, subchondral
Adjacent Subcutaneous Fat Signal	Inflammation, sinus tracts, abscess formation	Edematous
Deformity	Usually not seen	Midfoot collapse

Adapted from Ergen FB, Sanverdi SE, Oznur A[27] and Ertugrul BM, Lipsky BA, Savk.[31]

various isotypic labeling has been reported in the literature, though it has generally been considered less accurate than MRI or PET.[47] Bone scanning involving technetium99 methylene diphosphonate (99mTc-MDP) labels hydroxyapatite, a marker of bone turnover, whereas Indium-111 (In 111-WBC) marks white blood cells (WBCs). One recent meta-analysis demonstrated an 87% sensitivity and 29% specificity of 99mTc-MDP scintigraphy and a 79% sensitivity and 71% specificity of In 111-WBC scintigraphy in diagnosing osteomyelitis in those with diabetic foot ulcers,[47] values generally lower than those for MRI.

Methods of combined leukocyte/marrow scintigraphy, particularly using 99mTc sulfur colloid present in bone marrow cells, have also been researched. With osteomyelitis, the scan with the 99mTc sulfur colloid will have low uptake, while the In 111-WBC image will have high uptake, whereas in CN, a high 99mTc sulfur colloid uptake would be expected.[4,31,49] However, in a recent, rapidly progressing acute CN foot, In 111-WBC scan can be falsely positive due to localization of labeled WBCs at radiographically invisible microfractures,[31] thus limiting the ability of scintigraphy to differentiate the 2 processes.

Fluorodeoxyglucose (FDG) PET has also demonstrated usefulness in the diagnosis of CN. A low-grade diffuse FDG uptake is observed in CN, while intense focal areas of uptake are observed in osteomyelitis.[50] One prospective study demonstrated sensitivity and specificity of FDG PET in the diagnosis of CN to be 100% and 93%, respectively, both higher than the sensitivity of 76% and specificity of 75% for MRI.[50] In 1 prospective study comparing FDG PET and 99mTc-MDP scintigraphy, PET had a sensitivity and specificity of 87% and 71%, respectively, in diagnosing osteomyelitis, both higher than that of scintigraphy (81% and 28%%).[51] A sensitivity of 84% and specificity of 92% have been reported for diagnosing osteomyelitis using PET.[47]

A recently published multicenter retrospective study of 250 patients looking at MRI, WBC scintigraphy, and FDG-PET demonstrated that WBC scintigraphy was more specific (91% vs 70%) and accurate (86% vs 67%) than MRI in diagnosing osteomyelitis, while in CN, WBC scintigraphy had significantly higher specificity and accuracy (89%) than MRI (88%) and FDG-PET (62%).[52] The authors concluded that scintigraphy was the most reliable imaging modality to differentiate between infection and CN[52] The accessibility and cost associated with this imaging technique make this not as clinically applicable as other imaging techniques today, but future prospects of utilizing this in the commonplace diagnostic algorithm are promising.[4,38]

ADDITIONAL TESTING

Histopathology and Culture

Bone culture and biopsy can also be performed and are the gold standard and the only definitive way for discriminating between osteomyelitis and acute CN.[37] This should ideally be performed before initiating antibiotics or after a short antibiotic holiday.[34] Bone samples can be obtained using either an open operative procedure or via percutaneous biopsy, both of which should be performed using sterile technique guidance.[27] However, this invasive procedure does present with potential complications of infection, bleeding, pain, fracture, and the potential instigation of acute CN if not currently present and thus should only be performed if a diagnosis is inconclusive or osteomyelitis is strongly suspected.[37]

Culturing of bone allows for speciation and determination of antibiotic sensitivities if osteomyelitis is present; however, false positives, due to sampling of bacteria within the more superficial wound, and false negatives, due to prior antibiotic therapy, are still possibilities.[27,53] Bone culture alone is reported to have a sensitivity of 92% and a specificity of 60% in diagnosing osteomyelitis in those with diabetes.[27] Superficial swab cultures are not recommended as they do not identify the bone pathogens reliably.[34]

Histopathologic analysis should generally be performed in conjunction with culture, as several studies have shown that as high as 66% of histologically proven cases of osteomyelitis (OM) at surgery or biopsies of the foot and ankle had negative cultures.[54] Features of osteomyelitis include aggregates of inflammatory cells, bony erosion and bone marrow changes, and reactive bone formation.[40] Performing a bone biopsy in acute CN is not advised; however, an overabundance of osteoclasts to osteoblasts would be expected.[27]

Serum Analysis

Laboratory analyses are also impactful diagnostic tools when used in combination with other diagnostic tools. WBC counts, C-reactive protein (CRP), erythrocyte sedimentation rate (ESR), and procalcitonin are important laboratory analyses that should be obtained in any patient where infection needs to be ruled out. Uric acid level should also be obtained, especially if gout is on the differential diagnosis.[37]

WBC, CRP, ESR, and procalcitonin are also usually normal in acute CN, while they can be elevated in infection.[21,27,55] Studies have demonstrated that elevated ESR (>70 mm/hour) is strongly associated with osteomyelitis.[33,56] However, osteomyelitis may not present with elevated WBC and CRP due to the often chronic nature of bone infections, whereas associated soft tissue infections will have increased values.[1,57] Procalcitonin is elevated in those with osteomyelitis associated with diabetic foot ulcers.[58] Generally, markers of bone turnover, such as bone-specific alkaline phosphatase and urinary deoxypyridinoline, have been of little help in differentiating osteomyelitis and acute CN due to shared bone turnover characteristics[27,59]

RECOMMENDATIONS

Due to the challenge clinicians face in differentiating infection and CN, groups have been brought together to provide more strict diagnostic criteria that can help guide physicians.[1,56,60] The most recent was published by the Foot and Ankle Workgroup that was part of the Second International Consensus Meeting on Musculoskeletal Infection held in 2018.[61] This group attempted to provide answers to differentiate between acute CN and infection.[1] The group determined that moderate evidence was present to suggest that multiple diagnostic criteria are required to differentiate the 2. They stressed that CN is more likely with an absence of skin wounds and elimination of erythema and edema with elevation. Only in more unclear cases should laboratory testing, bone specimens, and advanced imaging be pursued. All members of the voting delegates agreed with this recommendation.[1]

In unclear cases, the senior author's diagnostic algorithm includes a detailed history and physical examination, specifically targeting areas that impact treatment-making decisions. For example, patients with poor social support and/or minimal baseline ambulatory status may not be candidates for multiplanar external fixation. Exhaustive imaging and laboratory workup may not be necessary as the treatment decision is unlikely to be impacted by the results. Aggressive bone resection and limb stabilization with internal fixation and/or amputation are likely to be pursued. In a patient where treatments including immobilization, acute versus delayed internal fixation, or external fixation are all possible treatments, laboratory testing with complete blood count, basic metabolic panel, ESR, and CRP is obtained. A contrast-enhanced MRI as well as weight-bearing CT scan provides sufficient imaging, along with plain radiographs, to aid in the treatment-making decisions in these complex patients.

DISCUSSION

The early diagnosis of CN and infection of the foot and ankle is essential in guiding treatment and guiding successful outcomes to prevent deformity, ulceration, impaired mobility, limb loss, and even mortality.[62] Up to an 80% to 95% rate of misdiagnosis has been reported in the literature.[36,46,63] Already with a lower quality of life than control patients,[64] the early diagnosis, referral to an orthopedic foot and ankle specialist, and treatment initiation for CN have shown to be vital in the prevention of further deformity.[65]

Early diagnosis and treatment have been demonstrated to have a significantly lower incidence of foot fractures and deformities.[36,46] Delayed diagnosis has also been demonstrated to have a much-increased complication rate (66% at 8 weeks) compared to early diagnosis (14% at 4 weeks), most commonly ulcers.[63]

Those with CN, with or without underlying infection, place a great economic burden on the health care system and opportunity costs.[2] Delayed diagnosis of CN can also lead to even higher excessive and unnecessary health care expenditures. One study has demonstrated that delayed diagnosis of CN in the inpatient setting led to 10% greater inpatient costs, largely due to more procedures performed, and a 12% longer length of inpatient stay.[66] Those with delayed diagnosis also had a greater rate of amputations, in turn leading to a 30% increase in costs and 31% longer inpatient stay.[66]

In terms of the effect on the patient with CN, a recent systematic review has demonstrated an 8% rate of amputation in patients with CN, which is similar to previously reported studies,[62,67] with 1 reporting a 20% rate of amputation.[18] This rate is even higher in those presenting with recurrent ulcers and a delayed diagnosis.[66,67] The life expectancy of those with acute CN has been shown to reduce by over 14 years in 1 observational study.[68] Another study has shown that 5-year mortality of those with CN was 28.3%.[69] Charcot neuropathy is associated with a significantly higher mortality risk than diabetes alone, and 1 study has shown that over 60% of patients with CN will experience a foot ulcer, leading to an even higher risk of mortality.[69]

Aside from CN, diabetics with foot infections also have very high morbidity. A large inpatient analysis has demonstrated that diabetics admitted for management of foot infections had a 30% rate of minor amputation and a 6% rate of major amputation.[70] Charcot feet with underlying osteomyelitis also had a reported amputation rate of 28%, significantly higher than the 13% rate of osteomyelitis in non-Charcot feet.[14]

With the importance of early accurate diagnosis and treatment for both infections of the foot and ankle region and CN, more prospective, high-quality research is needed to continue to guide clinicians in determining optimal diagnostic algorithms.

SUMMARY

Infection and acute CN are 2 very different disease processes present in those with neuropathic feet and ankles. The treatment of these is extremely different; thus making accurate and early diagnosis is extremely vital to these limb-threatening and life-threatening conditions.[45] With the continued rise of diabetes mellitus, these 2 conditions are expected to continue to be prevalent in patients.

Diagnosis should always be supported by multiple criteria. A detailed history and physical examination should always be performed of each patient, with key factors able to differentiate the conditions. Certain physical examination maneuvers, particularly the resolution of edema and erythema with elevation and the probe-to-bone test, should be performed. Standard radiographic imaging should be performed, followed by the liberal use of advanced imaging, particularly MRI, which is currently the most accessible and clinically applicable modality. Serum analysis can also act as a diagnostic tool and can track treatment efficacy. Histopathology with concomitant cultures should be performed if osteomyelitis is suspected, with prompt initiation of antibiotics if this diagnosis is confirmed. Timely referral to a foot and ankle specialist should be sought if CN is suspected or diagnosed, with nonoperative management being the first-line treatment.

CLINICS CARE POINTS

- Infection, both bony and soft tissue, and acute CN present with many shared characteristics in a similar patient population that often makes diagnosis difficult.

- Patient history, past medical history, and physical examination, including the resolution of edema and erythema with elevation and the probe-to-bone test, are key elements in differentiating infection and acute CN.

- Imaging, laboratory studies, and bone culture with histopathological analysis should be used to aid in the diagnosis, though using each as the sole method of diagnosis is not recommended.

- Bone culture with histopathological analysis is the gold standard of osteomyelitis diagnosis and guides treatment, but it should only be performed when high clinical suspicion of osteomyelitis is suspected due to potential complications.

- MRI is the currently recommended diagnostic imaging modality for differentiating between infection and acute CN, and clinicians should have a low threshold for its utilization, though nuclear imaging also may one day become part of the mainstream diagnostic algorithm.

- Incorrect or delayed diagnosis can cause adverse effects, including amputation and mortality, to patients and can have negative determinants on the entire health care system.

DISCLOSURE

The authors have nothing to disclose.

REFERENCES

1. Heidari N, Oh I, Li Y, et al. What Is the Best Method to Differentiate Acute Charcot Foot From Acute Infection? Foot Ankle Int 2019;40(1_suppl):39S–42S.
2. Hester T, Kavarthapu V. Etiology, Epidemiology, and Outcomes of Managing Charcot Arthropathy. Foot Ankle Clin 2022;27(3):583–94.
3. Frykberg RG, Belczyk R. Epidemiology of the Charcot foot. Clin Podiatr Med Surg 2008;25(1):17–28.
4. Strotman PK, Reif TJ, Pinzur MS. Charcot Arthropathy of the Foot and Ankle. Foot Ankle Int 2016;37(11):1255–63.
5. Lavery LA, Oz OK, Bhavan K, et al. Diabetic Foot Syndrome in the Twenty-First Century. Clin Podiatr Med Surg 2019;36(3):355–9.
6. Baumhauer JF, O'Keefe RJ, Schon LC, et al. Cytokine-induced osteoclastic bone resorption in charcot arthropathy: an immunohistochemical study. Foot Ankle Int 2006;27(10):797–800.
7. Kaynak G, Birsel O, Güven MF, et al. An overview of the Charcot foot pathophysiology. Diabet Foot Ankle 2013;4. https://doi.org/10.3402/dfa.v4i0.21117.

8. Schaper NC, Huijberts M, Pickwell K. Neurovascular control and neurogenic inflammation in diabetes. Diabetes Metab Res Rev 2008;24(Suppl 1): S40–4.

9. Chisholm KA, Gilchrist JM. The Charcot joint: a modern neurologic perspective. J Clin Neuromuscul Dis 2011;13(1):1–13.

10. Polk C, Sampson MM, Roshdy D, et al. Skin and Soft Tissue Infections in Patients with Diabetes Mellitus. Infect Dis Clin North Am 2021;35(1): 183–97.

11. Daryabor G, Atashzar MR, Kabelitz D, et al. The Effects of Type 2 Diabetes Mellitus on Organ Metabolism and the Immune System. Front Immunol 2020;11:1582.

12. Lavery LA, Armstrong DG, Wunderlich RP, et al. Risk factors for foot infections in individuals with diabetes. Diabetes Care 2006;29(6):1288–93.

13. Womack J. Charcot Arthropathy Versus Osteomyelitis: Evaluation and Management. Orthop Clin North Am 2017;48(2):241–7.

14. Waibel FW, Schöni M, Kronberger L, et al. Treatment Failures in Diabetic Foot Osteomyelitis Associated with Concomitant Charcot Arthropathy: The Role of Underlying Arteriopathy. Int J Infect Dis IJID 2022;114:15–20.

15. Mehlhorn AT, Illgner U, Lemperle S, et al. Histopathological assessment of a two-stage reconstructive procedure of the infected Charcot foot. Arch Orthop Trauma Surg 2023;143(3):1223–30.

16. Ramanujam CL, Stuto AC, Zgonis T. Surgical treatment of midfoot Charcot neuroarthropathy with osteomyelitis in patients with diabetes: a systematic review. J Wound Care 2020;29(Sup6): S19–28.

17. Galhoum AE, Abd-Ella MM, Zahlawy HE, et al. Infected unstable Charcot ankle neuroarthropathy, any hope before amputation? A prospective study. Int Orthop 2022;46(7):1481–8.

18. O'Loughlin A, Kellegher E, McCusker C, et al. Diabetic charcot neuroarthropathy: prevalence, demographics and outcome in a regional referral centre. Ir J Med Sci 2017;186(1):151–6.

19. Armstrong DG, Todd WF, Lavery LA, et al. The natural history of acute Charcot's arthropathy in a diabetic foot specialty clinic. J Am Podiatr Med Assoc 1997;87(6):272–8.

20. Trieb K. The Charcot foot: pathophysiology, diagnosis and classification. Bone Jt J 2016;98-B(9): 1155–9.

21. Petrova NL, Foster AVM, Edmonds ME. Difference in presentation of charcot osteoarthropathy in type 1 compared with type 2 diabetes. Diabetes Care 2004;27(5):1235–6.

22. Diabetes Statistics. DRIF. Available at: https://diabetesresearch.org/diabetes-statistics/. Accessed March 18, 2023.

23. Suaya JA, Eisenberg DF, Fang C, et al. Skin and soft tissue infections and associated complications among commercially insured patients aged 0-64 years with and without diabetes in the U.S. PLoS One 2013;8(4):e60057.

24. Game FL, Catlow R, Jones GR, et al. Audit of acute Charcot's disease in the UK: the CDUK study. Diabetologia 2012;55(1):32–5.

25. Ndip A, Jude EB, Whitehouse R, et al. Charcot neuroarthropathy triggered by osteomyelitis and/or surgery. Diabet Med J Br Diabet Assoc 2008; 25(12):1469–72.

26. Bariteau JT, Tenenbaum S, Rabinovich A, et al. Charcot arthropathy of the foot and ankle in patients with idiopathic neuropathy. Foot Ankle Int 2014;35(10):996–1001.

27. Ertugrul BM, Lipsky BA, Savk O. Osteomyelitis or Charcot neuro-osteoarthropathy? Differentiating these disorders in diabetic patients with a foot problem. Diabet Foot Ankle 2013;4. https://doi.org/10.3402/dfa.v4i0.21855.

28. Pakarinen TK, Laine HJ, Honkonen SE, et al. Charcot arthropathy of the diabetic foot. Current concepts and review of 36 cases. Scand J Surg SJS 2002;91(2):195–201.

29. Stuck RM, Sohn MW, Budiman-Mak E, et al. Charcot arthropathy risk elevation in the obese diabetic population. Am J Med 2008;121(11):1008–14.

30. Feng Y, Schlösser FJ, Sumpio BE. The Semmes Weinstein monofilament examination as a screening tool for diabetic peripheral neuropathy. J Vasc Surg 2009;50(3):675–82.

31. Ergen FB, Sanverdi SE, Oznur A. Charcot foot in diabetes and an update on imaging. Diabet Foot Ankle 2013;4. https://doi.org/10.3402/dfa.v4i0.21884.

32. Marmolejo VS, Arnold JF, Ponticello M, et al. Charcot Foot: Clinical Clues, Diagnostic Strategies, and Treatment Principles. Am Fam Physician 2018;97(9): 594–9.

33. Ertugrul BM, Oncul O, Tulek N, et al. A prospective, multi-center study: factors related to the management of diabetic foot infections. Eur J Clin Microbiol Infect Dis 2012;31(9):2345–52.

34. Butalia S, Palda VA, Sargeant RJ, et al. Does this patient with diabetes have osteomyelitis of the lower extremity? JAMA 2008;299(7):806–13.

35. Grayson ML, Gibbons GW, Balogh K, et al. Probing to bone in infected pedal ulcers. A clinical sign of underlying osteomyelitis in diabetic patients. JAMA 1995;273(9):721–3.

36. Chantelau EA, Richter A. The acute diabetic Charcot foot managed on the basis of magnetic resonance imaging–a review of 71 cases. Swiss Med Wkly 2013;143:w13831.

37. Milne TE, Rogers JR, Kinnear EM, et al. Developing an evidence-based clinical pathway for the

assessment, diagnosis and management of acute Charcot Neuro-Arthropathy: a systematic review. J Foot Ankle Res 2013;6(1):30.

38. Mautone M, Naidoo P. What the radiologist needs to know about Charcot foot. J Med Imaging Radiat Oncol 2015;59(4):395–402.

39. Shibata T, Tada K, Hashizume C. The results of arthrodesis of the ankle for leprotic neuroarthropathy. J Bone Joint Surg Am 1990;72(5):749–56.

40. Hartemann-Heurtier A, Senneville E. Diabetic foot osteomyelitis. Diabetes Metab 2008;34(2): 87–95.

41. Kapoor A, Page S, Lavalley M, et al. Magnetic resonance imaging for diagnosing foot osteomyelitis: a meta-analysis. Arch Intern Med 2007;167(2):125–32.

42. Ledermann HP, Morrison WB. Differential diagnosis of pedal osteomyelitis and diabetic neuroarthropathy: MR Imaging. Semin Musculoskelet Radiol 2005;9(3):272–83.

43. Toledano TR, Fatone EA, Weis A, et al. MRI evaluation of bone marrow changes in the diabetic foot: a practical approach. Semin Musculoskelet Radiol 2011;15(3):257–68.

44. Low KTA, Peh WCG. Magnetic resonance imaging of diabetic foot complications. Singapore Med J 2015;56(1):23–33. quiz 34.

45. Ahluwalia R, Armstrong DG, Petrova N, et al. Stage 0 Charcot Neuroarthropathy in the Diabetic Foot: An Emerging Narrow Window of Opportunity? Int J Low Extrem Wounds 2022;21(4):374–6.

46. Chantelau E. The perils of procrastination: effects of early vs. delayed detection and treatment of incipient Charcot fracture. Diabet Med J Br Diabet Assoc 2005;22(12):1707–12.

47. Llewellyn A, Kraft J, Holton C, et al. Imaging for detection of osteomyelitis in people with diabetic foot ulcers: A systematic review and meta-analysis. Eur J Radiol 2020;131:109215.

48. La Fontaine J, Bhavan K, Jupiter D, et al. Magnetic Resonance Imaging of Diabetic Foot Osteomyelitis: Imaging Accuracy in Biopsy-Proven Disease. J Foot Ankle Surg 2021;60(1):17–20.

49. Palestro CJ, Mehta HH, Patel M, et al. Marrow versus infection in the Charcot joint: indium-111 leukocyte and technetium-99m sulfur colloid scintigraphy. J Nucl Med 1998;39(2):346–50.

50. Basu S, Zhuang H, Alavi A. FDG PET and PET/CT Imaging in Complicated Diabetic Foot. Pet Clin 2012;7(2):151–60.

51. Shagos GS, Shanmugasundaram P, Varma AK, et al. 18-F flourodeoxy glucose positron emission tomography-computed tomography imaging: A viable alternative to three phase bone scan in evaluating diabetic foot complications? Indian J Nucl Med IJNM 2015;30(2):97–103.

52. Lauri C, Glaudemans AWJM, Campagna G, et al. Comparison of White Blood Cell Scintigraphy, FDG PET/CT and MRI in Suspected Diabetic Foot Infection: Results of a Large Retrospective Multicenter Study. J Clin Med 2020;9(6):1645.

53. Lipsky BA, Peters EJG, Senneville E, et al. Expert opinion on the management of infections in the diabetic foot. Diabetes Metab Res Rev 2012; 28(Suppl 1):163–78.

54. Wu JS, Gorbachova T, Morrison WB, et al. Imaging-guided bone biopsy for osteomyelitis: are there factors associated with positive or negative cultures? AJR Am J Roentgenol 2007; 188(6):1529–34.

55. Jeffcoate WJ, Lipsky BA. Controversies in diagnosing and managing osteomyelitis of the foot in diabetes. Clin Infect Dis 2004;39(Suppl 2): S115–22.

56. Berendt AR, Peters EJG, Bakker K, et al. Diabetic foot osteomyelitis: a progress report on diagnosis and a systematic review of treatment. Diabetes Metab Res Rev 2008;24(Suppl 1):S145–61.

57. Eneroth M, Larsson J, Apelqvist J. Deep foot infections in patients with diabetes and foot ulcer: an entity with different characteristics, treatments, and prognosis. J Diabetes Complications 1999; 13(5–6):254–63.

58. Van Asten SA, Nichols A, La Fontaine J, et al. The value of inflammatory markers to diagnose and monitor diabetic foot osteomyelitis. Int Wound J 2017;14(1):40–5.

59. Petrova NL, Dew TK, Musto RL, et al. Inflammatory and bone turnover markers in a cross-sectional and prospective study of acute Charcot osteoarthropathy. Diabet Med J Br Diabet Assoc 2015;32(2): 267–73.

60. Charcot's neuro-osteo-arthropathy - IWGDF Guidelines. Available at: https://iwgdfguidelines. org/charcot/. Accessed March 22, 2023.

61. Aiyer A, Raikin S, Parvizi J. 2018 International Consensus Meeting on Musculoskeletal Infection: Findings of the Foot and Ankle Work Group. Foot Ankle Int. 2019;40(1_suppl):1S. doi: 10.1177/10711 00719852356.

62. Schneekloth BJ, Lowery NJ, Wukich DK. Charcot Neuroarthropathy in Patients With Diabetes: An Updated Systematic Review of Surgical Management. J Foot Ankle Surg 2016;55(3):586–90.

63. Wukich DK, Sung W, Wipf SaM, et al. The consequences of complacency: managing the effects of unrecognized Charcot feet. Diabet Med J Br Diabet Assoc 2011;28(2):195–8.

64. Dhawan V, Spratt KF, Pinzur MS, et al. Reliability of AOFAS Diabetic Foot Questionnaire in Charcot Arthropathy: Stability, Internal Consistency, and Measurable Difference. Foot Ankle Int 2005;26(9): 717–31.

65. Shazadeh Safavi K, Janney C, Shazadeh Safavi P, et al. Inappropriate antibiotic administration in

the setting of Charcot arthropathy: A case series and literature review. Prim Care Diabetes 2022; 16(1):202–6.

66. Labovitz JM, Shapiro JM, Satterfield VK, et al. Excess Cost and Healthcare Resources Associated With Delayed Diagnosis of Charcot Foot. J Foot Ankle Surg 2018;57(5):952–6.

67. Saltzman CL, Hagy ML, Zimmerman B, et al. How Effective Is Intensive Nonoperative Initial Treatment of Patients with Diabetes and Charcot Arthropathy of the Feet? Clin Orthop Relat Res 2005;435:185.

68. van Baal J, Hubbard R, Game F, et al. Mortality Associated With Acute Charcot Foot and Neuropathic Foot Ulceration. Diabetes Care 2010;33(5): 1086–9.

69. Sohn MW, Lee TA, Stuck RM, et al. Mortality risk of Charcot arthropathy compared with that of diabetic foot ulcer and diabetes alone. Diabetes Care 2009;32(5):816–21.

70. Tan TW, Shih CD, Concha-Moore KC, et al. Disparities in outcomes of patients admitted with diabetic foot infections. PLoS One 2019;14(2):e0211481.

Moving?

Make sure your subscription moves with you!

To notify us of your new address, find your **Clinics Account Number** (located on your mailing label above your name), and contact customer service at:

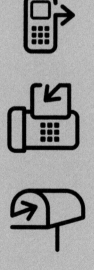

Email: **journalscustomerservice-usa@elsevier.com**

800-654-2452 (subscribers in the U.S. & Canada)
314-447-8871 (subscribers outside of the U.S. & Canada)

Fax number: **314-447-8029**

Elsevier Health Sciences Division
Subscription Customer Service
3251 Riverport Lane
Maryland Heights, MO 63043

ELSEVIER

Printed and bound by CPI Group (UK) Ltd, Croydon, CR0 4YY

08/05/2025

01864747-0018